T0260855

From Crisis to Catastrophe

Carework in a Changing World

Amy Armenia, Mignon Duffy, and
Kim Price-Glynn, Series Editors

The rise of scholarly attention to care has accompanied greater public concern about aging, health care, child care, and labor in a global world. Research on care is happening across disciplines—in sociology, economics, political science, philosophy, public health, social work, and others—with numerous research networks and conferences developing to showcase this work. Care scholarship brings into focus some of the most pressing social problems facing families today. To study care is also to study the future of work, as issues of carework are intertwined with the forces of globalization, technological development, and the changing dynamics of the labor force. Care scholarship is also at the cutting edge of intersectional analyses of inequality, as carework is often at the very core of understanding gender, race, migration, age, disability, class, and international inequalities.

From Crisis to Catastrophe

Care, COVID, and Pathways to Change

EDITED BY
MIGNON DUFFY
AMY ARMENIA
KIM PRICE-GLYNN

RUTGERS UNIVERSITY PRESS

NEW BRUNSWICK, CAMDEN, AND NEWARK, NEW JERSEY

LONDON AND OXFORD

Rutgers University Press is a department of Rutgers, The State University of New Jersey, one of the leading public research universities in the nation. By publishing worldwide, it furthers the University's mission of dedication to excellence in teaching, scholarship, research, and clinical care.

978-1-9788-2856-8 (paper)
978-1-9788-2857-5 (cloth)
978-1-9788-2858-2 (epub)

Cataloging-in-publication data is available from the Library of Congress.
LCCN 2022036825

A British Cataloging-in-Publication record for this book is available from the British Library.

References to internet websites (URLs) were accurate at the time of writing. Neither the author nor Rutgers University Press is responsible for URLs that may have expired or changed since the manuscript was prepared.

♾ The paper used in this publication meets the requirements of the American National Standard for Information Sciences—Permanence of Paper for Printed Library Materials, ANSI Z39.48-1992.

rutgersuniversitypress.org

For Debi Osnowitz

CONTENTS

Introduction   1

MIGNON DUFFY, AMY ARMENIA, AND
KIM PRICE-GLYNN

PART ONE   7
Crisis

1   Beyond Wealth-Care: Pandemic Dreams for a
    Just and Caring Future   11
    JOAN C. TRONTO

2   Latin America's Response to COVID-19: The Risk of
    Sealing an Unequal Care Regime   19
    JULIANA MARTÍNEZ FRANZONI AND
    VEENA SIDDHARTH

3   COVID-19, Global Care, and Migration   27
    ITO PENG

4   Black Lives Matter: Structural Racism, Sexism, and
    Carework in the United States   36
    ODICHINMA AKOSIONU, JANETTE DILL,
    MIGNON DUFFY, AND J'MAG KARBEAH

5   Disability, Ableism, and Care during COVID-19 in
    the United States   45
    LAURA MAULDIN

6   Unpaid Care in Public Places: Tensions in the Time
    of COVID-19   53
    PAT ARMSTRONG AND JANNA KLOSTERMANN

PART TWO   61
Catastrophe

7   The Right to Care at Stake: The Syndemic Emergency
     in Latin America   65
     MARÍA NIEVES RICO AND LAURA C. PAUTASSI

8   At the Crossroads of the Employment and the Care
     Crises: Care Workers during the COVID-19 Pandemic   73
     VALERIA ESQUIVEL

9   Caring for Children and the Economy: The Uneven
     Effects of the Pandemic on Childcare Workers, Primary
     School Teachers, and Unpaid Caregivers   82
     PILAR GONALONS-PONS AND JOHANNA S. QUINN

10   COVID-19 and Care for the Elderly People in Africa:
     An Analysis of South Africa's Mitigation Measures   94
     ZITHA MOKOMANE AND AMEETA JAGA

11   Transnational Family Caregiving during a
     Global Pandemic   102
     KEN CHIH-YAN SUN

PART THREE   111
Aftermath

12   Cheap Praise: Supplemental Pay for Essential Workers
     in the 2020 COVID-19 Pandemic   115
     FRANZISKA DORN, NANCY FOLBRE,
     LEILA GAUTHAM, AND MARTHA MACDONALD

13   Migrants in Europe's Domestic and Care Sector:
     The Institutional Response   134
     SABRINA MARCHETTI AND
     MERITA MESIÄISLEHTO

14   Budgeting Care Services during the COVID-19 Crisis   143
     ORLY BENJAMIN

15   Policy, Culture, and COVID-19: European Childcare
     Policies during the Pandemic   151
     THURID EGGERS, CHRISTOPHER GRAGES, AND
     BIRGIT PFAU-EFFINGER

PART FOUR
Transformation   159

16 Exposing Fault Lines, Flaring Tensions, and the Need
for New Alliances: Home Care in the Time of COVID-19
in Ontario, Canada   161
   CYNTHIA J. CRANFORD

17 End-of-Life Considerations during COVID-19   168
   CINDY L. CAIN

18 COVID-19 and the Rise of the Care Robots   176
   HELEN DICKINSON AND CATHERINE SMITH

19 Challenging Gender Regimes through Employee Voice
in Carework   183
   KATHERINE RAVENSWOOD

20 Building a Care Infrastructure in the United States 191
   JULIE KASHEN

Epilogue: Care in Crisis: Convergences and Divergences   199
   MIGNON DUFFY, AMY ARMENIA, AND
   KIM PRICE-GLYNN

Acknowledgments   203
References   205
Notes on Contributors   247
Index   255

From Crisis to Catastrophe

Introduction

MIGNON DUFFY, AMY ARMENIA, AND KIM PRICE-GLYNN

In a landmark 2018 report, the International Labour Organization warned of a worsening crisis in care stemming from demographic changes, existing inequalities of gender and labor, and inadequate social policy. They argued that "if not adequately addressed, current deficits in care service provision and its quality will create a severe and unsustainable global care crisis" (International Labour Organization 2018, v). They were not alone in sounding the alarm, as a small but growing group of advocates, academics, and policymakers had been warning about this care crisis for decades.

Then, in 2019, COVID-19 emerged rapidly in a context of secrecy, lack of information, and fortuitous communication. The World Health Organization (WHO) (2020a) has documented the chronology of events leading up to the global pandemic. The timeline began on the last day of 2019, when WHO learned that a novel coronavirus had been detected in Wuhan Hubei Province, China. Though "international law stipulates that new infectious disease outbreaks of global concern be reported to the World Health Organization within 24 hours," WHO learned of the outbreak not "through official notification" but through the diligence of one epidemiologist (McMullen 2021).

Dr. Marjorie Pollack, an infectious disease specialist and deputy editor of ProMed, a "surveillance system conducting global reporting of infectious disease outbreaks," heard about social media posts from an associate in Taiwan and sent an urgent message via ProMed notifying readers about the novel coronavirus. The following day, WHO established an emergency task force to address the virus. On January 4, WHO tweeted news of the novel coronavirus; there had been no fatalities at that point, and research was just beginning into the source of the virus (World Health Organization 2020b). One month later, WHO reported 7,818 infections and, though most were in China, the virus had already spread to eighteen other countries with a total of eighty-two persons infected. By March 11, 2020, 72 days after the WHO timeline began, WHO announced that it was "deeply concerned both by the alarming levels of spread and severity, and by the alarming levels of inaction." At this point WHO announced "that COVID-19 can be characterized as a pandemic" (World Health Organization 2020a)

Over one year, between May 2021 and 2022, deaths from COVID-19 around the world nearly doubled from at least 3.2 to 6.3 million people (World Health Organization 2021b, 2022), and in many places, those deaths continue unabated despite the increasing presence of vaccines in wealthy nations. Citizens of almost every country in the world spent the better part of 2020 in varying degrees of lockdown, creating unprecedented disruptions in everyday life. The lockdowns in most places included shutting down schools and childcare centers and decreased availability and safety of home-based care workers. Congregate care settings for older and disabled adults became some of the most dangerous places in the world, as death rates among residents and workers reached alarming rates.

In this historical moment, a care crisis became a catastrophe. The longstanding stresses, previously discussed in a few circles of academia and advocacy, were suddenly thrust into the spotlight of public dialogue and policy discourse. Talking about care as infrastructure enables us to think about care's vital importance to society, its policy scaffolding, the way it undergirds work and family life, and its human face. COVID-19 has revealed the connections and the gaps in the existing structure. The virus is like the dye that doctors use to see pathways in CT scans and MRIs; what was previously there but invisible suddenly lights up in fluorescent color.

In this volume, we ask a diverse group of care scholars to bring their expertise to bear on understanding the impact of the COVID-19 pandemic on care—our practice of care, our understanding of care, and our future vision for care. In doing so, they consider the ways in which the existing social organization of care in different countries around the globe amplified or mitigated the consequences of COVID-19. They also explore the impact of the global pandemic on already deteriorating conditions of care amid deeply rooted gender, race, migration, disability, and other inequalities. In addition, they analyze the insights gained from this crisis that deepen our overall understanding of care and enable us to imagine the opportunities for lasting change as we move forward.

Organization of the Book

The long-standing devaluation of care preceded the arrival of COVID-19. The pandemic has brought to light a system in which investment in care is shaped by legacies of inequality and long-term disinvestment in care systems. In part 1, Crisis, the authors highlight the historical and structural roots of the care crisis that intensified the catastrophe of COVID-19. At the center of these analyses, the authors consider why care infrastructures worldwide are so woefully inadequate and what structures marginalize care. Joan C. Tronto (chapter 1) introduces the concept of wealth-care to capture how the value of basic care is diminished when societies are organized around the accumulation of wealth as the top priority. Juliana Martínez Franzoni and Veena Siddharth (chapter 2) examine how preexisting Latin American care regimes that emphasized family solutions over public investment shaped pandemic policy responses to further increase women's unpaid labor. At a global level, Ito Peng (chapter 3) shows that the large global migration flows of care workers (interrupted by COVID-19) are connected to the intersection of the micro-level gender division of household labor and macrolevel economic inequalities among nation-states and regions. Odichinma Akosionu, Janette Dill, Mignon Duffy and J'Mag Karbeah (chapter 4) tie Black women's position at the epicenter of risk during much of the pandemic to a legacy of racial servitude and pervasive structural racism in the United States. Laura Mauldin (chapter 5) asks us to add a disability analytic to our intersectional analyses of class, race, and gender in order to get a full perspective on the care crisis before, during, and after COVID-19. Pat Armstrong and Janna Klostermann (chapter 6) lay bare the gaps in Canada's long-term care system that are in normal times filled by family members' unpaid work, which required military intervention during this emergency. Across all these chapters, we see the barriers to care infrastructure that both predate and continue through the pandemic. These chapters explain how interlocking systems of capitalism, sexism, racism, ableism, and global inequality set the stage for the pandemic catastrophe by undermining collective investment in care.

Part 2, Catastrophe, highlights the impact of COVID-19 and the accompanying mitigation measures on care processes, paid care workers, and families in different places around the world. Rooted in previous structures (as examined in part 1), the pandemic exacerbated what had already been crisis conditions and made them catastrophic. In Latin America, María Nieves Rico and Laura C. Pautassi (chapter 7) describe a syndemic emergency as the pandemic collided with preexisting structures of poverty and sexism that had pushed care into marginalization. Valeria Esquivel (chapter 8) characterizes the pandemic as a dual crisis of economics and care, with dire, although distinct, consequences for different groups of paid care workers. Pilar Gonalons-Pons and Johanna S. Quinn (chapter 9) compare the COVID-19 conditions of three groups who care for children—unpaid carers, paid childcare workers, and primary school teachers— and identify interdependencies between them that reproduce devaluation, invisibility, and stratification. Zitha Mokomane and Ameeta Jaga (chapter 10) examine the challenges South African elders and their families faced during the COVID-19 pandemic, as the mismatch between mitigation strategies and accepted norms exacerbated elder care burdens. Ken Chih-Yan Sun (chapter 11) explores the complexities of transnational caregiving during the COVID-19 pandemic, concluding that effective policies must address families who exist beyond state borders. Together, these chapters paint a rich picture of the real value of care across the globe, how that value is rendered invisible by a set of entrenched cultural assumptions and structural inequalities, and how the intersection of the devaluation of care with the arrival of COVID-19 had deadly consequences.

Part 3, Aftermath, examines the immediate fallout of the pandemic, and the range of policy responses as governments scrambled to fill the gaping holes in the care infrastructure laid bare by the emergency. These chapters consider what policy responses can teach us about the value of care. The authors interrogate how short-term policy measures in the face of a novel situation represent meaningful steps toward change and how they are rooted in old understandings of care, replicating historical inadequacies and inequalities. Franziska Dorn, Nancy Folbre, Leila Gautham, and Martha MacDonald (chapter 12) examine the sporadic attempts at "hazard pay" for care workers during the early stages of the pandemic as markers of value (or lack thereof). At the nexus of labor and immigration laws in Europe, migrant domestic workers face particular challenges, outlined by Sabrina Marchetti and Merita Mesiäislehto (chapter 13). Orly Benjamin (chapter 14) demonstrates how care can remain invisible in policy decision-making processes, even in the face of a public health disaster. Thurid Eggers, Christopher Grages, and Birgit Pfau-Effinger (chapter 15), compare emergency policy responses across Denmark, England, and Germany, emphasizing that a country's care arrangement is the result of a combination of policy and cultural norms. Understanding how governments reacted to the care crisis that emerged provides many lessons to help us move forward.

Part 4, Transformation, the final section of the book, looks to the future and considers how to move from emergency responses to creating long-term investments in care infrastructure. Authors consider the ideas that can help us emerge from the COVID-19 crisis with stronger care systems. There is no silver bullet, and many of our authors suggest that particular solutions may cause other dilemmas, but to the extent that emergency can catalyze change it is important to think about the possibilities. Cynthia J. Cranford (chapter 16) proposes a model of "intimate community unionism" that incorporates the collective voices of those doing care work and those being cared for into policy design and daily work routines. Cindy L. Cain (chapter 17) draws on the practices and principles of end-of-life care, identifying lessons for COVID-19 care and care systems moving forward. Helen Dickinson and Catherine Smith (chapter 18) write about the increase in discussion and use of robotic technologies in care, the potential for making care more accessible and safe, and the need to consider ethical and social consequences of these technologies. Katherine Ravenswood (chapter 19) examines the case of health care assistants in New Zealand/Aotearoa as an example of the successes and challenges of a collective employee voice for care and work conditions. Finally, Julie Kashen (chapter 20) makes a passionate case for robust public investment in a universal care infrastructure that recognizes long-term inequalities as it bridges groups of caregivers and receivers. Together, the authors in this final section of the book propose a multidimensional strategy for rebuilding and revaluing care as we move forward.

In the Epilogue, we endeavor to draw lessons from across these chapters, to identify consistent threads, tensions, and tradeoffs as well as pathways for progress. Examples from across the globe provide an opportunity to understand convergences—the universal characteristics of care systems—and divergences—where things are being done differently. We hope that this volume becomes part of a conversation about how to harness this catastrophic moment for real transformative change.

PART ONE

Crisis

When COVID-19 emerged, the virus found gaping holes not only in our immune responses but also in our care infrastructure around the globe. The inadequate systems of care that had created a crisis long before the pandemic are deeply embedded in structures of gender, economic, racial, and global inequalities. This first section examines how the pandemic exposed the values undergirding the crisis in care. These authors collectively demonstrate that building a robust care infrastructure is not simply a matter of implementing legislative and policy change; it requires us to rethink some of our core cultural values and dismantle a set of interlocking historical inequalities.

The news during the pandemic has been full of stories about shortages of what we need to fight off this disease—people around the world have not been able to get supplies like personal protective equipment, ventilators, and COVID tests, and health care facilities have struggled to keep basic staffing levels. Joan C. Tronto's concept of wealth-care helps us understand how these pandemic problems are reflections of a larger set of societal priorities that value the pursuit and preservation of wealth above all else. While her focus is the United States, this individualistic and wealth-centered value system is a worldwide export of the powerful Global North. Tronto argues that "the single-minded pursuit of more wealth to benefit the wealthy is not a responsible way to live together in a democratic society." Economic inequality undergirds the inadequacy and inequalities in the care structure that allowed the COVID-19 crisis to become a care catastrophe.

In their discussion of care regimes, Juliana Martínez Franzoni and Veena Siddharth paint a picture of what this focus on wealth-care looks like in Latin America. They describe how economic inequality among women undergirds a deeply embedded cultural and structural devaluation of women's care labor across the region. Ito Peng's chapter makes a similar argument at the global level, demonstrating how global stratification upholds a gendered division of care labor across the world by catalyzing the migration of women for care jobs. These care and migration regimes were disrupted by pandemic travel and work restrictions as well as by local shutdowns of schools and childcare centers. However, as both of these chapters argue, the policy responses (or lack thereof) threaten to reinscribe and further deepen preexisting fault lines of care between countries, between women, and between women and men.

Martínez Franzoni and Siddharth point out that the low-income women who perform the most invisible and difficult care labor are often "indigenous, migrant and/ or of African descent," emphasizing that these economic, gendered, and global divisions are also layered with the history of racism and colonialism. Odichinma Akosionu and her coauthors delve more deeply into the role of racism in the development of care systems in the United States. They demonstrate that there is a long history of the devaluation of Black women's bodies that is reflected in their overrepresentation in low-wage health care jobs, which were at the epicenter of risk during the pandemic. Laura Mauldin's chapter asks us to consider an additional axis of inequality in understanding care, exposing the ableism underlying the high rates of institutionalization of people with disabilities that allowed the virus to rip through this population with dizzying speed. Both of these chapters challenge us to dig beneath the surface of the disparate risks of this virus being fatal to understand that the structures of care— the care workforce, and care institutions—are built on differentially valuing these lives.

Finally, Pat Armstrong and Janna Klostermann detail a vivid illustration from the Canadian pandemic experience of the consequences of these intersecting value systems for care infrastructure. As labor shortages in nursing homes reached critical levels during the pandemic, the military was called in to fill some of the gaps. The impact of understaffing was exacerbated by the absence of labor usually provided by family members and community volunteers, who were shut out of institutions by pandemic restrictions. Armstrong and Klostermann argue that the emergency illuminated the previously invisible dependence of care institutions on this army of unpaid labor, which they explicitly name as coerced labor. The coercion of marginalized groups into unpaid and low-wage care labor is driven by the forces that Tronto names as wealth-care, and undergirded by the systems of sexism, racism, ableism, and global inequality described by the other authors in this section.

Taken together these chapters paint a powerful picture of the value systems and power imbalances that formed the foundation of the unsystematic patchwork of care infrastructure that was in place when the pandemic hit, exposing the gaps and inadequacies for what they were. These authors underscore not only how the pandemic exposed inequalities but in fact exacerbated them and threatened to further entrench the value systems underlying those inequalities in prepandemic days.

1

Beyond Wealth-Care

Pandemic Dreams for a Just and Caring Future

JOAN C. TRONTO

Who is responsible for the COVID-19 pandemic? On the one hand, this question makes little sense; a new virus is a natural occurrence, no one is responsible for it. On the other hand, to ask this simple question exposes layers of questions about how humans should respond to a novel health threat. Indeed, there are responsibilities aplenty to assign: from large-scale environmental concerns to human–animal interactions, to the profoundly entrenched inequities of opportunities and harms on a global level, to the role of political squabbles, to the activities of individuals who refuse to wear masks or observe rules about large-scale gatherings. To introduce the question of responsibility makes clear that this health crisis is also a crisis of justice. In a just world, we might expect those who are more vulnerable to be better protected from the harm (Goodin 1985). We might expect that those who take up dangerous risks on behalf of others receive greater protection. But these are not the realities. The pandemic has opened our eyes for a moment to the "essential" nature of care and care workers. It has also exposed, as the essays in this volume make clear, the realities of the vast inadequacy of contemporary care: that existing care infrastructures are barely worthy of the name; that care workers suffer economic penalties for doing the work that they do and try to do; that attempts to address paid and unpaid care have been halting and grudging and inadequate; that caring exacerbates inequalities of class, race, and gender; and that those who give and receive care locally and globally and transnationally are treated with disregard. The pandemic has exposed how people in different social and economic situations in contemporary societies are able—or not able—to care adequately for themselves, those near to them, and those in their communities and societies. Some essential workers are forced to risk their lives for their livelihood, while others boast of their special status as they receive special care, early access to vaccines, and so forth.[1]

Knowing about the unjust distribution of burdens of care does not correct them. Since we live in a world in which virtually all nations remain profoundly antidemocratic (if democracy bears any relationship to the claim that people are equal), it will not be difficult for the pandemic and its unjust burdens to be brushed aside as a self-contained health crisis, despite mounting evidence that its devastating effects on bodies, lives, communities, governments, and democratic norms will continue for decades. Even worse, we can imagine a future triumphant narrative that ignores many of these harsh realities and instead insists that "we won" through sacrifice and care and beat back this threat and resumed "normal" life. Such a congratulatory narrative is surely possible, accompanied by a great deal of what The Care Collective have called carewashing (The Care Collective et al. 2020) as corporations and governments spin the tale of their own heroic activities, ignoring some of the permanent damage they have done. And the patterns of these harmful effects will, if current reality is any indication, follow historical patterns of entrenched injustices; the hardest hit will be racialized groups, the elderly, people with disabilities, and (mainly women) workers who provide paid and unpaid care.

Scholars such as Rico and Pautassi (chapter 7) have begun to refer to these intersecting systems of gross inequality and the human tragedy they create as a syndemic, but we might also use a moral and political frame and call this *injustice in itself*. John Stuart Mill wrote that "the great error of reformers and philanthropists" was "to nibble at the consequences of unjust power instead of redressing the injustice in itself" (Mill quoted in Ackerly 2018, 71). If injustice in itself is, as the political theorist Brooke Ackerly claims, "a power relation, not merely the consequence of a power relation," (72) then to root out injustice we need to see its complex causes, the inequalities of power it produces, and how "the workings of injustice itself are self-concealing" (73).

Scholars have noted for decades that caregivers and care receivers receive short shrift in economic rewards, and their efforts are rarely in the public eye. This essay seeks to name "wealth-care" as the "injustice in itself" that makes other forms of care—care for humans as well as care for other creatures and care for the planet—seem less important than the pursuit and preservation of wealth. If this argument is correct, then it will help to reframe how to make the argument to take care more seriously. If we can persuade people to reconsider their commitment not to an economic system but to wealth-care, we can refocus public attention on care so that perhaps we can finally be rid of the idea that care just happens naturally, requires only minimal public attention, and is not worthy of being our highest collective value.[2]

Wealth-Care

Wealth-care is meant as a clarifying concept that allows us to make sense out of the question of responsibility with which this chapter began. At the most general level every society must create institutions and practices for care. Indeed, it might make sense to categorize societies by exploring what the philosopher Harry

Frankfurt called "the importance of what we care about" (1988). Increasingly, American[3] society focuses not on the importance it attaches to the everyday lives and thus the everyday care of citizens, not even on hard work, but on the accumulation and preservation of wealth. Surely the creation of wealth is important for all human societies; without wealth there would be no way to respond to health emergencies. But there is a difference between what Joshua Preiss has recently noted is the growth of wealth in a well-ordered society and the pursuit of wealth to the exclusion of all other goals, which Preiss denotes as "winner take all" capitalism (2021) and which I call here wealth-care. Although neologisms are not always welcome, I describe our current political economy as a system of wealth-care rather than as a "free market" or as "neoliberal" because it highlights the fact that wealth-care is a set of *fundamental values* as well as an account of economic structures. Many scholars writing about the limits of the neoliberal political economy have spoken of its broader harms to human flourishing through its distortion of rationality and political life, and its exploitation of the natural world and its inhumane treatment of workers (Brown 2015, 2019; Fraser 2016; Giroux 2005; Harvey 2005; Mohanty 2013; Pellandini-Simányi, Hammer, and Vargha 2015; Tronto 2017; Williams 2018). This critique of wealth-care follows many of these lines. Using the language of wealth-care clarifies its status as a normative claim about what matters in society, and what constitutes justice in such a society. Wealth-care is a set of values which posit that the growth of wealth is the central value, activity, and purpose of society, and that society's rewards should go to those who create and grow wealth since they are the worthiest members of society. To its adherents, justice in a wealth-care society centers on the preservation of property and "freedom," especially the freedom of those with great amounts of property to use their property to accumulate ever more property and wealth.

Wealth-care functions as a kind of injustice in itself because proponents of wealth-care control the rules for regulating wealth and make certain that those rules always redound to their own benefit.[4] Furthermore, because an important component of wealth-care is passing wealth on to the appropriate heirs (Harrington 2016), the effects of accumulated wealth are deepened through time. The injustices of the past, for example, in the United States, the injustices of slavery, dispossession of Indigenous peoples, and distribution of federal wealth that excluded people of color (Merritt 2017), are deepened and made to appear "natural" through the accumulation of wealth over time.[5] Furthermore, wealth-care seeks to extract wealth from the state itself. When the government needs goods to carry out its functions, for example, providing the military with equipment, such trade produces enormous wealth for contractors in the private sector. Increasingly, the state generates wealth for private individuals, when, for example, "private" prisons or schools perform what might have previously been public functions. Indeed, functions of the state that seem remote from large sources of wealth have become a part of "predatory capitalism," (Friedman 2020; Page, Piehowski, and Soss 2019), described in the United Kingdom by Alan White as a "shadow state" (2016).

When wealth itself becomes the focus of care, people are enlisted to care for it and to protect it against diminution. A whole range of practices and institutions exist to care for wealth in the world, not the least of which is the legal order that recognizes property rights and wealth (Pistor 2019). As Jeffrey Winters argued in his book *Oligarchy* (2010), in addition to the people who live off of wealth itself, many well-to-do members of modern societies work in what he called "The Income Defense Industry," protecting wealth through the manipulation and construction of tax codes, banking regulations, and so forth. As Brooke Harrington argues, wealth managers are significant international actors in their interactions with fundamental social institutions, such as families, markets, and states (2016).

Wealth produces injustice vis-à-vis care in a number of ways. In the first place, when a society focuses so much of its efforts and wealth on preserving and extracting wealth, "investment" becomes the way to think of care; how much does one actually need to invest in people, especially those conceived as "surplus" or "poor," to keep wealth intact? This has certainly been the case in some of the world's highest-income countries, such as the United States, where despite soaring wealth in recent decades, there has been a disinvestment in public education, public health, public higher education, physical infrastructure, and so forth. But public disinvestment from institutions and other forms of care is only a part of this problem. Another problem is that it is difficult to extract wealth from the time-intensive basic care that people need. By its nature, care requires hands-on attention that requires a great deal of time. From the standpoint of wealth, such care is both too expensive and too resistant to greater wealth-generating efficiencies.

The main solution to this problem of the wealth-resisting costly nature of care is to leave it outside the economy, or to include it only on the edges of the economy in the informal economy or in poorly paid positions at the bottom of the economic ladder. Indeed, in the perfect logic of wealth-care, care dwells in a "private" realm of family that contains its costs, and is only visible publicly when some of that care appears on the market. Care is an individual responsibility, or a family responsibility, and beyond that, care can be allocated through the market; anyone who needs care can purchase it (and if they cannot afford it, then they are at fault because they do not have enough wealth to do so). The end result is that this process "invisibilizes" the process of shifting care responsibilities increasingly back on individuals; a process made clear by the amount of economic activity that relies on unpaid care work (see Gonalons-Pons and Quinn, chapter 9 this volume). This shift has been accelerating throughout the past decades in higher-income countries. In the United States, for example, as June Carbone and Naomi Cahn have argued (2014), increasingly marriage is reserved for upper-class individuals; others cohabit because the economic stakes of sharing accumulated debt are too great. In wealth-care society, people's real energies should be focused on their investments, which leads to a way of thinking about the relationship of parents and children in investment terms; indeed Lundberg and Pollak now see "investments in children as a principal motive for marriage" (2013, 27). But if marriage is primarily about investments in children, what happens to the care needs of elderly people, people who have an illness or disability, and people who just need others to help them take care of themselves? During the pandemic, this situation has grown even worse. The hard-won gains made for women in Latin America, for example, have been reversed (Martínez Franzoni and Siddarth, chapter 2 this volume), and while wage-earning people are thrown back on themselves to try to provide care, the fortunes of the wealthy continue to grow (McCarthy 2020). In this "new normal," some, especially women, are taking on additional caring burdens that place them at a disadvantage vis-à-vis the rest of the economic realm.[6]

Wealth-care not only privatizes care in households it also affects how care practices operate in other institutional settings. Stories appear daily about how basic health supplies—personal protective equipment (PPE), hospital beds, oxygen—are in short supply in country after country. As the pandemic took its first heavy toll in the United States, it might have seemed paradoxical that the most expensive health care system in the world did not have enough PPE available for hospital staff to conduct their work. On another level, though, insofar as providing health care has also become a site for the extraction of wealth, it makes sense that the investment decisions in health care did not consider shortages in cheap basic supplies as a fundamental concern (though public health officials had warned of this possibility) (Kunzmann 2020; Slack and Voyles Pulver 2020). Faced with ventilator shortages, the public learned that a large manufacturer of "full-service" expensive ventilators had bought a smaller company that had had a government contract to produce less expensive machines and killed off the project (Kulish, Kliff, and Silver-Greenberg 2020). That health care provision is skewed toward producing medications, devices, and procedures that are more profitable while curtailing spending on expensive commodities, such as staffing, reflects the priorities not of good health care but of wealth-care.[7]

The dogma that public services are too expensive is part of a larger argument to undermine all forms of public life, since when suffering publics become engaged they often demand support that will redistribute wealth. Thus wealth-care protects itself through an ongoing attack on all forms of public institutions, as Nancy MacLean has demonstrated in her book on the history of public-choice economics, *Democracy in Chains* (2017). There she quotes Pierre Lemieux, a historian of that movement, "The public choice revolution rings the death knell of the political 'we'" (ix).

The final dimension of the "injustice itself" of wealth-care reveals itself here. Not only does it block out the realities of disinvestment in the public sphere but it changes the ways in which people will think about their responsibilities. Citizens might be thought to have responsibilities beyond themselves—at minimum, to obey the laws, pay taxes. But the strange world of wealth-care evacuates citizenship roles of all meaning and presumes a world in which there is only the household and economic activity. Karl Polanyi, the critic of an earlier generation of market fundamentalists, foresaw the consequence of such a wealth-care worldview in 1945.

He wrote that "neither voters, nor owners, neither producers, nor consumers could be held responsible" for any decisions of government that were meant to reflect a public end. In this way, freedom started with economic activity and ended with being able to cast aside all forms of "compulsion on the part of a state" or for responsibility for "economic suffering in society from which he, personally, had not benefitted." Indeed, such a person came to view himself as outside politics and economically produced structures of inequality, and *"he denied their reality in the name of his freedom"* (Polanyi [1944] 2001, 266; emphasis added). Injustices that do not exist cannot be addressed. If there is no public health crisis, then one bears no responsibility for it. If those who are poor just made poor choices for themselves, then others owe them nothing. With the false promise that proper investment can make everyone wealthy, wealth-care forces individuals to presume that they are their own failures.

If we look at the economic harms wrought by the pandemic, it becomes clear that they do nothing to disrupt the forms of injustice and irresponsibility that underpin wealth-care. In economic terms, the most affected are the least well off. Much of the first U.S. bailout went to already wealthy firms and individuals, with little transparency about where and how that money was spent (Holden and Strauss 2020). Those most likely to lose their jobs were the people—especially women and men of color—in low-paying services and marginal positions. This pattern perpetuates the privileged irresponsibility entailed by the wealth-care worldview. As Polanyi observed, this "lack of responsibility for [these consequences] seemed so evident that he denied their reality in the name of his [*sic*] freedom." Declaring the virus a hoax and refusing to follow public health guidelines are signs of people unwilling to admit to any form of responsibility, and such COVID-deniers have been organized and vocal in many countries.

An Alternative

On one level, it is not difficult to conceptualize what an alternative worldview requires. We can recite already the steps that would make the social provision of care better, more equitable, and more fair.[8] It begins with providing adequate support to care workers, providing for their basic needs and for their abilities to care for their families. Care also exceeds the capacities of families to provide it, so better education, health care, public transit, affordable housing, are also necessary. Care institutions need adequate resources and close monitoring. All of this forms a "care economy." Good social and economic policies are not sufficient, then; we need a global political awakening to the need to think about responsibilities for care.

But to make such arguments in the face of the entrenched injustice in itself is to whistle in the wind; the logic of wealth-care makes any proposal that seems to diminish wealth a nonstarter. This knee-jerk reaction is in part a result of the debasement of the capacities of citizens to make judgments, part and parcel of relying on beneficiaries of wealth-care to shape public judgment, a condition Sheldon

Wolin called "managed democracy" (2008). So to change our values to better reflect the centrality of all forms of care, we need to turn to the people. Providing extended care so that individuals can provide care for all is, in the final analysis, the end goal of the democratic expansion that began centuries ago. Without democratic institutions, there is no way to ensure that everyone and everybody is cared for well, and that everyone is doing their fair share of care.

Thus care must be democratic in order for democracy to become caring (Tronto 2013). There is a tremendous amount of wealth in the world; I daresay there is enough to meet every human's basic direct care needs and to provide care for the rest of the natural world. Seeing wealth-care for what it is, a form of injustice in itself—a set of practices and institutions that misdirect our care toward the objects of wealth rather than toward the more important needs of people, animals, plants, the biosphere, and the geosphere—invites us to switch our worldview. It does not mean that there is no value to the pursuit of wealth or growth, but that, as with all needs in a just and caring society, the needs for further wealth need to be weighed against other competing needs and responsibilities to meet these needs fairly and equitably distributed. The single-minded pursuit of more wealth to benefit the wealthy is not a responsible way to live together in a democratic society. The capacity to discuss such questions, though, depends on a level of equality in meeting people's care needs as well as limiting the excessive power over others that comes from too much concentrated wealth. Nothing short of such a radical rethinking, though, can transform the world to be more just and caring. Each day, a new pandemic story appears that sharpens our awareness of the profound injustices of the present order. Will this pandemic help us to see this reality more clearly? Such clarity is at the heart of our pandemic dreams.

NOTES

1. On the special status of some, see, Stolberg (2020). "Vaccine nationalism" will benefit wealthier countries. On February 1, 2021, the 16 percent of the world's population in high income countries had secured 60 percent of vaccine doses (Attiah 2021). Inequities exist within nations as well; on the United States see Jean-Jacques and Bauchner (2021).

2. Building upon Diane Elson's "three Rs" (recognize, reduce, and redistribute) for care, Ito Peng adds a fourth R, "revalue," in discussing unpaid care work in chapter 3 of this volume.

3. Wealth-care is not limited to the United States; indeed, the global nature of wealth is one of its important qualities because wealth managers use international movement as an important means to preserve and enhance wealth (Harrington 2016). In this chapter I shall primarily draw on the U.S. case because it is the one that I know well.

4. One of the clearest statements I know of the ways in which the powerful construct gendered and racialized hierarchies to retain their power appears in the work of Barbara Reskin (1988, 2012).

5. The unequal distribution of wealth by race in the United States is an example of this effect; in general, "the net worth of a typical white family is nearly ten times greater than that of a Black family" (McIntosh et al. 2020).

6. On the situation in the United States and India, for example, see Schultz and Raj (2020). Globally, UN Women summarize the picture (2020a).

7. Dr. Vijay Prasad, a medical doctor, makes the point this way: "We will always prioritize interventions that consolidate money in the hands of the few, over interventions that disperse money to the hands of many, with the same levels of evidence" (2019). For a discussion of this idea see Smith (2019).

8. A series of excellent sets of recommendations on a "caring economy" have appeared within the past year; among others, readers can consult Oxfam's *Time to Care* report (Coffey et al. 2020), UN Women's 2020 Report (Razavi 2020), a report by German-speaking scholars of care (care-macht-mehr.com 2020), the Women's Budget Group, UK (Commission on a Gender Equal Economy 2020), and (The Care Collective et al. 2020).

2

Latin America's Response to COVID-19

The Risk of Sealing an Unequal Care Regime

JULIANA MARTÍNEZ FRANZONI AND VEENA SIDDHARTH

Women's[1] entry into the labor market is a critical marker and driver of economic growth and poverty reduction (Folbre 1994; Fraser 1994; Iversen and Rosenbluth 2013; Novta and Wong 2017; Therborn 2004; UN Women 2015). Yet simply increasing the numbers of working women is not enough. The quality of their jobs also matters (Verick 2014). Women have greater work quality and stability when there are social policies to assist with their unpaid care responsibilities (UN Women 2017).

The COVID-19 pandemic caused an unprecedented number of women around the world to leave their jobs (Carli 2020; Eggers, Grages, and Pfau-Effinger, chapter 15, this volume).[2] The pandemic has disproportionately harmed sectors where women predominate, such as health, services, tourism, and the informal sector[3] (ILO 2021a), and increased care responsibilities have fallen on women far more than men. The economies that undervalue carework have had even greater costs to female employment, children, and families (Madgavkar et al. 2020). A 2020 study of six industrialized countries showed that women were 24 percent more likely to permanently lose their jobs during the pandemic than men (Dang and Nguyen 2020).

Without urgently restructuring and redressing the inequalities inherent in all "care regimes" (Bettio and Plantenga 2004),[4] the pandemic's adverse effects will outlast the actual epidemic for years to come (Alon et al. 2020), harming not only female employment possibilities and the welfare of families but also the resilience of economies to external shocks.

This chapter examines how the COVID-19 pandemic has intensified the racial, gender, and ethnic inequalities already existing in Latin America's care regime (Bango 2020; Bastides Aliaga 2021; ILO 2020d). While the region made progress in the last decade in instituting paid parental leave, flexible work arrangements, and affordable, high-quality childcare as protective elements of essential "social" infrastructure (ILO/UNDP 2009; Martínez Franzoni and Camacho 2007; OECD 2018), the pandemic demonstrated the insufficiency and fragility of these measures.

Latin America's Unequal Care Regime

More than half of all women in Latin America entered the labor force since the early 1990s. Among women in their prime working age (24 to 54 years of age), the proportion is considerably higher: labor participation increased from 47.2 percent in 1990 to 66.7 percent in 2014 (ECLAC 2014).[5] During the 2000s, however, despite the continued growth of economies, jobs, and wages, female labor participation stagnated (Filgueira and Martínez Franzoni 2017). The invisibility of care is one reason why. The failure of governments to collectively address care responsibilities stunts the social protection and earning capacities of women at all levels.

Indeed, the increase in women in the labor force did not alter a solid sexual division of labor (World Bank 2012, 35). Time-use surveys in Latin America show that the hours men spend in carework is highly inelastic across time, income levels, age, family responsibilities, and family arrangements (UN Women 2017). At the end of 2019, on average, unpaid work in Latin America accounted for 46 percent of all worked hours: 76 of every 100 hours of this work were in women's hands—8 hours of carework a day compared to 2.4 hours for men (Filgueira and Martínez Franzoni 2019). Intertwined with this gender gap in carework was a high level of income inequality. Before the pandemic, eighteen of the thirty most unequal countries in the world were in Latin America, with an average Gini coefficient of 0.54 (ECLAC 2019). While women in the upper end of the income distribution spend less than 4 hours per day on unpaid carework—and can therefore devote time to paid work—those at the lowest levels spent, on average, 8 hours per day on unpaid carework (UN Women 2017).

In the absence of universal care services, the low wage and unprotected jobs of poor women in Latin America sustain advances in upper-income women's labor participation, while allowing the division of care responsibilities within the family to remain unchanged (Filgueira and Martínez Franzoni 2019). An entrenched sexual division of labor is coupled with high income inequality and a care regime that relies largely on domestic workers. Domestic workers account for about 14 percent of women's total employment (ILO 2020d, 4)—which leaves the care needs of poor women unmet. Of this predominantly female and low-income workforce, 78 percent work informally without benefits and little possibility of advancement (Rico and Pautassi, chapter 7, this volume), resulting in greater inequality among women (ILO 2013). Latin America's extreme income inequality along with other structural dimensions of inequality, such as race and ethnicity, creates a trap that further skews gender inequality and care arrangements.

Sticky Floors, Broken Ladders, and Glass Ceilings

"Sticky floors," "broken ladders," and "glass ceilings" constitute a typology of women's experience in the labor force, documented in the UN Women's 2017 regional report

(UN Women 2017) on Latin America. As such, it highlights primary prepandemic care arrangements and experiences of motherhood that vary depending on women's potential for advancement and job security.[6]

Under sticky floors women face the greatest instability and poverty. They have primary education at best and reside in low-income households. Their labor force participation rates are lower than those of men with equal education. As described earlier, when they do enter the labor market, they are often trapped in insecure and unprotected work, such as paid domestic service. Women in this group cope with a heavy burden of unpaid carework, exacerbated by persistently high rates of early motherhood, which they frequently face alone (Blofield et al. 2021).

At the other end are women with tertiary education and high household incomes. These women took advantage of the region's economic expansion from 2000 to 2015, yet still face glass ceilings that limit their professional advancement, as reflected in the gender pay gap and labor segregation. The burden of unpaid work for this group is lower than it is for women in the other two scenarios, reflecting their greater capacity to buy carework instead of negotiating to share these duties with men in their households.

Between these two scenarios are the women who struggle with broken ladders. These women participate in the labor force at a higher rate than their sticky floors sisters, even with small children. Without policy protections to work steadily while managing care responsibilities, they are highly sensitive to shocks, creating volatility in their work lives that hinders their advancement (UN Women 2017).

Although there are wide cross-national variations in women's economic empowerment and care arrangements, Latin America's absence of universal care services generally coexists with low-paid and unprotected domestic carework across the board.

During the 15 years of expansionary social policy that took place between 2000 and 2015, feminist academics and some governments instigated progress to address carework in order to support women in the workforce. First, paid time for care as reflected in maternity leave reached beyond formal salaried workers to include self-employed, temporary, and domestic workers. For example, in Brazil and Argentina, domestic workers gained the right to maternity leave, as did rural and temporary workers in Brazil. At the peak of the expansionary period of formal employment and social policy reforms, circa 2013, the proportion of female *salaried* workers in Latin America entitled to maternity leave was 41 percent. This proportion went up to 48 percent when self-employed and domestic workers were included in the count. Thus the incorporation of domestic workers and the self-employed increased coverage by more than 6 percentage points (feminist economist Soledad Salvador, estimate upon request, pers. comm., email, October 25, 2019). Still, many women were not included. Of the more than 18 million domestic workers in the region, mostly women, Indigenous peoples, and migrants, 77.5 percent were informal workers and less than 11 percent had social security, parental leave, or other benefits (ILO 2020d, 4–5).

Second, beyond paid time to care within the family, during the expansionary phase of social policy from 2000 to 2013, carework entered the public agenda as a matter calling for state efforts, largely as a result of international agencies, state actors, and, to a lesser degree, feminist social movements (Esquivel and Kaufmann 2017; Staab 2012). Under this new framing, states faced the need to improve leave at birth, expand more quality care services, and rely on sound programs aimed at the care-dependent elderly population—which is fast growing across the region. Several countries moved in this direction and created care systems (Uruguay), care networks (Costa Rica), or care programs (Chile) (Arza and Martínez Franzoni 2018; Rico and Robles 2016).

Despite these measures, carework is still seen in the region as a private, family concern. In most countries state-sponsored services are not explicitly or primarily aimed at providing care, with schools as one example. Costa Rica's failure to provide fathers with paternity leave points to the limitations of even robust social policy when care is considered an exclusively female responsibility.

Uruguay is a rare example of a state that recognizes fathers as caregivers, addressing it as a paternal *right*, not one that comes along with the status of husband or partner. Uruguay defines the provision of leave at birth as a measure to help strengthen bonds between father and child, and to promote a caregiving fatherhood (Martínez Franzoni 2021b). The sanctioning of parental leave in Chile is another example of moving to coresponsibility between women and men. This expansive view of fathers is distinct from the more typical view in the region of paternal leave as merely a means to assist mothers following child delivery.

Indeed, whether social protection is weak or robust, it is typical for Latin American governments to see a limited role for men as carers, with half of all countries still lacking paternity leave and most of the rest having just a few—3 to 5—days (Blofield and Touchton 2019; Lupica 2016). As indicated earlier, the only two countries that have taken steps to address maternalism are Chile and Uruguay, with shareable parental leaves, acknowledging that either parent could be the primary caregiver. Yet neither has to date introduced a "daddy quota" that makes the leave nontransferable from fathers to mothers (Blofield and Touchton 2019).

The truncated (in terms of the sexual division of labor) and unequal (in terms of income inequality) care regime depicted here (Filgueira and Martínez Franzoni 2019) is largely responsible for the stagnation of female labor participation in Latin America. By 2017, only half of women were in the workforce (Novta and Wong 2017). While for men the main reasons to exit the labor force are studies, sickness, or disability, for women it is family responsibilities (ILO 2018; OECD 2018). As a result, as in most of the world, the formal sector continues to operate without fully recognizing care needs and assumes that for at least 8 hours a day and 365 days of the year, workers need not pay attention to family responsibilities.

A configuration of work that fails to recognize care harms women in a myriad of ways. At the macrolevel, it limits women's working capacities, with economic costs for the individual and the economy as a whole. At the individual level, women experience strain on their mental and physical health. These multiple burdens make it difficult for women to engage socially and politically in civic life (Bango 2020). And finally, societies lose when women do not participate in shaping laws, policies, and institutions; when their exclusion is the norm; and when economic interpretations exclude women's experience and needs (Kabeer 2020).

Facing the Pandemic with Rapid Yet Gender-Blind Responses

By June 2021, Latin America, with 8 percent of the global population, accounted for over 30 percent of COVID-19 deaths. The simultaneous health, financial, labor, and care crises created by the pandemic (i.e., a syndemic) (Rico and Pautassi, chapter 7, this volume) intensified the already highly unequal distribution of resources. As of February 2021, state-financed schools had been closed for almost a year. Childcare centers and services for the elderly were reduced or shut down altogether, increasing the demands on women as families struggled to secure income, pay bills, and provide care. As elsewhere, women multitasked by simultaneously taking the role of teachers, nurses, cooks, therapists, entertainers, and more. This compression of roles within the family and in women's hands is grounded on the truncated and unequal care regime depicted in the previous section.

While worldwide, women tend to work in sectors worst affected by pandemic lockdowns, in Latin America, 79 percent of all female work is concentrated in ten occupations that include retail, domestic services, education, and hospitality services (Martínez Franzoni 2021a). Women also predominate in essential services, especially the health sector, where they represent nine out of ten nurses and 57 percent of doctors. There, at the start of the pandemic the largely female workers were compelled to keep working, even in the absence of public support networks that ensured access to quality care services for their care-dependent family members (ILO 2020h).

Cross-national variations depend on the strictness of the lockdown (with implications for social services, including schools and care services) as well as on policy legacies (with implications for the scope and generosity of policy responses to support individuals and families). The latter made a difference between countries with and without robust social policies as families transition to home-schooling, remote health care assistance, and cash transfers to compensate for the loss of jobs.

The loss of earnings during the pandemic has been inconsistent across the income distribution, disproportionately affecting those in the middle (Lustig et al. 2020). In terms of the typologies of economic empowerment, the pandemic has had the heaviest toll for women with broken ladders due to the combination of precarious labor participation and care demands that they faced. These women risked losing jobs, earnings, and all the gains they had achieved since 2000.

Women with glass ceilings face a different challenge: they must adapt to more work demands as essential workers or remotely from home, while responding to the explosion of care needs. These women operate in labor markets that are gender blind, regulated by state policy that views labor productivity as separate from family responsibilities. These women risk falling behind their careers yet not necessarily losing their jobs and income altogether.

Women with sticky floors are trapped in a vicious circle of job losses and lack of care services. Even more than women in broken ladders, they cannot purchase care services adapted to the pandemic (e.g., school pods where a group of families form a bubble to educate their children together).

Since the start of the pandemic, governments in Latin America have most commonly employed cash transfers to address the adverse impacts. In addition to relying on existing programs, both contributory (e.g., unemployment insurance aimed at the unemployed) and noncontributory (e.g., social assistance aimed at the poor), they instituted arrangements for informal workers left out of existing schemes, benefiting female workers in the informal sector without other resources. Although coverage and services did not match the needs generated by the pandemic (Blofield, Giambruno, and Filgueira 2020), the measures made it clear that even in national contexts where state capacity is limited, governments can act and even improve such capacities along the way.

The pandemic has appeared to have erased women, gender, and carework from the significant yet still fragile visibility that had been gained since 2000. Families—and women within them—seem to have retreated again to an all-encompassing, taken-for-granted role. Overall, policies related to recovery and economic growth do not incorporate carework as an essential component. Remarkable exceptions are policies to maintain public care services (Costa Rica), to extend parental leave during the duration of the emergency for parents of newborns (Chile), and to create leave for parents of young children (Argentina) (ECLAC 2020a, 2020c; Martínez Franzoni 2021a; UNDP 2020). More typical were pandemic efforts that ignored the sexual division of labor and women's roles as caregivers. These gender-blind policies and measures fail to address the extra care burdens women have faced and continue to face.

Prospects

If Latin America does not reverse the significant drop in the quantity and quality of women's labor participation during the pandemic, the risks are threefold: for labor markets, the loss of human talent in a region where, unlike other regions of the Global South, women have more formal education than men; for social protection systems, a widening gap between social needs and the amount and quality of state supply of transfers and services; and for societies, an increase in poverty and inequality of women and their families. As Rico and Pautassi say in chapter 7 (this volume), if the multiple crises worsened by the pandemic are not dealt with in an integrated fashion, there will be greater fragility and risk for the region.

Strengthening social protections builds resilience and addresses inequality when building back from crises (Stiglitz 2009). Giving greater value and prominence to paid and unpaid carework would help the region face future economic and social stress. Solutions would have to address women at all income levels, as it is the poorer women (sticky floors) whose care needs are often ignored. Governments and key social and political actors would need to place carework at the center of social, labor, and economic policies. Carework needs to be an intrinsic element of all social policies, from cash transfers that reward unpaid carework (e.g., eligibility criteria to retire from paid work at old age), to the timetable for school services and the very existence of universal quality care services for young children. In addition, the expansion of "decent care jobs"—in ILO's terms—enables carework to be a key component of building more distributive market economies. Acting on these points would potentially create cross-class coalitions around a matter that affects most women and families.

Reorganization of carework cannot happen without addressing fiscal policy (Bárcena 2020). Doing so is challenging in a region where the fiscal space is narrow, partly due to a minimal taxation of wealth and property (ECLAC 2020b).[7] Yet there is evidence that investing in care can expand the tax base while expanding formal employment for women (Ilkkaracan 2016). Making care services a central element of "social infrastructure" (Braunstein, Seguino, and Altringer 2019; Martínez Franzoni and Camacho 2007; Seguino 2020) rather than a temporary measure avoids the danger of it being seen as a luxury for emergencies. It is also essential to normalize carer roles for men, both in unpaid and paid work. One way forward is paternal leave as well as transfers that reach men in the informal economy.

Continuing with the status quo of treating carework as outside the realm of economic and social policy will come at great cost to the region's growth, welfare, and well-being for years to come. Simply being aware of the unjust distribution of burdens of care does not solve the issue (Tronto, chapter 1, this volume). Before the pandemic, progress in women's labor participation was precarious; state efforts to address carework were still incipient; and policy decision making was and is embedded in a strong familialistic culture that assumes that families, and within them women, bear the brunt of caregiving demands. Eggers, Grages, and Pfau-Effinger (chapter 15, this volume) describe how the pandemic's lockdowns have encouraged a "retraditionalization" of childcare roles, mediated by the degree of state support to alternate forms of care and society's attitudes toward childcare outside the home. Populist and authoritarian voices in the region that view women as primarily caretakers also hinder women's full economic participation and sexual and reproductive rights.

Acknowledgments

Ideas in this chapter owe much to previous collaboration with Fernando Filgueira. We are also indebted to Sarah Gammage, editors, and authors of this book for their valuable comments. Any errors remain ours.

NOTES

1. Throughout this chapter we refer to women and men, but we recognize that transgender women and nonbinary individuals also face particular care and work constraints during COVID-19.

2. A survey conducted in the United States during 2020 indicated that one of four women who reported becoming unemployed during the pandemic said it was because of a lack of childcare—twice the rate among men (Sasser Modestino 2020).

3. Globally, by June 2020, almost 510 million, or 40 percent of all employed women, work in hard-hit sectors. The proportion of Central and South American women working in hard-hit sectors was above the average (58.9 and 45.5 percent, respectively) (ILO 2021a, 8–9).

4. Other terms used are the "social arrangement of care" (Jenson 1997) and the "care diamond" (Razavi 2007).

5. As in other regions, women disproportionately occupy jobs in the lowest-paid sectors and earn lower incomes than men with similar experience and education. Peculiar to Latin America is that women have reached gender parity at all levels of education, yet income gaps detrimental to women persist and are higher among the most educated women (UN Women 2017).

6. Economic empowerment as women's threefold capacity to hold and control property in conditions equal to those of men; access to their own income to a similar extent as men; and, last but not least, have a balanced distribution of unpaid care and domestic work with men. Of the three dimensions, this chapter concerns itself with the organization of carework, which, in turn, has a two-way relationship with access to income.

7. Tax collection in Latin America is currently 23.1 percent of GDP on average for the region's national governments, compared with the 34.3 percent seen among countries of the Organization for Economic Cooperation and Development (ECLAC 2020b).

3

COVID-19, Global Care, and Migration

ITO PENG

COVID-19 has put the spotlight on the importance of care and highlighted the preexisting inequalities delineated by carework. As older people and frontline care workers succumb to the coronavirus and parents struggle to manage work and childcare under lockdown conditions, we are reminded of the human costs of unmet care, the deleterious consequences of work–family imbalances, and the hazards and hardship associated with carework. We are also reminded of carework's utter invisibility. Throughout the world, older people have overwhelmingly fallen victim, and along with them frontline care workers. In Canada, over 80 percent of all COVID-related deaths in 2020 were people living in long-term care (LTC) homes (CIHI 2020). The situation was so bad that the federal government had to call in the military for help (Canada-National Defence 2020; Armstrong and Klostermann, chapter 6, this volume). While deaths of older people have received much media attention, less attention is paid to the rising infection rate and deaths among frontline care workers (CTV News 2021).

Carework has been invisible, partly because it happens out of sight, in places like LTC homes, daycare centers, and private homes, and partly because much of this work is done by women, immigrants, and people of color—people who are less likely or able to speak out. In addition to this traditional labor pool, higher-income countries' incessant demand for care has propelled the migration of care workers (most of whom are women) from lower-income countries, thus intensifying a web of global care interdependence. As the pandemic continues, we are seeing more clearly an underlying problem associated with the existing global care interdependence: at the core, it is premised on pervasive gender inequality structured by unequal gender division of labor, low value given to carework, and high social and economic inequalities. This chapter shows how global care interdependence rests on the pervasive gender inequality, the devaluation of carework, and the exploitation of global inequality. To the extent a pandemic can serve as an important lesson, COVID-19 has made us aware of and driven to reassess the value of care and carework and to find ways to create healthier and more sustainable global care migration.

Global Care Interdependence: Recent Data

The rapid population aging, increased maternal employment, and changing norms and expectations about childcare and education in many higher-income countries have created a huge demand for care and a growing shortage of care workers. But because carework is largely considered an extension of women's unpaid familial obligations, it is generally assigned low wages and low status in the labor market, and most middle-class, native-born women will not take the job if they have other options (Dwyer 2013; England 2005; England et al. 2002). Consequently, the work is often filled by immigrant women and women of color and, increasingly, by foreign migrant care workers (Duffy 2005; Glenn 1992; Peng 2021).[1]

Across the globe, women make up over 70 percent of the care workforce (ILO 2018; UN Women 2020d). In the United States, over 85 percent of health care and childcare workers are women; in Canada they account for 82 percent of the total health care and social assistance workforce (BLS 2021; Moyser 2017). Within this imbalanced gender representation, immigrant women and women of color are prominent, particularly in the low-wage care sector. As illustrated in table 3.1, in the United States, Black/African Americans and Hispanic/Latinos are disproportionately represented in low-wage carework (BLS 2021).

In the United States, immigrants make up 38 percent of home health aides, even though they account for only 17 percent of the overall workforce (MPI 2020). In Canada, immigrants account for 35 percent of nurse aides and related workers (Bhaskar 2020), while the foreign-born population represents only 22 percent of the total population, and new immigrants (those arriving in Canada within the last 10 years) account for 8 percent of the total labor force (Statistics Canada n.d.; K. Wong 2020). The large number of immigrant and foreign-born workers in low-wage carework is not a reflection of their lower skill level, however. In the United States, immigrants aged 25 and over working in the health care sector—particularly those working as home health aides, personal care aides, and nursing assistants—are more likely to hold a bachelor's degree or higher than their native-born counterparts (MPI 2020). In Canada, nearly 60 percent of foreign live-in-caregivers have a bachelor's or higher degree[2] (Banerjee et al. 2017; Tungohan 2020).

In addition to the extensive use of immigrant women and women of color, the huge care demand in higher-income countries has drawn a large number of migrant women into the global care market. The International Labour Organization (ILO) estimates that of approximately 11.5 million migrant workers employed in domestic service globally, 73.4 percent (8.5 million) are women, and their work often involves caring for young, old, or disabled persons—in other words, they are care

TABLE 3.1

**Employed persons (16 years+) by occupation, sex, race/ethnicity
[numbers in thousands]**

			% of total employed			
Occupation	Total employed	Women	White	Black/ African American	Asian	Hispanic/ Latino
	152,581	47	77.5	12.3	6.6	18
Health care support occupations	4,887	85.1	64.5	24.5	6.8	20.9
Home health aides	570	87	56.3	32	8.9	25.9
Personal care aides	1,411	80.4	61.6	24.9	8.5	21.5
Nursing assistants	1,248	88.9	58.3	33.2	4.8	14.8
Orderlies and psychiatric aides	55	52.9	60.2	32.3	2.7	16.9
Maids and housekeeping cleaners	1,357	88.7	74.9	15.2	5.2	48.2
Childcare workers	974	94.6	77.6	14	4.4	24.4

Source: BLS 2021.

workers (ILO 2015; Peng 2017c; WHO 2017).[3] In Latin America and the Caribbean, 93 percent of the 750,000 migrant domestic workers are women (ILO 2015; Rico and Pautassi, chapter 7, this volume).

In Europe, the demand for care, particularly LTC, is so acute that the World Health Organization (WHO 2017) estimates a shortage of 2.3 million formal LTC workers in the region alone. Foreign-born workers already make up 29 percent of the home-based caregiver workforce[4] across Organization for Economic Cooperation and Development countries; in some, they make up more than half of that workforce: 89 percent in Italy, 75 percent in Greece, 67 percent in Spain, and 50 percent in Luxembourg. These migrant care workers come from neighboring countries, such as Romania, Ukraine, Moldova, and Bulgaria, but also from other parts of the world, such as Peru, Bolivia, Ecuador, and Colombia (OECD 2015; Marchetti and Mesiäislehto, chapter 13, this volume). In short, many EU countries simply would not be able to sustain their LTC systems without foreign migrant care workers.

Migration's Wrong Turn in Global Care

Studies based on the concept of the global care chain have revealed a complex interplay of individual agencies, national policies, and global political economic forces shaping global care migrations. At the individual/household level, the unequal gender division of labor despite changing postindustrial contexts has led to the outsourcing of carework by middle-class families (Duffy, Armenia, and Stacey 2015a; Michel and Peng 2017); while at national and global levels, neoliberal policy emphasis on privatization and marketization of care and economic growth through competition and productivity gain have reinforced carework's low market valuation and rationalized the use of immigrants, women of color, and foreign migrant workers in care services (Lutz 2018; Michel and Peng 2012, 2017; Parreñas 2012; Razavi and Staab 2012). Indeed, the combination of unequal gender division of labor and neoliberal market logic has stimulated global care migration and deepened global care interdependence (Belanger and Silvey 2020; Gottfried and Chun 2018). There are two problems with this phenomenon.

First, the current format of global care interdependence does little to solve the global care crisis because it remains blind to the root cause of the problem—the unequal gender division of labor. The global care crisis stems from two interrelated dynamics: in higher-income countries, the combination of an aging population, increased expectations for childcare, and women's increased paid employment has resulted in a greater demand for care; in lower-income countries, the out-migration of women has left growing numbers of children and elderly persons without adequate care. While migrant care workers might alleviate some of the concerns of middle-class women in higher-income countries, they cannot solve the global care crisis problem because populations in both higher- and lower-income countries will continue to age, and women will continue to join the paid labor force (Peng 2017a). Similarly, as more women from lower-income countries out-migrate, it will create more demand for care in the sending countries that are already losing their most important caregivers.

The global care interdependence in its current format is not only unsustainable but also induces and reinforces inequality. Outsourcing carework to women from lower socioeconomic class, immigrant women, and women of color through domestic or global care chains thus perpetuates and underscores the problem of unequal gender division of labor faced by women across the world, and it highlights the sharp divide among women along racial, class, and citizenship status lines (Duffy, Armenia, and Stacey 2015a; Ehrenreich and Hochschild 2003). The global care chain is an expedient solution for middle-class families to meet their care needs without having to address and change the unequal gender division of labor at home. Left in its current format, it will only serve to privilege middle-class men.

Second, the direction in which the global care interdependence is currently moving is premised on low valuation of care and the exploitation of gender, class, race, and global inequalities. As I noted earlier, the low labor market valuation of care results from the continuing acceptance of the unequal gender division of labor within the household; it sustains the historical and cultural bias that sees care as a woman's family obligation and hence of little or no market value (Dwyer 2013; England 2005). Added to this, the dominant neoliberal macroeconomic theory sees the outsourcing of care and global care migration largely as a value-neutral, and even potentially a positive-sum proposition (OECD 2014; World Bank 2018). According to this perspective, global care migration will benefit women in receiving countries because higher-wage-earning women outsourcing their carework to other women at a lower wage will achieve greater economic efficiency and create employment opportunities for "less-skilled" (women) care workers. At the same time, families and employers will also benefit from the in-migration of foreign care workers because they supply services that are in demand and fill a labor shortage. For the sending countries, the global care migration will benefit the foreign migrant care workers, their families, and the government because the migrants can potentially earn more money abroad than if they stay in the country, and they send back remittances.[5]

Yet the mechanism of global interdependence works precisely because the low value given to carework and multiple layers of social and economic inequalities that exist between men and women, among women of different race and socioeconomic classes, and between countries serve to reinforce one another. As the ILO report points out, the precarity and the availability of migrant care workers allow employers to suppress wages for certain types of carework: "In labour markets with wide earnings inequality or high levels of unemployment, certain care workers might be placed at the bottom of the pay hierarchy, putting pressure on care workers' pay" (ILO 2018, 174). What neoliberal macroeconomic theory does not consider is the systemic market devaluation of carework; gender-, race-, and citizenship status–biased wage structures; poor working conditions; and potential human rights abuses associated with carework, or the physical, mental, and social costs associated with family separation, employment insecurity, and liminality for foreign migrant care workers (Sun, chapter 11, this volume).

COVID-19 as an Opportunity for Transformation

The COVID-19 pandemic has made explicit the importance of care, our deepening global care interdependence, and its inequality-inducing potential. But the pandemic also gives us an opportunity to make transformative changes. I suggest a two-pronged strategy to achieving these changes: first, apply Elson's (2017) three Rs of unpaid carework in research, policy, and civil society activism; second, restructure global care migration through more equality-inducing political and policy actions.

Elson (2017) attributes the stalled progress in the gender wage gap since the 2010s to women's disproportionately greater unpaid care and domestic work. To fix this, she suggests three Rs—recognize, reduce, and redistribute unpaid carework. To this I add a fourth R—revalue. The pandemic has helped achieve the first R. The importance of both paid and unpaid carework has been recognized by all sectors of society: parents are raising issues about school closures and mental health impacts of work–care imbalance; communities have come together to cheer frontline care workers; some employers are giving carework wage enhancements; and some governments have begun to invest in the care economy. At the societal level, the pandemic has made people appreciate the importance of care in ensuring a healthy and productive economy. These recognitions have led to calls for more public investment in social and health care, better wages and working conditions for frontline care workers, and more equitable and quality social and health care systems across the globe.

To reduce unpaid carework, the second R, more public investments in care and social infrastructure are necessary. Some governments are beginning to move in this direction. For example, the Canadian government is beginning to invest in childcare and LTC systems (Canada 2020). In the United States, the Biden administration is investing in care infrastructure (New York Times 2020), and the work on this has already begun. Of course, politicians may be motivated by political opportunities and imperatives, but the recent initiatives to invest in care and social infrastructure suggest a step toward reducing unpaid carework. The next step is to ensure that these plans are implemented and investments continue.

The third R, redistributing unpaid carework between men and women, may be more challenging. It will involve cognitive/behavioral as well as cultural/institutional changes. For care to be redistributed equally, men will have to increase their share of unpaid carework within the household.[6] Women and men must commit to share unpaid carework equally, and employers and businesses must change their practices to enable workers to do unpaid carework. Policies such as equal paid parental leaves for both men and women are important, but nontransferable paid paternity leave will encourage more men to take a parental leave. Employers must also actively change their work and organizational cultures to include respecting and supporting workers' right and need to give care and ensuring that they will not be penalized in pay and career advancement. Governments must anchor workers' right to provide care and gender equal practices in social and economic policies. As more men engage in carework at home, individual mindsets and employment and business cultures will begin to change.

These are, however, not an easy ask as these involve ideational as well as structural changes, and social norms about gender division of carework are deeply rooted in our societies and tied to individual identities, and they are often intergenerationally transmitted (Kleven et al. 2018; Kremer 2007; Pfau-Effinger 2005a; Sevilla-Sanz et al. 2010). Indeed, recent studies show that across the globe, while both men and women have increased the amount of their unpaid carework within households since COVID-19, women continue to take on a much greater share compared to men (Adams-Prassl et al. 2020; Peng and Jun 2022; Sevilla and Smith 2020; UN Women 2020c). These suggest the intractable nature of gender division of carework, and the resilience of that normative practice even in the face of an unprecedented and monumental socioeconomic crisis such as COVID-19. In short, while the pandemic might serve as a catalyst for better redistribution of carework, it might also reinforce and intensify the preexisting unequal distribution of unpaid carework. The process of societal normative changes could be very slow.

However, even if the redistribution of care between men and women happens, this will not necessarily reduce the need for care services. An aging population and increased women's employment mean that the demand for care will continue, and sustained public investments in care and social infrastructure will be necessary. This also means that global care migration will continue. This leads to my fourth R: with more public investment in care and social infrastructure, and with our recognition of its importance, we must seriously revalue carework. Some countries have begun to do this. In Canada, most provinces have raised the wages of care workers in recognition of their importance. In the province of British Columbia, the government has reclassified all frontline care workers in the LTC sector as public sector employees and raised their wages to union level (Armstrong et al. 2020). Raising wages and formalizing care workers' employment will lead to positive employment and have economic outcomes. Macroeconomic simulations show that public investments in care and social infrastructure can lead to significant employment generation and positive economic growth, and this is particularly important in the context of the COVID-19 pandemic (UK Women's Budget Group 2020).

Finally, the four Rs must be complemented by the second prong of the two-prong strategy for transformative changes—the restructuring of global care migration through equality-inducing political and policy actions. While redistributing and revaluing paid and unpaid carework might help reduce excessive outsourcing of care—and its concomitant dependence on migrant care workers—we must also restructure the current form of global care interdependence to ensure that this will not reinforce inequalities. This will require putting pressures on both sending and receiving countries to revalue carework and raise the wages and improve the working conditions of all care workers regardless of immigration status. Both sending and receiving countries can begin this process by ratifying the ILO Convention C-189 on international employment standards and the human rights of migrant domestic and care workers. This Convention sets a baseline employment standard for migrant care workers, and is *not* a high barrier for receiving countries to agree to. Yet, so far, only thirty countries have ratified the Convention, most of them sending countries, while most of the receiving countries, including the United States, United Kingdom, and Canada, remain silent on the issue. Receiving countries also need to reform their immigration and employment policies to preclude conscious and unconscious bias in the assessment of foreign migrant care workers' skills and accreditations, to provide protection under national employment legislation, to ensure that employers do not violate workers' human rights, and to provide pathways to long-term residency. For their part, sending countries must reform their economic and labor policies to protect the rights of their citizens working abroad and regulate intermediary agencies to prevent human rights violations. They must also revise their development strategy from human capital export to domestic human capital investment and development through social infrastructures, such as health care and public education. As Chami et al. (2018, 45) point out, while remittances might help lift millions of families in sending countries out of poverty, in the long run it could also create "a remittance trap that causes economies to get stuck on a lower-growth, higher-emigration treadmill," thus draining these countries of their precious human capital and suppressing long-term positive social and economic development.

Conclusion

The COVID-19 pandemic has shaken the world awake to the importance of care and carework, and the reality of the global care interdependence hinged on multidimensional gender and global inequalities unlike any other crises of the past century. But because of this, it has also created an opening for us to rethink care and migration, and to push for transformative changes. As we move beyond the second year of the pandemic we must learn from this experience and seize this opportunity to institute the four R principles in our daily lives and to push for institutional and policy changes and more equality-inducing policies for global care migration.

NOTES

1. It is important to point out that although the majority of care workers are women, some men also participate in both paid and unpaid carework. See Hussein and Christensen (2017) and Locke (2017) on male care workers and how carework intersects with gender, race, class, and migration status.

2. Canada's Live-in-Caregiver program was terminated and replaced by the Caregiver program in 2014. The conservative government feared that the program, which offers a pathway to long-term residency after 2 years of employment, will result in too many people abusing this system as a means of gaining family reunification (CBC 2014). The Caregiver program removed the automatic pathway to long-term residency.

3. In countries like Canada and the United States, immigrant workers are normally considered those who have been accepted to the country with a long-term/permanent residency visa and the right to citizenship following a required residency period, whereas migrant workers are foreign-born workers who are formally or informally working in the country on a temporary basis, and who do not have long-term/permanent residency or a right to citizenship.

4. OECD defines "home-based caregiver" as a care worker in a private home providing personal care services for children and, increasingly, elderly and disabled people. Many also perform domestic labor as part of their caregiving work.

5. Studies show that migrant women workers make significant contributions to their families' well-being and to their countries' economic development. In fact, the UN Women argues that half of the World Bank's estimated $601 billion in global remittance is made by migrant women workers, and "in countries such as Nepal, women migrant

workers—mostly domestic workers—contribute about 50 per cent of migrant workers' remittances, or around 23 per cent to Gross Domestic Product (GDP) (UN Women n.d., 2; Chami et al. 2018).

6. A recent opinion poll survey conducted in the UK found that men want to do more care and to have more time to care, and most people support more public investment in care (UK Women's Budget Group 2020).

4

Black Lives Matter

Structural Racism, Sexism, and Carework in the United States

ODICHINMA AKOSIONU, JANETTE DILL, MIGNON DUFFY,
AND J'MAG KARBEAH

Facing simultaneous crises of COVID-19 and nationwide protests in response to the high-profile police killings of Breonna Taylor, George Floyd, and many others—the continued impact of anti-Black racism in the United States was laid bare during the pandemic. There was widespread media attention to racial disparities in infection and mortality rates, with the Centers for Disease Control and Prevention reporting in August 2020 that Black non-Hispanic Americans were 2.6 times as likely to contract the virus as white non-Hispanic Americans. Even more alarming, Black women in the United States were 4.7 times more likely to be hospitalized for COVID-19, and their risk of death was more than double that of white Americans (Centers for Disease Control and Prevention 2020a). This chapter argues that these differential impacts must be understood in the context of Black women's unique position in the health care workforce, a product of structural racism and sexism.

Leading into the pandemic, 23 percent of all Black women in the U.S. labor force worked in health care, meaning that almost one in four Black women were at the epicenter of risk during the COVID-19 crisis.[1] Black women are more over-represented than any other demographic group in health care, and within the sector they are most heavily concentrated in some of its lowest-wage and most hazardous jobs. The position of Black women in health care has its roots in the same devaluation of Black bodies that is reflected in police brutality and killings of Black men and women.

Importantly, the risks to Black women working in hazardous low-wage health care jobs that lack benefits such as paid sick days did not begin or end with the pandemic. Solutions must reach beyond the impact of the COVID-19 virus to directly address the underlying inequities and inadequacies stemming from the intersections of structural racism and sexism. Public and private investment in the carework infrastructure in the United States is therefore key to creating racial and gender justice as well as to providing safe and high-quality care to all beyond the public health crisis of COVID-19.

Black Women, Health Care, and COVID-19

As Julie Kashen argues (chapter 20, this volume), paid carework in the United States reflects a hierarchy of human value in which we value the lives and contributions of some people over those of others. The intersection of anti-Black racism and sexism has led Black women to be particularly affected by these racialized and gendered hierarchies.

The racialized division of labor between white and Black women in the performance of overwhelmingly feminized carework has its roots as far back as chattel slavery. Scholars note that throughout history this division of labor channeled white women to become masters of the emotional, more performative aspects of carework, whereas Black women were forced to engage in more invisible "backroom" and physically intensive tasks (Duffy 2011; Glenn 1992, 2010). In the context of slavery, white women of means were the hostesses and mistresses of the home, while Black enslaved women often did the backbreaking and never-ending work of cleaning houses and outhouses, laundering and maintaining clothing, and procuring, preparing and serving food. Domestic servitude in the North in the pre–Civil War era mirrored this gendered and racialized division of care labor, despite the different economic structure, and Black women were heavily overrepresented in the expanding ranks of domestic servants across the nation in the second half of the nineteenth century (Duffy 2011; Glenn 1992, 2010).

As the ranks of domestic servants began to decline in the early twentieth century, the modern health care system was being created in the United States. The professionalization of medicine meant that physician jobs were increasingly closed to women (Ehrenreich and English 1979). White women activists carved out the niche of trained nursing as a "feminine" domain by focusing rhetorically on the moral and spiritual caring aspects of the job (despite the reality of hard physical labor for many nurses at that time), and Black women were largely excluded from professional nursing well into the 1960s (Hine 1989; Reverby 1987). The development and explosive growth of a wide range of low-wage health care support roles began in earnest in the second half of the twentieth century, and these jobs have been disproportionately held by women (and smaller numbers of men) of color as well as immigrant workers (Duffy 2007). Women of color are heavily concentrated in these roles that constitute the "dirty work" of care—direct care for older, disabled, and ill bodies and bodily functions as well as cleaning and food preparation and serving in hospitals and long-term care institutions. The gendered and racialized stratification of health care, created by an interplay of structural exclusion and cultural association, mirrors the division of labor first created during slavery, and places Black women in a very particular high-risk position.

TABLE 4.1

Health care industry by sex

Industry	Total number of workers	% Male	% Female
Labor force	166,063,647	52.7	47.3
Total health care	18,562,557	23.0	77.0
Home health care services	1,543,212	13.7	86.3
Hospitals (except psych)	7,398,455	25.0	75.0
Nursing care facilities (skilled nursing)	1,875,203	17.2	82.8
Residential care (except skilled nursing)	1,165,336	24.7	75.3
Medical offices, outpatient centers, and other health care services	6,580,351	24.4	75.6

Note: Calculated by authors from American Community Survey 2018 (Ruggles et al. 2022). Includes only workers in the labor force.

Going into the pandemic, women were heavily overrepresented across the health care sector, making up 77 percent of health care workers overall, 83 percent of workers in skilled nursing facilities, and 86 percent of home health workers (table 4.1). Within this extremely female dominated workforce, Black women were overrepresented at higher rates than any other group. While Black women made up only 6 percent of the overall labor force in 2018, they made up almost 13 percent of the health care industry overall and 22–23 percent of workers in home health care services and nursing care facilities (table 4.2). These rates of representation are more than 3.5 times their rate of representation in the labor force. So, although white women are the numerical majority in health care, Black women workers are more highly concentrated in these low-wage, high-risk jobs. In fact, as mentioned earlier, almost one-quarter of Black women worked in health care in the years directly preceding the pandemic.

It should be noted that other groups of women of color are also overrepresented in the health care sector. For example, Hispanic women are overrepresented at a rate of about 1.3 times their representation in the labor force in the health care sector (10.1% of health care workers compared to 7.8% of the labor force). Asian women are overrepresented at a rate of about 1.7 times their representation in the labor force (5.2% of health care workers compared to 3.0% of the labor force). While women from other racial groups are overrepresented it is not to the same degree that Black women are concentrated in the industry, and not with the same kind of widespread representation across subsectors and occupations. The

TABLE 4.2

Health care industry by sex and race

Industry	% Black female	% White female	% Black male	% White male
Labor force	6.3	28.9	5.6	32.6
Total health care	12.8 (2.0×)*	46.9 (1.6×)	3.3	13.7
Home health care services	23.7 (3.8×)	38.9 (1.3×)	3.1	6.1
Hospitals (except psych)	11.2 (1.7×)	47.7 (1.7×)	3.6	14.5
Nursing care facilities (skilled nursing)	22.5 (3.5×)	45.9 (1.6×)	4.5	8.8
Residential care (except skilled nursing)	18.5 (2.9×)	42.0 (1.5×)	6.2 (1.1×)	13.7
Medical offices, outpatient centers, and other health care services	8.3 (1.3×)	49.0 (1.7×)	2.2	15.9

Note: Calculated by authors from American Community Survey 2018 (Ruggles et al. 2022). Includes only workers in the labor force. Note that percentages do not add to 100 because not all groups are included in the table. These racial categories include only Black non-Hispanic and white non-Hispanic workers.

* Represents rate of overrepresentation.

health care sector is further gendered and racialized in the distribution of jobs within the industry (table 4.3). Black women and white women are overrepresented in almost every major occupational category in health care, with only two exceptions. Women overall are underrepresented among physicians and surgeons, where white men make up a large segment of the workforce. And white women are also underrepresented among janitorial and housekeeping workers, a heavily racialized sector where Black men are also overrepresented.

The three occupations in which Black women are most heavily concentrated are licensed practical nurses; nursing, psychiatric, and home health aides; and personal care aides (see table 4.3). This is a group of jobs that is often referred to as direct care, emphasizing the hands-on nature of the care provided by these workers to older adults and people with disabilities in private homes and in institutional settings. In the first waves of the pandemic, nursing home workers were considered to have "the most dangerous jobs in America" because of the high incidence of COVID-19 cases and deaths (McGarry, Porter, and Grabowski 2020).

TABLE 4.3

Occupational breakdown within health care by sex and race

Occupation	% Black female	% White female	% Black male	% White male
Labor force	*6.3*	*28.9*	*5.6*	*32.6*
Medical and health services managers	9.7 (1.5×)*	47.6 (1.6×)	3.3	19.3
Physicians and surgeons	2.7	21.8	2.6	42.3 (1.3×)
Registered nurses	9.8 (1.6×)	62.4 (2.1×)	1.4	7.4
Licensed practical nurses	22.5 (3.6×)	46.8 (1.6×)	3.8	5.9
Nursing, psychiatric and home health aides	29.5 (4.7×)	37.1 (1.2×)	4.0	5.1
Medical assistants and health support	14.1 (2.2×)	43.6 (1.5×)	2.8	5.8
Personal care aides	23.6 (3.7×)	35.7 (1.2×)	4.9	6.7
Food service and preparation	16.3 (2.6×)	33.5 (1.2×)	10.1 (1.8×)	16.6
Janitorial and housekeeping	17.5 (2.8×)	24.1	11.9 (2.1×)	17.5
Receptionists and information clerks	11.9 (1.9×)	55.9 (1.9×)	1.2	2.7
Secretaries and admin assistants	10.8 (1.7×)	65.2 (2.3×)	0.7	2.3

Note: Calculated by authors from American Community Survey 2018 (Ruggles et al. 2022). Includes only workers in the labor force. Note that percentages do not add to 100 because not all groups are included in the table. These racial categories include only Black non-Hispanic and white non-Hispanic workers. These occupational groups were chosen because they are some of the largest numerically within the field of health care.

*Represents rate of overrepresentation.

While workers in these institutions were sometimes lauded as heroes, staff who held jobs at multiple facilities were often painted as vectors of disease (Freytas-Tamura 2020), racialized narratives that are similar to those used against immigrant laborers decades earlier (Molina 2011). During the first waves of the crisis, many workers in long-term care facilities did not have access to adequate personal protective equipment, and risks were exacerbated by chronic understaffing (Grabowski and Mor 2020). Home health care workers were also identified as at high risk for infection, as lacking in appropriate protections, and as potential vectors of transmission as they traveled between clients' homes (Penton 2020).

The other two types of jobs where Black women are most overrepresented are in the "back-room" positions in food service and preparation and janitorial and housekeeping (see table 4.3). These workers clean hospital rooms, serve food in nursing homes, and do laundry in long-term care facilities. Despite also being deemed essential, the labor of these workers and their role in a pandemic world of care have been less visible and received even less attention than the work of direct care. Housekeeping staff at a hospital have been exposed to COVID-19 but may have received differential access to appropriate personal protective equipment (Hong 2020).

New Virus, Old Problems

While COVID-19 changed almost every aspect of work and life for people around the globe, the risks faced by Black women working in health care during this crisis were a direct result of existing inequities and inadequacies. The labor of workers in care is devalued, meaning that workers earn less in these occupations as compared to occupations that require the same level of education and skill but do not involve carework (England, Budig, and Folbre 2002; Levanon, England, and Allison 2009). This is especially true for direct care and other low-wage care workers, where Black women are overrepresented, while professionalized nurturant care occupations like nursing that are more likely to have a higher proportion of white women are less likely to incur a wage penalty (Budig, Hodges, and England 2019). Additionally, studies of carework in the health care sector demonstrate that Black and other women of color experience the largest wage penalties of all women in these occupations (Dill and Hodges 2019).

The long-term care sector is where Black women are most overrepresented and where we also find the lowest wages. The mean hourly wage in 2019 for home care workers was $12.12, residential care earned average wages of $12.69 per hour, and nursing assistants in nursing homes earned $13.90 per hour (PHI International 2020). Low incomes lead to high poverty among long-term care workers: one in six home care workers live below the federal poverty line and nearly half live in low-income households. More than half of home care workers receive some form of public assistance, and nearly half rely on means-tested Medicaid coverage for health insurance. Direct care workers in institutional settings (either residential care or nursing homes) are slightly more advantaged than home care workers, but nearly half of these workers live in low-income households, more than a third receive some form of public assistance, and around a quarter rely on Medicaid for health insurance (PHI International 2020). A recent research study found that among Black and Latina female direct care workers specifically, about 50 percent earn less than $15 per hour, and only 10 percent have employer-based health insurance coverage (Himmelstein and Venkataramani 2019). Direct care and cleaning and food workers also fall into the low-wage group that has the least access to paid leave, with estimates ranging from one-fifth to one-third having any access to paid leave for illness or to care for a loved one (Kinder 2020). In fact, some health care workers were even exempt from the emergency COVID-19 paid sick leave passed by Congress because of worker shortages (Long and Rae 2020).

Low wages and lack of benefits are deeply problematic for Black women and others working in direct care and other low-wage jobs in the health care sector (True et al. 2020). Living in poverty increases the risk for many chronic diseases as well as exposure during a pandemic like COVID-19 (Conway 2015; Kinder 2020; Nguyen et al. 2020). Workers in this labor force often work multiple jobs to cobble a living wage together, which became a barrier to containment during the crisis (Baughman, Stanley, and Smith 2020; Van Houtven, DePasquale, and Coe 2020). And lack of access to appropriate medical insurance and adequate paid leave policies both cripple individual workers and undermine larger public health efforts.

Direct care and cleaning and food service jobs in health care were hazardous long before the pandemic brought the dangers into public view. Health care workers have the highest rates of workplace-related injuries compared to other sectors in the United States (Gomaa et al. 2015). Within the workforce, nurse aides and nurses, who are overwhelmingly women, are much more likely to experience workplace-related injuries and stress compared to other health care workers (D'Arcy, Sasai, and Stearns 2012). In addition to being exposed to biological agents, such as viruses, direct care and reproductive workers in health care are exposed to toxic chemicals used in cleaning and sanitizing, heavy lifting of equipment and patients, physical and verbal assault, and a range of high-stress conditions, including long hours and night shift work (Kurowski, Boyer, and Punnett 2015). Black women are more likely to work in nursing homes and other long-term care settings that are understaffed and underresourced, leading to greater risk and exposure to injury or infection (Barnett and Grabowski 2020; Grabowski and Mor 2020). Despite this increased risk, the unique vulnerabilities of Black women in these sectors are often overlooked and necessary protections delayed—a pattern that is also mirrored in national conversations about police violence.

Transforming Care, Dismantling Racism

Kimberlé Crenshaw has noted that movements against police violence often highlight cases involving Black men and that similar cases of police violence against

Black women are largely ignored (https://www.aapf.org/sayhername). Care is another critical arena in which Black women are located at the intersections of racism and sexism, and their experiences are central yet underappreciated. Investing in Black women through targeted investment in care infrastructure can begin to undermine some of the ideological constructions and structural barriers that have devalued both. There are a number of immediate steps the United States can and should take to address the inequities and inadequacies in the care infrastructure highlighted by the COVID-19 pandemic.

First, we need policy to raise wages in the direct care, cleaning, and food service segments of the health care sector where workers are currently most grossly underpaid (Dill et al. 2020; Hess and Hegewisch 2019). This should start with a federal minimum wage increase that is inclusive of all workers (in the United States as in many other countries workers who work in private homes have often been excluded from fair labor legislation). A recent study estimated that increasing the minimum wage to $15 would result in a reduction of household poverty rates among female health care workers by up to 27 percent (Himmelstein and Venkataramani 2019). In the United States, many long-term care facilities and home health care programs are funded by federal and state governments through Medicaid and other programs. In order to ensure that wage increases do not further exacerbate staffing shortages, the rate at which facilities are reimbursed for patient care in these programs must also be adjusted accordingly. Increasing wage levels is a critical component of reimagining health care workforce policies to center social justice (Hess and Hegewisch 2019).

Second, we need public policy that addresses the problematic working conditions of low-wage jobs in the health care sector in which Black women are concentrated. Protective equipment, including not only infection control but also lifting assist devices and other interventions, must be provided to workers across occupational categories, and workers should have access to predictable schedules and reliable hours (Harknett, Schneider, and Luhr 2022). All health care workers, including those who work in private homes, must be fully integrated into federal and state worker safety standards. Health systems currently lack incentives to address the quick turnovers that happen due to these high-stress, low-wage jobs that have inconsistent work hours (McDermott and Goger 2020; True et al. 2020). Direct care and other low-wage workers in hospitals and long-term care facilities need better career growth pipelines. In addition, Black workers who oftentimes provide culturally sensitive care should be compensated for the extra care they provide, in addition to creating a healthy work environment, free from experiences of discrimination and microaggressions, where they can thrive (Travers et al. 2020).

Finally, health care workers at all levels, including those who work behind the scenes in kitchens and housekeeping, must be provided with sufficient paid sick leave and paid care leave (Addati et al. 2018; Hess and Hegewisch 2019). The United States lags far behind other countries in the provision of paid leave to workers across the board, and this pandemic has highlighted the costs to all of us of workers not being able to stay home when they are ill or caring for an ill family member.

All of these interventions will cost money. But this pandemic has shown us that public and private sector investment in care infrastructure is not only important but imperative (Poo and Shah 2020). Black women and others who do these essential jobs in health care deserve to be paid fairly and protected fully. Beyond that, we have seen more starkly than ever during this public health crisis that we are all compromised in terms of our health and well-being when health care workers are not adequately paid and protected. And, finally, the national reckoning with systemic racism in the United States that has emerged simultaneous to the pandemic requires us to address the gendered and racialized inequities in care to move toward gender and racial justice.

NOTE

1.   Unless otherwise cited, all statistics were calculated by the authors using the 2018 American Community Survey (Ruggles et al. 2022). Note that we define health care broadly to include long-term care services for older and disabled adults, both in institutions and in homes.

5

Disability, Ableism, and Care during COVID-19 in the United States

LAURA MAULDIN

COVID-19 has unequal effects on disabled, chronically ill, and elderly people across the globe. In the United States (the focus of this chapter), this is evidenced by the fact that more than 41 percent of all COVID-19 deaths were at one point linked to nursing home residents or care workers (CMS 2020b). Congregate settings—a broad category including sites of long-term care, such as nursing homes, rehabilitation facilities, as well as some types of elderly housing, homeless shelters, and even prisons—were hit hardest because of residents' proximity to each other. On its face, this may seem explainable through biological factors. After all, many individuals occupying the high-risk categories identified by the Centers for Disease Control and Prevention (CDC) (over the age of 65 and having prior chronic illnesses or disabilities) primarily live in nursing homes and other long-term care facilities and residences. (Though to be sure, young disabled people[1] are often subject to being warehoused in nursing homes because the United States lacks adequate home care supports.) But the premise of this chapter is that ableism, or the systematic discrimination against and devaluation of disabled people, must be better recognized as a key social process and more centered in our analyses.

Prior care scholarship is based on the foundational tenets that systems of care are raced and gendered, but the way that disability and ableism figure into such systems is less discussed. Yet the devaluation of ill or disabled lives profoundly shapes how our care systems are structured in the first place. Rather than attributing higher COVID-19 rates in disability communities to biological factors, a sociological perspective on disability turns analysis toward social factors. Rather than accept COVID-19's decimation of these populations as "self-evident" or based on a "health status" that is somehow inevitable, a *disability analytic* opens up a new way of thinking about disabled people as a category (Mauldin and Brown 2021) and the systems shaping and constraining their lives, especially during COVID-19. Ableism is also intertwined with sexism and racism. For example, care workers are primarily Black and immigrant women, and nursing homes with higher populations of residents who are people of color have fared worse than those with primarily white residents (Gebeloff et al. 2020; Kim 2020).

I use the term "disability" to refer broadly to a heterogeneous category of disabled, chronically ill, and elderly people in order to engage in strategic universalizing (Mauldin and Brown 2021; Thomson 1997). A universalizing approach, inclusive of those with chronic illnesses and the elderly, recognizes that disability is not "special," but rather a typical and expectable part of life, though to be sure particular impairments take unique and diverse forms and vary in onset and effects. Nearly one quarter of the U.S. population has a disability, and half of adults live with one or more chronic conditions (Centers for Disease Control and Prevention 2019; National Health Council 2019). Additionally, various U.S. laws, as well as national and global health and disability organizations, define disability in relation to both physical and mental bodily functions, which would clearly include chronic illness (Thomas 2007). Sociological literature on conceptualizing the category of disability also engages with measurement and type of impairment (Altman 2016). And most of these categorizations that are adopted by governmental agencies rely on definitions of disability and impairment that would indeed include chronic illness and elderly individuals with impairments. Finally, "As people with impairment, those living with declared or readily apparent characteristics of chronic illnesses share in forms of social exclusion and disadvantage experienced by those whose impairments have other qualities and features" (Thomas 2007, 50).

My framing is not necessarily new; more than 30 years ago, British sociologist Michael Oliver posed the social model of disability (Shakespeare 2013), arguing that disability is socially produced through structural and cultural arrangements that exclude or otherwise oppress individuals with various types of impairments. Oliver states that the social model goes "beyond the personal limitations that impaired individuals may face, to social restrictions imposed by an unthinking society. Disability is understood as a social and political issue rather than a medical one" (Oliver 1998, 1446). More recently, sociologists contend that disabled people on the whole are subjected to marginalizing processes, though the specificities of their conditions give them their particular shape, and the intersection of other social locations will exacerbate or ease these processes. In other words, disability is more than just a "health status," it is an axis of inequality for which we need an analytic (Frederick and Shifrer 2018; Mauldin and Brown 2021; Naples, Mauldin, and Dillaway 2019).

By considering disability as an axis of inequality, we can better understand ableism, a value system characterized by discrimination against disability and the devaluation of certain bodies (Lewis 2019; Wolbring 2008). Ableism is behind hostility toward a class of individuals considered "unproductive," which is rooted in eugenics and clearly reflected in U.S. neoliberal policies related to a lack of health care and home care supports for ill and disabled people (Wolbring 2008). Furthermore, the ideology of ableism, particularly in the United States, is rooted in racism. As Lewis (2019) writes, ableism is "a system that places value on people's bodies and minds based on societally constructed ideas of normalcy, intelligence, and excellence . . . [these are] deeply rooted in anti-Blackness, eugenics, and capitalism." Integrating the critical work of disability scholars who take up the issue of ableism complements much of the work already being done in care scholarship and shows how multiply marginalized individuals experience care receiving or giving at the intersection of sexism, racism, *and* ableism. Inadequate public funding (especially for Medicaid, the social safety net for disabled people in the United States), crumbling care infrastructure, transnational and migrant care chains, and so on, have all been analyzed and understood as rooted in capitalism and racism. But the interlocking system of ableism is often not engaged within care scholarship more broadly. The critical work of disability scholars on the issue of ableism and disability as an axis of inequality would deepen central threads of inquiry in care scholarship on the COVID-19 pandemic, and beyond.

The tragedy of nursing homes and COVID-19 with which I began this chapter reveals how congregate care settings can be deadly for disabled people. But we can look at this from a structural angle: a damning report from AARP (Eaton 2020) cites the main problems as outdated laws, the nursing home industry's lax adherence to regulations, and the lack of oversight and accountability, as well as de-prioritization by government officials. Disability rights organizations cite persistent institutional bias in long-term services and supports as a result of policies that devalue disabled people and their integration into communities. Underfunding home care creates a situation where disabled people are pushed into congregate care settings instead of being provided with home- and community-based services (Center for Public Representation 2020). Meanwhile, "At least 18 states have laws or governor's orders that protect nursing homes from lawsuits and/or criminal prosecution related to the pandemic. New York and New Jersey so far are the only two states to provide immunity to corporate officials from the nursing home industry from civil lawsuits and some forms of criminal prosecution" (A. Wong 2020).

Beyond Nursing Homes: Ableism and COVID-19

The vast majority of disabled people and those who fit CDC high-risk categories for COVID-19—80 percent—live in private homes in the community (Congressional Budget Office 2015). In this context, paid carework is performed by home health aides. However, again, we see how resource allocation for serving disabled people in their homes intersects with raced and gendered carework. As Cranford (chapter 16, this volume) explains, home care workers in Canada have long worked in harmful conditions (earning minimum wage, possibly working for multiple agencies or in multiple homes), and COVID-19 has only exacerbated this. The situation is similar in the United States, where racist labor policies embedded in Roosevelt's New Deal continue to affect working conditions[2] and the conditions in which disabled people receive home care (Kim 2020; MacDonald 2020). During the pandemic, many disabled people chose to suspend care services to avoid being exposed to COVID-19. In my own research, this led to drastic effects on family caregivers and resulted in deteriorating health for disabled people in their homes (Mauldin 2021).

Elsewhere, younger disabled residents (and their care workers) in smaller congregate care settings like group homes are also "dying from the virus at a higher rate than the wider populations" (MacDonald 2020), but not all states are keeping statistics on these locations (Knezevich 2020). According to some available data, "Congregate housing for disabled people in New York other than nursing homes also shows infection and death rates far above average that may equal or even exceed those of nursing facilities" (Tsaplina and Stramondo 2020). No matter where they reside, disabled persons who acquire COVID-19 may be taken to the hospital, another site where they experience discrimination. Multiple states released "triage plans" for rationing care during the crisis, and disabled people as a category were targeted for denying treatment because of their disability status (Ne'eman 2020). This is evidenced by "Alabama's Emergency Operations Plan that would deny ventilators to folks with severe or profound intellectual disabilities, or Tennessee, where those with spinal muscular atrophy who require help with activities of daily living would be denied treatment in a pandemic" (Stramondo 2020).

This kind of discrimination in health care is not new; it has been long known that medical providers assume that disabled people have worse "quality of life" and make care decisions based on such assumptions (Gitlow and Flecky 2005; Goering 2008; Longmore 1995). One COVID-19 case caught national attention when a disabled Black man was denied a ventilator; his wife had captured the physician on video saying it was because he had a disability and therefore a poor quality of life (Cha 2020). In popular culture and discourse there is evident disdain for providing care for disabled and elderly people. Disabled and elderly people in the United States have been specifically targeted as "disposable" members of society when it comes to the possibility of rationing medical care. This is evidenced by instances of government officials arguing that disabled and elderly people are disposable and that care for them does not matter and should not be prioritized. The lieutenant governor of Texas suggested that older people should sacrifice themselves so the economy does not get destroyed (Levin 2020). Elsewhere, a California official suggested that the virus be left to take its natural course on "the sick, the old, the injured" (Ormseth 2020).

The Necessity of Ableism for Understanding COVID-19

Through a lens of ableism, it is clear that deadly flaws in the U.S. health and home care systems existed prior to COVID-19, but its arrival has unmasked these flaws. As outlined earlier, statistics related to COVID-19 infection rates and deaths have exposed that disabled people are subjected to the pandemic in ways that are unequal compared to nondisabled people. At the macrolevel, the entire design of a health care system tied to work and being "productive" is arguably ableist. Disability theorists Mitchell and Snyder (2015) deploy the term "ablenationalism" as a defining feature of the biopolitics of disability, and this can be useful in reflecting back on how ableism shapes care infrastructure in the United States. They merge together features of nationalism to capture the ways in which some parts of the population are deemed worthy of care and protection by the state, while others are considered disposable.

Scholarship rooted in a disability analytic provides tools for better understanding how these larger patterns in U.S. care systems carry over into the specific phenomenon of COVID-19. A disability analytic reveals how ableism and ablenationalism are central to the design of care infrastructures and policy. Ablenationalism is one of the reasons disabled people are far more likely to be institutionalized in some way than nondisabled people, whether in a nursing home, a rehabilitation center, a smaller congregate care setting, and so on. For example, the institutional bias in U.S. long-term care has meant long-term services and supports provided by Medicaid have largely gone to institutions rather than to funding home and community-based services (HCBSs) (Friedman and VanPuymbrouck 2019; Schulson 2020). On the one hand, deinstitutionalization in the United States is at an all-time high compared to before the disability rights movement in the United States in the 1970s and 1980s (Friedman and VanPuymbrouck 2019; Nielsen 2013; Shapiro 1994). On the other hand, these gains are slow: "Despite research indicating community living has more benefits than institutions, even for those with more severe impairments, a sizable proportion of people with disabilities still live in institutions in the US" (Friedman and VanPuymbrouck 2019, 360). The Center for Public Representation has been fighting to extend funding for the Money Follows the Person program, which helps Medicaid-funded congregate care residents to move to their communities. But the program expired in 2018, having suffered from only short-term and small funding extensions, resulting in significant drops in people being able to switch to HCBS. These social arrangements, informed by entrenched ableism, have a direct impact on the resources allocated to disabled people, their caregivers, and families.

A view of how COVID-19 affects disabled people across a variety of sites reveals the lack of a "disability lens on decision-making. . . . Especially in the areas of equality of access to health care and supports; access to information; and the lack of an emergency response plan for people with disabilities" (Wolbring 2020). Bioethicists and other scholars point out that "people who rely on long-term care can be especially vulnerable in a public health crisis, and fairly constructed and implemented crisis standards of care must account for this vulnerability" (Guidry-Grimes et al. 2020). This section highlights just some of the ways that a disability analytic can deepen how we analyze the organization of care infrastructure in the United States. Concepts like ablenationalism, vulnerability, the intersection of racism and ableism, deinstitutionalization and its roots in disability activism can better inform our COVID-19 scholarship as we seek social change.

Disability Activism: Dreaming of Lasting Change

I have tried to link ableism and the devaluation of disabled and ill people as part and parcel of why we also devalue care workers in these sectors. The plight of care workers and caregivers is a product of our devaluation of disability more broadly. In this final section, in thinking about how to make change, I highlight ways that disability communities, especially disabled communities of color, have responded to ableism and the COVID-19 pandemic and some of the ideas they have put forward for addressing these issues. How might looking to these communities for ideas contribute to our work as care scholars? I also consider some of the opportunities for lasting change that can occur when scholars integrate a disability analytic into research.

Scholarship on disability and scholarship on disability activism have long been intertwined. Yet care scholarship and disability scholarship have not historically been in conversation, though there are two excellent examples of times when they have converged. Kelly's (2016) book *Disability and the Politics of Care* expertly outlines the antagonism between disability movements and care issues, outlining how the disability rights movement has historically de-emphasized the need for care as a strategy to reject notions of disabled people as passive. Cranford (2020) comprehensively researched the tensions and interlocking interests between disability communities and care workers. While disabled people push for home and community-based care instead of congregate care, home care workers are needed. Yet disability studies have rarely engaged these workers (again Kelly is an exception with her focus on disabled people employing home care workers), and Cranford's work examines where and how the interests of care workers and disabled people employing them might diverge and converge. There is opportunity within our field to build on this kind of exciting work. A long-standing motto of the disability rights movement has been "Nothing about us without us." As I consider how care scholars might find opportunities to ignite lasting change with their work, I think about using COVID-19 as a moment to consider how engaging disability and critiques of ableism can better inform our work.

One critique of care in critical disability scholarship is the assumption that care recipients only "take" and care workers only "give." Critical disability scholarship argues instead that care is not a binary and that ableism shapes our view on care into binaries that perpetuate views of disabled people as passive (Kröger 2009; Piepzna-Samarasinha 2018). Relatedly, disability scholarship also emphasizes that care work is itself disabling, and that many care workers are themselves disabled (Institute of Medicine 2008). How might greater attention to disability and ableism's effects on all people (disabled or not) lead to care scholarship that can find new alliances and dialogue? Critical disability scholarship links capitalism, neoliberalism, racism, and ableism (Goodley and Lawthom 2019; Mitchell and Snyder 2015; Piepzna-Samarasinha 2018) and offers much analysis that could be engaged by care scholars.

Beyond reflecting on our own work as care scholars, we can also better engage disability scholarship and activism. Care scholars could look to disability communities putting theories to practice in their activism. This work has long been happening, particularly in disabled communities of color. One of the preeminent organizations is Sins Invalid (sinsinvalid.org), a disability justice performance project that has led to scholarly work on defining the disability justice movement in their primer *Skin, Tooth, and Bone* (2019). They have been instrumental in shifting conversations on the ground about care, emphasizing collective care outside state programs (as the state is seen as unreliable) and interdependence as a key value (eschewing goals of independence, long associated with the disability rights movement). Moreover, long before this pandemic, "disability justice communities have been steadfastly organizing . . . groups like the Disability Justice Culture Club in the San Francisco Bay Area and Crip Fund have been providing direct assistance and money to those facing serious needs. Disability rights organizations such as the American Association of People with Disabilities and the National Council of Independent Living have mobilized nationally to advocate for the passage of legislation that ensures that the needs of people with disabilities are included in every aspect of social and political response to the pandemic" (Mauldin et al. 2020,15). More recently, disability communities have come together to form #NoBodyIsDisposable (nobodyisdisposable.org) in response to the discriminatory triage plans for rationing COVID-19 care mentioned previously. Such grassroots campaigns against discrimination in triage deserve our scholarly attention and can push care scholars to ask new questions in the work we do and reveal new angles on the policy changes we recommend. Many disability justice groups have put forward plans for care collectives and more HCBS supports instead of congregate settings. With the pandemic laying bare how clear it is that disability is an axis of inequality, perhaps care scholarship can more explicitly connect with disability activists and include them in our research and framing.

Conclusion

I have argued that the devaluation of care is a product of our devaluation of disability more broadly, and that this has been made clear in the unequal effects of COVID-19 on disability communities and the dangers that disabled people face across different sites, from congregate to home settings to hospitals. One of the key ideas of disability justice movements is the belief that the state will not value or save disabled people. This is based on generations of neglect by the state in the United States, particularly with respect to people of color. In response, many have put forth care collectives and care pods, ones that transcend traditional family ties and expand outward enough to form supportive networks in the absence of a welfare state (Piepzna-Samarasinha 2018). Certainly, disability justice movements are not monolithic. Many work in concert with more disability rights–oriented groups that focus on state recognition and expansion of benefits, but in general there is little faith that this can be depended on as the sole answer to the neglect disabled people face. Meanwhile, care scholars are working to increase care infrastructure investment and address labor issues. There are different approaches, from dismantling our current for-profit system to increasing state-funded support and tightening oversight in congregate care settings. Overall, paying attention to disability communities during the COVID-19 crisis is crucial for being more attuned to disability in our research and strategic in our collaboration to capitalize on the opportunity to create lasting change in U.S. care infrastructures.

NOTES

1. So-called person-first language has its origins in service providers rather than disability communities. Please see Emily Ladau on why identity-first language is often preferred by disabled people: https://www.thinkinclusive.us/post/why-person-first-language-doesnt -always-put-the-person-first.

2. As I have reported elsewhere, "Racism is built into our care infrastructure. When Roosevelt's New Deal was passed in 1933, domestic and farmworkers were specifically excluded from labor protections precisely because these were jobs that were largely filled by people of color, and Southern Democrats wouldn't vote to improve the circumstances of a Black workforce. Many of these exclusions still apply" (Mauldin 2022).

6

Unpaid Care in Public Places

Tensions in the Time of COVID-19

PAT ARMSTRONG AND JANNA KLOSTERMANN

During a March 2020 Ontario lockdown that prevented all nonstaff from entering nursing homes, the Canadian Armed Forces were sent to provide support in seven homes. At the time, more than four out of five deaths in the province were in nursing homes where most of the residents and workers are women, many of them racialized or newcomers (Bowden 2020). When they marched out, the military took the unprecedented move of publicly publishing a report documenting the horrific conditions and indicating their shock at what they found. The report provided examples of abuse, neglect, and inadequate care (Mialkowski 2020). It detailed how residents were being sedated and were "scared and feel alone like they're in jail." Direct personal care also went missing, with "residents not having been bathed for several weeks," with rushed routines or "aggressive transfers." In one home, "patients [were] observed crying for help with staff not responding (30 minutes to over 2 hours)." According to the report, some residents did not receive meals, some were missing meals, and some who were unable to feed themselves were left without assistance. Laundry was left undone, residents were left undressed or in soiled garments, and linen shortages "led to residents sleeping on beds with no linens, leading to increased skin breakdown." The report described a "general culture of fear to use supplies because they cost money" and the prohibition against extra soaker pads. Staff had no time to provide basic care, find extra supplies, or offer social or psychological support.

This chapter locates the gaps in care highlighted by the military report within the state's continuing efforts to privatize care. Informed by our decade of international research that is based on methods detailed in our book *Creative Teamwork* (Armstrong and Lowndes 2018; see also Doucet and Armstrong 2021), we focus primarily on one form of this privatization, namely the shift to unpaid care. The pandemic prevented much of this work, in the process making more visible the ways unpaid care has filled gaps in paid care. This exploration allows us to critically reflect on feminist care scholars' questions, namely, assuming a right to care or to have one's care needs met, what are our collective, familial, and individual responsibilities to provide care? How do we navigate the tensions between structure and agency and among collective, family, and individual responsibilities in providing or not providing care? And what are the skills required? COVID-19 has highlighted and intensified tensions in care, emphasizing the need to unpack these questions. Here we use the specific example of nursing homes in Ontario, Canada's most populous province, to set out the full range of care provided by families—broadly defined, and to analyze the context in which such care was provided pre-pandemic. We then revisit the military report written during the pandemic to consider what it tells us about family care. To close, we critically reflect on struggles related to the right to care, elaborating promising policy suggestions

The "Right to Care"

Our understanding of the "right to care" is informed by the work of care ethicists who assume people deserve to have their care needs met (see Tronto, chapter 1, this volume), and by others who attend to how women are conscripted or coerced into caring (Armstrong et al. 2002). Glenn (2010, 5) writes, "The social organization of care has been rooted in diverse forms of coercion that have induced women to assume responsibility for caring for family members." In keeping with her thesis and our feminist political economy approach, we elaborate the historically specific social organization of Ontario long-term care and the forces that often serve to coerce women into unpaid family care. We also stress structures and agency, autonomy, and resistance that complicate our understanding of caring responsibilities.

Ontario's long-term care sector offers a fitting case study for thinking through the "right to care." Health care is primarily a provincial/territorial responsibility in Canada, although the federal Canada Health Act makes funding dependent on these jurisdictions providing universal access to medically necessary doctor and hospital care without any direct cost to the patient (Armstrong and Armstrong 2016). Nursing homes are not covered by this federal legislation, although all jurisdictions provide some public funding for nursing homes and cover medical care within them. Given the resulting variability across the country and the importance of attending to a historically and socially specific context, we focus here on Ontario nursing homes, defined as those with extensive public funding that provide 24-hour nursing care, primarily to older adults.

Locating Long-Term Care

We understand the growing reliance on unpaid care within public services as one form of neoliberal privatization strategies (Armstrong and Armstrong 2020; Armstrong, Armstrong, and Connelly 1997; Armstrong et al. 2002). By privatization, we mean a process that can involve any or all of moving away not only from public delivery and public payment for health services and health workers but also from a commitment to shared responsibility, democratic decision making, and the idea that the public sector operates according to a logic of service to all.

Historically, care for the older population relied mainly on coercing women into providing unpaid family care, in part by failing to provide alternatives, or on poorly paid women servants. Public involvement in Ontario nursing homes carried the legacy of the poorhouse and only accommodated those "without family or friends" to provide care (Struthers 2017, 285). In the context of the post–World War II welfare state development and a booming economy, Ontario required all municipalities to provide a home for the aged. It was a response to a growing older population, the exposure of terrible care in unsupervised commercial services, and women moving into the paid labor force in large numbers (Struthers 2017, 287).

But the energy crisis in the 1970s marked the end of the postwar profit boom, sparking a new international search for profit that included public services. As part of an austerity agenda (Whiteside 2016), the public sector was reorganized so that governments would steer markets, not row by providing services (Osborne and Gaebler 1992) and so that any remaining public services would be managed like for-profit ones. Once again, family, which usually means women, were held responsible for care.

In trade talks, Canada's health care was described as an "unopened oyster" (Nelson 1995), ripe for profit-making. And this was particularly the case for residential care. The aging population offered a golden opportunity for profit, given insufficient public alternatives for care. But investment opportunities were not restricted to what in Ontario are called retirement homes. They also extended to nursing homes primarily funded and regulated by the state. To "address" long wait times for nursing homes, then owned by municipalities, charitable organizations and small, private companies, the Conservative government expanded supply by setting up a competition that favored for-profit chains. It was an attractive opportunity for investors who were guaranteed payment and customers (Armstrong and Armstrong 2020).

In Ontario today, nearly 60 percent of nursing homes are owned by for-profit companies, and many of the not-for-profit ones are managed by for-profit corporations or have contracted out other services to corporations (Daly 2015; Hsu et al. 2016). Despite homes being highly regulated, there are no staffing minimums, and staffing levels are lowest in for-profit homes. While most homes are unionized, unions have not been as successful in raising staffing levels and full-time employment or in preventing services being subcontracted to nonunionized staff. Most care is provided by female personal support workers, many of whom are racialized or newcomers or both (Turcotte and Savage 2020) and have little required formal training. Injury and illness rates are high (Ontario Health Coalition 2020), further lowering staffing levels and limiting continuity in care that allows staff to respond to individual needs and develop care relationships. For-profit strategies focused on just-enough care or on minimally defined task-based care mean many workers have part-time jobs and work in multiple nursing homes (Hsu et al. 2016). Contracted services for food, laundry, and cleaning also bring in workers who are not part of the care team and who often move among workplaces.

All this has profound implications for the right to care and for the pressure on families to provide care, as well as on infection rates. People can wait up to 3 years to get a publicly funded nursing home bed. By the time someone gets admitted, they often have very complex care needs. And by the time they do, the women who provide most of the unpaid care at home have reached the breaking point. That said, obtaining a place in a nursing home does not end the demand for unpaid care. As a result of for-profit managerial strategies to provide just-enough care, much care is left undone. Gaps are left to be filled—or not—by families or by companions paid-for by families that can afford to do so (Daly, Armstrong, and Lowndes 2015). This was the case pre-pandemic, as we explain in the next section.

Families at Work: Gendered Coercion in Nursing Homes

As we saw in our research, family members' work is central to the care of residents and to the operation of Ontario nursing homes. By family, we mainly mean women. Well before the pandemic, we had women tell us that it would be "impossible" for their relative's basic care needs to be met without family involvement. Their work goes well beyond social care to include other essential care and management work. Families, and especially women, do a lot of unpaid work and unpaid worrying.

Certainly, families chat and provide forms of social support like listening and asking. Speaking about her mother, one woman joked, "Well, first of all I go in and I listen to all her complaints." But families do much more than that. They cook, shop, clothe, do laundry, assist with walking, offer activities, and celebrate holidays. They help their relatives and other residents eat, brush their teeth, comb and wash their hair, or even bathe them. Some described mopping floors, making beds, and assisting with physical therapy, while others detailed portering multiple residents to and from meals, putting on bibs and helping to serve dinner nightly. It is common for families to purchase necessities, such as soaker pads or run small shops within the home where residents can purchase these supplies. They also organize other family members to visit or do other kinds of carework. This work is especially necessary when the home is organized around the dominant culture, requiring families to serve as cultural and language interpreters and to provide food and appropriate body care.

There is no question that many women felt coerced to provide unpaid care. We heard repeatedly that otherwise the work would not be done. They reported lots of unpaid worries, ranging from worrying that relatives would not be dressed appropriately or turned to prevent bedsores or would be left in a wheelchair, to worrying that they would become dehydrated, be left unfed, or be given inappropriate medications. They felt responsible as daughters and wives. As one woman put it, "There's a lot of things I prevent myself from doing [such as travelling] because of guilt and worry" about what would happen in her absence. Women are often held responsible by both their relatives and the home. One woman described her husband as always "high maintenance" and noted that he expects her to be there all day long. Another handled her guilt and the gaps in care by privately paying companions to be with her husband 24/7, an option only available to those with economic resources. In Sweden, by contrast, where there is a stronger commitment to collective care along with nonprofit approaches with higher staffing levels and more supportive conditions, workers told us that it is their job to relieve the family of responsibility for care (Daly and Szebehely, 2012). On paid time, they even did shopping for residents.

Many families do not simply passively accept the private responsibility for care. They educate themselves about the system and about particular care needs in order to shape the collective care. Their advocacy work ranges from seeking help for their relatives or other residents when call bells are not answered to ensuring residents have appropriate medications and demanding that the government increase funding for care and stop funding for-profit care. In one home, the Family Council worked to cancel the corporate food contract, successfully bringing the food services back in house.

Unpaid care is not without tensions. While we heard from family care providers who saw themselves as "part of the team," emphasizing their strong relationships with workers and insisting that they weren't "watching over" them, we also noted that advocacy work can put families in conflict with staff. They do not have the same training as staff and struggle to understand the work of staff, resulting in inappropriate demands for care (Armstrong and Lowndes 2018). Moreover, demands for more collective care and better conditions can be undermined by unpaid care that hides the gaps in care and the skills required in the work.

Structural conditions serve to coerce women into providing unpaid care. Yet some relatives found their involvement rewarding, and described the pleasures of visiting, reading, going for walks, going on outings, accompanying relatives to activities or special events, sneaking in pizza or beer, and spending time with them as well as with other residents, staff, or visitors who became "like family." Individually, they supported residents on the units, around the facility and collectively, through family councils. One woman took pride in the "good things that they had done" as part of the family council, including creating community space. This satisfaction also depends on adequate conditions for paid work that allow families to participate meaningfully.

While fixed, low fees mean economic barriers do not limit access to care in Ontario, the limited number of spaces available does, as do the staffing levels and other conditions that create gaps in care that women in particular are pressured to fill. This pressure to provide care that comes from staff working conditions and the responsibilities assigned to women especially can undermine women's health. Women talk about exhaustion and stress caused by the unpaid work and worries. Long travel times add to the health consequences. Those who have paid jobs talk about the difficulty of balancing job demands, while others report that they had to quit their jobs to provide care. The way nursing homes are organized doesn't just put women in vulnerable positions, it puts care home residents in vulnerable situations, as the COVID-19 pandemic revealed.

The Military Marches In: Privatization and Women's Unpaid Carework

The COVID-19 pandemic exposed and exaggerated many of the already well documented weaknesses in nursing homes. As death rates rose alarmingly, families could no longer provide care within the home or monitor managerial practices. The military report revealed the disastrous conditions made worse by the absence of the unpaid care that had become critical as a result of privatization.

Six of the seven homes identified as requiring military support were for-profit, one was not-for-profit, and none were government owned. Indeed, for-profit homes had 78 percent more deaths than nonprofit homes and nearly twice as many people infected (Ferguson 2021). Across Ontario, the care gaps are most obvious in for-profit homes, although market principles for organizing work infect them all. The report reveals the absence of direct personal care to support with bathing and independence, food and meals, laundry (including clothes and linens), and access both to care supplies (such as soaker pads) and to personal supplies (such as shampoo, snacks, or magazines), but our research indicates this absence was not only the result of missing staff and pandemic times. It was also about missing unpaid care. Although the critical absence of unpaid care was implicit in the military report, some media have made the absence explicit and advocated for family members as "essential caregivers," often emphasizing the negative consequences of missing social support and connections that are essential components in care. The military reports were about care in a crisis, but they served to expose structural weakness in working conditions, paid staffing levels, and training as well as the dependency on unpaid care, especially when it comes to social support.

Public Outrage and Promising Policy Suggestions

Our research highlights the need for organizational and social policy changes. Earlier scandals, along with pressure from community organizations and unions, have resulted in more regulation in nursing homes as well as in family and residents' councils intended to provide regular monitoring and advice (Lloyd et al. 2014). Nursing homes are *already* highly regulated but, to date, regulations have focused primarily on monitoring workers or the care delivered rather than on structural changes, such as minimum staffing levels, working conditions, and ownership.

Although the response to COVID-19 was slow, the Ontario government eventually restricted most staff to working in one home to limit spread among homes, but it failed to ensure that they had full-time work or pay. The government also temporarily added four dollars an hour to staff wages to keep people at work.

Recognizing that most health care workers are women and that many women need childcare in order to work, it allowed some childcare centers to open but did not fund them from provincial coffers. It was too little too late.

In Ontario, families individually and collectively protested. While some demanded that families be let in to provide essential care, in the process supporting assumptions about unskilled work, additional responses galvanized demands for structural change. Advocates have successfully fought for innovative communications strategies in individual homes and the right for families to provide care. They documented the importance of social care and won the right to be called essential workers (Payne 2020). But they also demanded public responsibility for ensuring the right for care. They filed multiple class action and other lawsuits against individual homes and one against the government itself, alleging that the province breached the *Canadian Charter of Rights and Freedoms* (Ontario Health Coalition 2020) in failing to provide adequate care, and especially adequate staff. The government responded by introducing legislation limiting lawsuits. Public outrage has forced the establishment of formal investigations, and family councils have united with unions, employers, and community organizations to demand that the government initiate structural change (Doolittle 2020).

Our research speaks to the need for massive public investments and major changes in the social organization of long-term care, working to reverse privatization in all its forms. In the short term, this means increasing staffing immediately by training more people quickly at public expense, as the province of Quebec did by immediately educating 10,000 care aides. It also means paying higher wages, providing full-time jobs to attract those who already have training, and improving other working conditions, including "day care facilities for children and the elderly onsite" (De Henau and Himmelweit, 2020, 9). Increasing staff would help reduce the coercion of women into unpaid care, as would the recognition that paid care includes social care.

In the longer term, access to care must be increased by providing more public spaces in nursing homes. This also means moving to eliminate for-profit homes and the contracting out of services within nonprofit ones, shifting the focus from profit to care and recognizing how food, laundry, and cleaning are all central both to care and to teamwork in providing that care. Management models should be care models that include in decision making all those who live in, work in, and visit long-term care and that recognize our collective responsibility for care. Expanding and investing in public care can help reduce socioeconomic inequalities while boosting the economy and reducing the demand for unpaid care.

Continuing Tensions

There is little question that even within public services, women are coerced into providing unpaid care. Neoliberalism reinforces this coercion that holds women especially responsible for family care, in large measure through structural means that reduce the right to care provided collectively while also limiting their right not to care. Although many women have developed skills through providing care and through educating themselves, and although many derive satisfaction from applying those skills, the assignment of so much carework to those without formal training can render the skills invisible and undervalued. At the same time as those providing family care are demanding the right to provide unpaid care during COVID-19, they are also demanding structural changes to ensure that care is collectively provided by those trained and paid appropriately for the job. Recognizing how paid care and unpaid workers alike are picking up the slack in organizations stretched thin (Klostermann 2020) can also foster mutual empathy and solidarity. Situating tensions in more extended social and historical relations is equally important in promoting the right to care.

PART TWO

Catastrophe

The chapters in this section highlight the impact of the pandemic and the accompanying mitigation measures on care processes, paid care workers, and families. In response to the emergence of COVID-19 as a major health threat, governments across the globe enacted lockdowns, closed borders, banned international and domestic travel, shut down schools and public gatherings, and recommended use of face masks and social distancing when in public (WHO; CDC). The exceptions to these policies were "essential workers," who were compelled to remain accessible, providing in-person direct care to address the pandemic. The essential workers most often identified in the media were public health first responders, including technicians, nurses, and doctors. However, this category of essential workers also included emergency personnel, like police officers and firefighters, food distribution employees, grocery store workers, and workers overseeing safe drinking water (CDC). The mitigation measures most important for these workers included providing personal protective equipment that was in desperately short supply early in the pandemic.

This approach to mitigation had contradictory impacts for different populations of workers and families. Lockdown policies included broad home confinement and remote learning measures. Home confinement meant that nonfamilial care services were immediately halted, and institutionally based care sites were closed to outside access. The accessibility of frontline workers combined with inadequate resources resulted in long hours, uncertain health risks, and burnout.

María Nieves Rico and Laura C. Pautassi conceptualize the COVID-19 global pandemic as a syndemic, emphasizing that the arrival of the virus collided with not only a preexisting care crisis but also concurrent crises in health, poverty, and discrimination. Valeria Esquivel also points to the ways in which the public health crisis emerged at the crossroads of health and economic challenges. These authors describe how variations in economic power and labor protection structured the consequences of the virus for different groups of paid care workers. Health care workers across the board were exposed to high levels of risk due to inadequate protections, and domestic workers were particularly vulnerable to the extremes of job loss on the one hand and forced confinement with their employer on the other.

Lockdowns limited many families to their households, increasing social isolation, exacerbating the invisibility of unpaid care labor, and expanding the unpaid care labor performed by women. Women faced unsustainable work–family conflicts, as they did their best to absorb disproportionate increases in unpaid household caregiving alongside paid employment. As Rico and Pautassi describe, across Latin America women who engaged in telework, designed as a mitigation strategy, experienced accumulating demands that increased their overall workloads. Pilar Gonalons-Pons and Johanna S. Quinn found that in the United States, employed mothers provided greater care and supervision for their children's remote learning than did fathers. And Zitha Mokomane and Ameeta Jaga explain how, within the extended family households of essential workers in South Africa, grandmothers faced increased carework as adult parents were called into essential work.

Travel bans disrupted the lives of those who migrate for work or family. In South Africa, Mokomane and Jaga describe the gaps in elder care left in the wake of mitigation measures as many older adults were not able to receive their usual care from their nonresident migrant children who visited regularly in pre-pandemic times. Ken Chih-Yan Sun also describes the impact on transnational families, who faced mitigation strategies that blocked access to extended visits within host countries and reentry into their home countries; these circumstances made communication, care, and financial provision across national borders considerably more challenging. There were also transnational workers who benefited from their status, namely those whose affluence and family supports enabled them to maximize strategic choices across countries.

In contexts where elders are a primary source of care in multigenerational households, as in Mokomane and Jaga's research on South Africa, caring for grandchildren increased elders' risk of exposure to the virus. Elders' caregiving was further challenged by mitigation measures that did not take into consideration their reliance on family networks.

These chapters show how the pandemic catastrophe is rooted in previous structures, misunderstandings, and devaluation of care. As the chapters in part 1 examined, the pandemic was exacerbated by historical inequalities and systematic discrimination around the world. Most locations were woefully unprepared to address the concomitant economic, health, and care crises simultaneously due to prolonged underinvestment in care. Rather than conceptualizing care as a public good that needs recognition, protection, and investment, around the world we commonly see a global disregard for unpaid care and a chronic devaluation of paid care workers that have left care workers and those they serve especially vulnerable.

When access to caregivers and care sites closed down and women took on the bulk of the expanded unpaid labor that resulted, underlying racial and economic inequalities shaped differential outcomes for women. Employed mothers precariously maintained paid and unpaid work, facing demands that were difficult to reconcile, in particular in the wake of different understandings of childcare. Gonalons-Pons and Quinn find that in the United States, childcare is cast simultaneously as a luxury service for affluent mothers and dependence-producing for poor mothers, and that the pandemic conditions intensified these racial and class inequalities among women.

As Esquivel explains, policies to support paid care have been precarious at best, facing a history of underinvestment, further cuts during periods of economic crisis, and further deterioration under threats of current austerity measures. Rico and Pautassi echo that there has been ongoing silence in the policy realm surrounding care and its organization. An underinvestment in care services around the world meant that most places lacked the policies and care infrastructure to address pre-pandemic problems, let alone the even more dangerous working conditions at home and in places of employment that have emerged within the pandemic.

It is important to point out that some mechanisms helped provide protection to some groups of workers. Gonalons-Pons and Quinn find that workers with access to unions and collective bargaining, like U.S. elementary school teachers, were in a somewhat better position for self-advocacy than nonunionized childcare workers.

The groundwork for this crisis was laid long before today, through a history of structural inequalities. Mitigation measures laid bare how crisis conditions confronted by care workers around the world were exacerbated by the COVID-19 pandemic. Underlying this catastrophe is a deep lack of acknowledgment of the critical role care plays in social reproduction and the paid workforce's interdependence on paid and unpaid care workers' crucial labor. As a result, we saw conflict over pandemic priorities. These conflicts include economic policies—stimulus and investment versus austerity; understandings of work and family; public versus private responsibility; the sovereignty of national borders; social versus epidemiological responses; and how to address groups with seemingly oppositional needs.

Across so much of this pandemic, taking a more syndemic approach toward understanding care might have mitigated negative outcomes. For example, drawing together the complexities of transnational caregiving during the COVID-19 pandemic demonstrates that effective policies to halt pandemic transmission must address families that exist beyond state borders. Likewise, epidemiological solutions must account for social factors—mitigation strategies may mean very different things depending on the context, the population, and available resources. Finally, the pandemic has made painfully clear the ways in which groups' needs, when not considered through a broader care framework, can pit people against each other. With a broader care lens we can see transnational caregiving through the needs and experiences of both citizens and migrants; we can see education through the importance of both teachers' health and students' learning; and we can see the interrelated needs of paid and unpaid caregivers.

7

The Right to Care at Stake

The Syndemic Emergency in Latin America

MARÍA NIEVES RICO AND LAURA C. PAUTASSI

The COVID-19 pandemic appeared in a time and place marked by the existence of depleted natural resources that led to a historic environmental emergency, and a predatory form of capitalism, promoting segregation and inequality. Latin America faced the unprecedented health crisis of COVID-19 together with a financial crisis that prevented growth and increased poverty. These crises, together with the loss of jobs, aggravated the preexisting crisis in care and its social organization, which feminists have been warning about for years. In Latin America, women perform about 80 percent of unremunerated carework[1] and constitute a majority (over 93%) of paid care workers.[2]

Focusing on gender and human rights, we analyze some consequences of certain policies implemented during the pandemic and their impact on the right to care (Pautassi 2007) and on women's autonomy (Rico 2014). We apply the notion of a *syndemic* (Horton 2020; Singer 2009), a concept that addresses the synergies of the care crisis, the crisis in health and poverty, and social and cultural conditions, such as discrimination based on sex and age. The notion of a syndemic (Singer 2009), derives from epidemiology and extends to medical anthropology and the social sciences in general, making it possible to identify interconnected issues that shape the near future. The notion of a syndemic has larger, systemic implications. It reveals the convergence of risks that affect a society at a specific time in history. Unless such risks are handled together, the effects of a syndemic multiply and increase vulnerability for large sectors of the population. The notion of syndemic points to the interaction of health and social factors that affect people's lives and exacerbate disease in specific groups.

These simultaneous threats aggravate the risks and adverse consequences of COVID-19 and demand alternative policies through which care can become a tool for achieving greater social equality. The current organization of carework in Latin America is unbalanced as to the role, responsibility, and costs involved for the family, the government, the market, and the community, and it is unfair as to the distribution and workload between women and men. This is yet another threat that exacerbates poverty and inequality.

The Pandemic in Latin America: Is Care the Focus?

COVID-19 sounded an alarm, but its long-term effects will depend on the capacity of social actors to cause change. As a source of conflict, the pandemic put pressure on all levels of the social, financial, and political systems, including patriarchy and its corollary, the sexual division of labor and care, that are both strongly heteronormative. The pandemic, thus, intensified preexisting systems of discrimination and oppression. For this reason, an intersectional approach is vital, both to understand the experience of this crisis as it affected both groups and individuals and to explain the injustice of a response that has generated greater asymmetry of carework in daily life.

At the beginning, the lack of a vaccine and the need to provide support as infections spread led Latin American governments to make decisions without considering their broader impact. Home confinement during lockdowns, for example, led to loss of social contact, reduced mobility, impeded education, caused economic losses, and increased the possibility of domestic violence. Strategies for infection control that kept people at home also promoted the traditional sexual division of labor, and the measures taken are far from gender neutral. Joan Tronto asserts, "The risk would be seen differently if society was organized following a reference to care" (2020, 32). A balance between needs and rights is required as a substantive part of political debates.

Considering simultaneous threats, we base our analysis on rights and gender, which together go beyond a single focus on the cause and effects of the pandemic. We propose a dynamic approach to analyzing this syndemic and its effects on structural inequalities. To explain interdependencies in the case of COVID-19, we analyze relational phenomena conditioned by gender and by financial and political arrangements in which persistent inequalities and disregard for individual rights affect the daily lives of individuals and communities. Women were especially affected by the COVID-19 crisis, particularly domestic workers, women in poverty with no income of their own, and remunerated and unremunerated care workers. Confined to their homes, if they had homes, these people had little opportunity to enjoy rights and autonomy.

Latin American countries have high levels of inequality, with social gaps that leave many material needs unsatisfied and systems where relations of power promote multiple forms of discrimination. At the same time, neoliberal programs have rendered redistribution policies fragile, reflecting governments' limited capacity to provide solutions to long-term poverty, labor informality, and insufficient public utilities. A concentrating economy, however, requires regulation to safeguard social, cultural, and economic rights, including the rights of women and of sexual minorities. The syndemic thus revealed contradictions, forcing a dialogue to consider the scope of care, both as essential work and as a human right.

Carework in the Broader Economy

The COVID-19 crisis led to serious consequences for labor markets and economies more broadly. It weakened the economy, which had expanded in the preceding 5 years. The Economic Commission for Latin America and the Caribbean (ECLAC 2020a) considered that the share of the population in poverty would increase to 37.3 percent and the population in extreme poverty could reach 15.5 percent. In the preceding decades, the poverty femininity index for Latin America persistently showed values above 100 in both urban and rural areas, indicating more women in impoverished households.[3] Greater poverty predicted aggravated effects of the pandemic. Indeed, more poor women of working and reproductive age, many with children, were unable to avoid carework, exacerbating a vicious cycle of ongoing poverty.

The health effects and socioeconomic impact of COVID-19 differed across social groups. If we consider nonmonetary poverty, we see more adverse effects of the pandemic and its lockdowns on those who lacked access to food or water, who lacked jobs or stable homes, or who were forced to take care of others or work to survive. These are the people who cannot readily comply with lockdown measures, the people governments often ignore. More than 6 months after the pandemic was declared in Latin American countries, many productive sectors showed evidence of a sharp fall in business. Demand for carework, however, increased, underscoring the relevance of the nonmonetary economy.

Several analyses have assessed the value of unremunerated carework and domestic work. Though they apply different methods, these studies all find that such work represents between 15 and 24 percent of the GDP in each Latin American country (ECLAC 2017).[4] The last of these analyses was conducted by Argentina and estimated that the economic contribution of women's unremunerated work represents 15.9 percent of the GDP, making it the sector with the largest economic contribution; greater than industry, which represents 13.2 percent, and trade, which represents 13 percent (MECON 2020). As Eisler (2007) argues, care may be invisible to many and may be socially and economically undervalued everywhere, but societies require an "invisible hand" facilitating and establishing order. Rather than the market, this hand comes from women's unremunerated work. Although revealed by the pandemic, the need for a focus on care produced little evidence that men or governments were assuming responsibility or attempting to rebalance the distribution of care. Care workers, disproportionately women, remained largely invisible.

The Labor Market and Female Caretakers

Another myth that the pandemic made clear is related to labor market conditions in Latin America;[5] across the region, structural inequalities limit access to formal jobs and social security. These conditions reproduce poverty, especially for women and for rural and Indigenous peoples. In the 5 years preceding the pandemic, unemployment rates in Latin America had already shown signs for concern, particularly for women and young people, but COVID-19 caused a material destruction of jobs, leaving unemployed workers, especially women, discouraged from seeking new employment. In Chile, for example, nine out of ten unemployed women stopped trying to enter the labor market (Comunidad Mujer 2020). The impact on their financial autonomy and the welfare of their families was detrimental.

In trade and tourism, two sectors employing a large number of women, high unemployment comes with an increase in the precariousness of informal and low-productivity jobs. In these sectors, almost 80 percent of working women experience high labor market uncertainty, together with low salaries and insufficient social security protection (ILO 2019). Government measures during the pandemic exacerbated these problems. Lockdowns and home confinement particularly punish those who depend on a daily income. For example, women street vendors, many of whom are Indigenous people, have no choice but to take care of their children while they work; for them, the closing of street markets meant a lack of demand and the loss of street trade.

Informal labor also encompasses paid domestic work, where 93 percent of workers (about 18 million) are women. Here the rate of informal employment (defined as no or insufficient registration) is 77.5 percent (ILO 2019). The COVID-19 emergency, however, revealed the vulnerability of home care, both for children and for dependent elders. In this sector, multiple infringements of labor rights included forced confinement, mistreatment, termination without compensation or severance payment, and exposure to the virus due to inadequate biosafety measures. All had an impact on the health of women workers, and insufficient government control meant that women, once again, experienced the highest costs of the crisis.

For "essential" workers, the situation was similar. For example, women health care workers, both public and private, represent more than 70 percent of the workforce in health care worldwide (Boniol et al. 2019). These workers include doctors, nurses, assistants, technicians, administrators, and cleaning staff, and the overrepresentation of women in these occupations exposes them to the virus and to infection in greater numbers than their male peers. Increasing demands for patient care during the crisis also led to longer shifts, with adverse effects on workers' physical and mental health, as well as on their families, who often lacked support. No Latin American country heeded the call for safe, affordable care services for children and elder parents of essential workers (Staab 2020).

The sudden appearance of COVID-19 led to the fast, massive implementation of telework in both public and private sectors. These measures were aimed at preventing physical contact and reducing mobility—hence limiting infection—while keeping organizations and businesses operating. Registered, salaried women with professional positions and those with access to technology became teleworkers, though arrangements remained subject to conditions negotiated with employers. Telework, however, often required simultaneous attention to care and education of children, who were not attending school, or to care for elders, who have limited mobility. Rather than redistribute carework, therefore, telework concentrates paid and unpaid work in domestic space, accumulating the demands on women. Nonetheless, both governments and market actors transferred labor to workers' homes with little attention to the costs for individuals and their families (Rico and Marco Navarro 2020).

During the months of confinement, some Latin American countries did regulate telework. Among these regulations were those applied to the costs of equipment in Chile and technological platforms in Costa Rica. Beginning in August 2020, an Argentinian law also included carework in delineating the right to disconnect. Yet any acknowledgment of care as a human right—the right to self-care, the right to receive care, and the right to care for others—remained absent (Pautassi 2007). Even where issues regarding care were expressly addressed with government actions that provided support for households, the work that care required continued to fall to women.

Regression in the Right to Care

One structural marker that made the crisis a syndemic is the intersection of multiple interdependencies constituting the right to care. For example, during the syndemic, millions of children and teenagers suffered an impact on their right to education. According to UNESCO (2020a), as of March 30, 2020, thirty-seven Latin American countries had canceled in-person classes. The closing of educational facilities and the shift to online classes for approximately 113 million home-based children brought new challenges for families, particularly mothers, who traditionally have monitored schoolwork. They became responsible for their children's attendance online and, with new requirements, had little room for self-care.

The right to health and the right to care are in tension within homes. Care that women traditionally provide their families constitutes an invisible health care system (Durán 2008). Ensuring preventive measures against COVID-19 was necessary so that women not only contributed to the economy but also deployed core strategies for curbing the pandemic. They fed and cleaned sick individuals and dealt with the formal health care system. Some women left social isolation to cover the care needs of their relatives, generally elders who lived elsewhere, thereby putting themselves at risk. When governments' crisis management transferred responsibility for health care to families, therefore, women assumed its obligations, typically without acknowledgment.

For elders and persons with disabilities, who often require permanent care, interdependence appeared more extreme. In both cases, the right to receive care and the right to self-care were acknowledged, but these rights were then largely ignored. Instead, stereotypes of aging underlaid the government's confinement measures. People in specialized centers were left collectively to suffer the consequences of infection, even death, without support from their families, and those living in their own homes were left unable to go out, even while taking safety measures, thereby violating their rights to remain self-sufficient and socially and economically active. Those living alone, most of them women, lost contact with support networks, restricting the possibility of providing and receiving care. Crisis measures thus promoted an image of extreme fragility and dependence while ignoring a range of needs.

The right to a decent home and to internet connectivity were also ignored. Many homes are too small to accommodate the combination of teleworking parents, children connected to schools, and young people connected to universities. Although a serious social issue before the pandemic, overcrowding was worsened by the digital gap affecting the poorest homes.

As a syndemic perspective thus reveals, domestic space reproduces gender inequalities, together with social reproduction and support for the labor force. These inequalities are sometimes enforced through violence. Mandatory isolation, in particular, forces some women to cohabit with their aggressors 24 hours a day, causing them serious difficulties and sometimes punishment if they try to leave (Gherardi 2020).

Postsyndemic Scenarios

The effects of COVID-19 will be deeply felt beyond health concerns, and long-term outcomes remain uncertain. The short-term effects, however, reveal immediate concerns. Care was central during the pandemic crisis, but its status as work was ignored, and rights to enjoy and provide care remained overlooked. The pandemic, thus, revealed the ongoing silence surrounding care and its organization. Also missing from public discourse was the relationship of care as to politics and the economy, including long-standing gender inequalities that cost both women's time and their physical and mental health. For children and young people, both self-care and care of others encompass not only health but also the social and economic value of care. Including these dimensions of care in school curricula—together with the need for its redistribution—would establish a basis for the future of care-work beyond the pandemic.

In addition, the syndemic aspect of COVID-19 is evidenced in vaccines. First, science showed its capacity and speed for developing them, while public policies proved insufficient to achieve the required scope and distribution. The relation is not linear because, among other reasons, the Global North, far from complying with their commitments in the field of human rights, accumulated doses and patents and fostered disputes over vaccine approval, giving rise to geopolitics with new human mobility criteria for exclusion/inclusion. For example, in July 2021, 46.3 percent of the population in the United States and Canada had completed their vaccination schedule, followed by 34.9 percent of the European Union, while in Latin America and the Caribbean only 13.6 percent of the population had been vaccinated, resulting in 11.3 percent of the world population being vaccinated (ECLAC 2021). In October 2021, the average for countries in Latin America and the Caribbean had increased vaccination rates to 30 percent of the population, but the possibility for expansion depends on international suppliers, which, in many cases, discontinued supplies as most high-income countries accumulated their own supplies (ECLAC and PAHO 2021). There are also interregional and intracountry differences, showing once again the inequality of preexisting structures.

With strategies for social protection vital to controlling COVID-19, a syndemic perspective that encompasses gender and human rights is even more imperative. Social security and systems of protection must ensure a minimum level of well-being for everyone. These universal guarantees should include access to basic services, protection of income and employment, and care policies that promote the provision of services. Standards and principles of human rights require a mandatory minimum floor, together with progressive increases to extend the scope and ensure the enjoyment of care. Deeper reflection should also consider today's dynamic social reality. For example, neither labor regulations nor legal theory has acknowledged specific rights for women in charge of carework. Rather, their access to rights is still derived from paid work or from a legal relationship with a worker. Law and policy need to value women as caretakers and acknowledge their full personhood, both socially and economically. These redistributive measures can then operate not only in their interests but also in the broader interests of society.

With the future in dispute, no inevitable logic will define a new scenario. The echoes of the syndemic may lead to a reconsideration of the market as the community's central organizing principle, or the same conditions may promote a return to a dysfunctional normality marked by the gender inequalities endemic in Latin America and elsewhere. Data, however, point to high risks for societies not organized on the right to care (Tronto 2020). On a smaller scale, cities are also inadequate in care provision (Rico and Segovia 2017). Defining the COVID-19 crisis as a syndemic allows us to highlight the need for an integrated approach, but any solution requires guarantees inherent in human rights: civil, social, cultural, political, and environmental.

With life at stake in the twenty-first century, rights and their enjoyment must provide protection. Safety at work and access to care can mitigate risk but only after cultural change that promotes a redistribution of care undergirded by the sexual division of labor. Latin America has the opportunity to transform the "new normality" wrought by COVID-19 into a new scenario marked by greater equity. Such change, however, will happen only to the extent that care, as a public good, is distributed equally. With care at their core, public policies can address interrelated goals, such as overcoming poverty, achieving autonomy of women, and providing decent, universal care.

NOTES

1. According to time-use surveys conducted in nineteen countries in the region, women over age 15 spend between one-fifth and one-third of their days or weeks, respectively, on domestic work and carework. For men the time spent is around 10 percent. This indicator is calculated as follows: average time = (time spent in unpaid domestic work + time spent in unpaid carework) / population. If the average time is shown in week-hours, it is divided by 7 working days to arrive at the day's average time. To calculate the proportion, the day's average time is divided by 24 hours (ECLAC 2016).

2. Occupations are placed in three branches of activity: education, health and social work, and household services. For further analysis refer to ECLAC (2013, 131–170).

3. The femininity index is calculated as follows: quotient between (number of women in poor households between ages 20 and 59 / number of men in poor households between ages 20 and 59) / (number of women between ages 20 and 59 in total number of households / number of men between ages 20 and 59 in total number of households)×100. For more information, see https://estadisticas.cepal.org/cepalstat/tabulador/SisGen_MuestraFicha _puntual.asp?id_aplicacion=17&id_estudio=221&indicador=3330&idioma=e.

4. Colombia's analysis dates from 2012; Costa Rica's from 2011; Ecuador's from 2012; El Salvador's from 2010; Guatemala's from 2014; Mexico's from 2014; Peru's from 2010; and Uruguay's from 2013 (ECLAC 2017).

5. For an analysis on Latin America, see Martínez Franzoni and Siddharth (chapter 2, this volume).

8

At the Crossroads of the Employment and the Care Crises

Care Workers during the COVID-19 Pandemic

VALERIA ESQUIVEL

The COVID-19 pandemic is both a health and an economic crisis—or, in other words, a crisis at the crossroads of employment and care. Measures to contain the spread of the virus aimed at alleviating the pressure on health care systems or at gaining time to expand them were put in place almost universally as the pandemic spread, first around northern and then southern countries. Containment measures, particularly stringent at first, brought economies to a halt, threatening employment and livelihoods. By April 2020, 94 percent of workers were living in countries with some sort of workplace closure measures in place (ILO 2020f). At the end of the year 2020, 8.8 percent of global working hours had been lost relative to the fourth quarter of 2019, the equivalent of 255 million full-time jobs (ILO 2021b). By the end of 2021, the COVID-19 employment recovery had already started but was incomplete and uneven (ILO 2022).

Not all economies were equally hard-hit by the pandemic, and their recovery paths are divergent (IMF 2021). There are many reasons for these differences—most notably among them the relative strengths or fragilities of the economies to face the multiple shocks that emerged, the level and distribution of social infrastructure, the functioning of labor markets, and the extent and timeliness of the social and economic policies put in place. Crucially, the preparedness of care services and the working conditions of care workers not only defined how well the health crisis was tackled but also acted as transmission mechanisms between the care and the employment crises. Indeed, when health systems risked collapse, second- and third-wave lockdowns were put in place. The trade-offs between "the economy" and lives lost due to inadequate health care were already well known and were behind the delays in imposing more stringent measures—or in some contexts, not imposing them at all. School closures were among the most effective measures to control the spread of the virus (Haug et al. 2020), but they brought with them costs in terms of the social development and the welfare of children and adolescents (OECD 2021).

School reopening was a prerequisite for parents (particularly mothers) to reenter the labor market.

Women were particularly hit by the employment crisis, as the sectors most severely hit—like retail, tourism, or labor-intensive manufacturing—are dominated by them (ILO 2020e). Most care sectors across the world, broadly defined as health and social work, education and domestic work, also dominated by women, experienced the opposite effect: in median high-income countries, employment in care sectors increased from 19 percent to 19.3 percent of total employment, and in median upper-middle-income countries this proportion went from 15.3 to 16.2 percent of total employment. In lower-middle-income countries, however, employment in care sectors experienced a contraction, from 12.1 to 10.4 percent of total employment.[1] Health and social work, including long-term care, were at the center of the COVID-19 response, and as we shall see, health care workers and personal care workers in institutional care settings bore the brunt of the health crisis. Following childcare and school closures, teachers faced the challenge of moving to online teaching, though that was not always possible. Keeping schools open brought increased health risks to teachers and other school personnel before vaccination was widely available (Gurdasani et al. 2021). Personal care workers and domestic workers faced different challenges. Some continued to work in countries in the South, also facing high contagion risks, as they typically work unprotected. Many in the informal care sector lost their jobs, and their incomes if no policy was envisioned for them.

The pandemic made visible and exacerbated another preexisting trade-off— that between paid work and unpaid carework, which, in the absence of redistribution between women and men, only care services help bridge. Indeed, unpaid carers, most of them women, bore the brunt of the collapse of care services. Women who remained in employment juggled work and care, and their greater care obligations sometimes forced them to cut down on paid working hours or to extend total working hours (paid and unpaid) to unsustainable levels (ILO 2021c). Others lost their jobs as a result.

This chapter takes a bird's-eye view of how the crisis unfolded in the main care sectors, showing the relationship between the impacts of the COVID-19 crisis, the institutional arrangements that govern care sectors, and the situation of care workers in them. In the second part, this chapter elaborates on a progressive care agenda in which investments in the provision of public care service take center stage in the recovery strategy, spurring decent employment, restoring caring capabilities, and building resilience, averting future health and economic crises of the magnitude of the ones we are barely emerging from.

Care Workers during the COVID-19 Pandemic

Health Care Workers

Health workers are the backbone of health care systems. Globally, before the onset of the COVID-19 pandemic, employment in health and social work amounted to

4.5 percent of total employment and 8.4 percent of total women's employment. On average, women represented more than 70 percent of those employed in the sector. In developed regions, women reached close to 80 percent of the health workforce, and health and social work accounted for almost 10 percent of total employment—indeed, the greater the employment in the sector, the more feminized it is. The proportion of women is even higher among nurses and personal care workers, 90 percent of whom are women (Addati et al. 2018). In turn, women tend to be engaged in lower-skilled and lower-paid jobs in this sector, which are associated with larger gender pay gaps (26% in high-income countries and 29% in upper-middle-income countries) (ILO 2020c). Employment in health and social work remained constant or slightly increased as a proportion of women's and men's employment, before and after the onset of COVID-19 (table 8.1).

The COVID-19 pandemic made blatantly evident the already known relationship between the working conditions of care workers and the care provided. Long working hours in intensive care units, insufficient personal protective equipment, and resource-constrained environments were associated with a deterioration of the working conditions of health workers, and to higher-risk work injuries, accidents, and infection. They were also testimony to health care systems unable to cope with the pandemic.

TABLE 8.1

Employment in health and social work, in education and in households as a proportion of total employment, before and after onset of COVID-19

		Pre-COVID		Post-COVID	
		Women	Men	Women	Men
Health and social work	Lower-middle income	5.0	1.9	5.4	2.2
	Upper-middle income	8.7	3.2	9.3	3.0
	High income	16.0	3.7	15.9	3.9
Domestic workers	Lower-middle income	3.0	0.2	2.0	0.2
	Upper-middle income	5.9	0.6	5.1	0.4
	High income	1.2	0.1	1.1	0.1
Education	Lower-middle income	7.1	3.1	7.0	2.4
	Upper-middle income	10.3	3.3	11.6	3.6
	High income	12.9	4.3	13.8	4.4

Source: Author's calculations based on microdata for forty countries. Median values.

Figures of infections among health care workers vary, but the World Health Organization (WHO) has indicated that they were greater than those in the general population. While health workers represent less than 3 percent of the population in the large majority of countries and less than 2 percent in almost all low- and middle-income countries, around 14 percent of COVID-19 cases reported to WHO were among health workers in 2020 (WHO 2020c). These high rates of infections among health care workers, in turn, lead to lack of availability of trained personnel, and hence to the redeployment of clinical staff to frontline positions (intensive care units or COVID-19 patient care rooms) and to the recruitment of less experienced personnel (i.e., recent graduates or health care workers from unrelated specialties) (PAHO 2020). These workers were at higher risk of infection, and they also amplified outbreaks within health care facilities when they became ill (CDC 2020b). In other cases, retired health workers were brought in to help colleagues overwhelmed by the pandemic, but their advanced age put them at a higher risk of infection, hospitalization, and death (Franklin 2020). In early September 2020, Amnesty International reported that at least 7,000 health workers had died around the world after contracting COVID-19 (Amnesty International 2020). As of August 2020, 2,500 of these deaths had taken place in the Americas. Of those death, 72 percent were women care workers (PAHO 2020). WHO's latest figures, based on the overall health and social work employment figures from the International Labour Organization and the overall death data suggest that between 80,000 and 180,000 health and social workers could have died of COVID-19 in the period between January 2020 and May 2021, with a medium scenario of 115,500 deaths (WHO 2021a).

Such a critical context led to depression and anxiety among health care workers. Reports have found that at least one in five health care professionals reported symptoms of depression and anxiety, and almost four in ten health care workers experienced sleeping difficulties or insomnia, and that rates of anxiety and depression were higher for female health care workers and nursing staff (Pappa et al. 2020). Young health workers (18–29 years old) have been hit even harder by burnout (Kirzinger et al. 2021).

There is also anecdotal evidence that women working in health care occupations were more likely to report increases in their unpaid care and domestic work than other workers during the pandemic (Oxfam 2020). Moreover, the postponement and rescheduling of nonurgent health care visits during the first COVID-19 wave created a backlog of unfulfilled care demands, putting continued strain on the health system and its workers and jeopardizing second-wave preparedness (Franklin 2020).

The situation of health care workers is also crucially dependent on how prepared care systems were to respond to the crisis. It is well documented, for example, that the crisis in Lombardy, the initial and worst-affected Italian region, is related to the fragmentation of privatized medical services and the lack of support of frontline health workers (Lal et al. 2021). More generally, weak health systems constrained the ability of governments to respond to the pandemic, and certain systems, in particular those with greater dominance of the private sector, were less able to cope (Ortiz and Stubbs 2020).

First-wave lockdowns and containment measures were used to gain time to expand the capacity of intensive care units and COVID-19 beds, to train health care workers until vaccines could be deployed. In Argentina, for example, this expansion was combined with bonuses for public health care workers, in an attempt to compensate their meager pay. In many countries, including Canada, France, and Italy, schools remained open to care for the children of health care workers, and in the United States emergency lodging was provided to protect their families from the risk of contagion. We know little of how extended or sustained in time these measures were, but anecdotal evidence suggests that they were put in place only in rich countries, and only when public investment was utilized to ramp-up public health services provision. The exigencies and risks facing health care workers in the Global South must certainly have been greater.

Care Workers in Institution-Based Care

Elders were particularly vulnerable to the worst effects of COVID-19, and first-wave figures indicated that on average 46 percent of all COVID-19 deaths were care home residents in developed countries. Disaggregated data on infection rates and COVID-19-related deaths among care workers providing home-based care are, however, unavailable for most of these countries (Comas-Herrera et al. 2020). Beyond infections and deaths, however, COVID-19 had a deleterious impact on care workers providing institution-based care, given their preexisting precarious labor conditions.

Care workers in institutions are considered "low skilled" and typically receive low pay. Cultural values relating to aging and to work that involves touching the human body—often considered "dirty work"—contribute to the lack of recognition of these workers, ignoring the emotional skills and empathy required to do this work (Austen et al. 2016; Molinier 2012). Institutional settings also explain the working conditions of these workers. For example, their median hourly wage is €9, compared to €14 for workers in the same occupation in hospital settings (OECD 2020b). Care workers in institutions are often employed under part-time or temporary working arrangements, leading to unpredictable or excessive working hours, job insecurity, and limited access to labor rights and social protection benefits (ILO 2020b).

The COVID-19 crisis put the spotlight on institutional care in terms of both older persons, their risks and rights, and their care workers. An initial unawareness of how rapidly COVID-19 was spreading in care homes and the cultural norms mentioned earlier delayed the identification of care workers in institutions as frontline workers, denying them personal protective equipment and testing. This was all the more risky as these workers' work entails activities that impede their physical distancing from care recipients, making them particularly vulnerable to COVID-19 exposure in the workplace (ILO 2020b; Klarok 2021).

Also, the lack of social protection benefits, including paid sick leave and health coverage, among these care workers have made some of them continue to work while unwell because they could not afford to lose their income. Some of them worked in multiple facilities, increasing the risk of contracting and transmitting the virus (ILO 2020c). The crisis also brought higher work intensity and increased working hours, and therefore shorter rest periods. This sometimes led to increased absenteeism and in some cases to greater conflict between care workers and care recipients (Hoffman et al. 2020 cited in ILO 2020b).

The COVID-19 crisis hit a highly fragmented care sector, dominated by private (for-profit) and community (not-for-profit) service providers, with the public sector usually playing a subsidiary role and, perhaps more worryingly, a weak regulatory role. The marketization and outsourcing of long-term care services, with the objective of lowering costs, has led to lower wages, high rotation, and minimum staffing levels even before the crisis (Klarok 2021; OECD 2020b). Cutbacks in public spending have translated into lower fees being paid to private providers, further exacerbating these trends. In turn, higher out-of-pocket costs for older persons mean unequal access and varying service quality. In extreme but unfortunately not uncommon cases, these differences have had enormous human costs (Ortiz 2020).

Care Workers Providing Home-Based Care and Domestic Workers

Care workers providing home-based care and domestic workers, whose work combines domestic chores and personal care activities, accounted for 2.1 percent of global employment and 3.8 percent of women's global employment just before the onset of the crisis. Seventy percent of them were women, and they accounted for almost a fifth (18%) of the total care workforce; their role in care provision cannot be underestimated (Addati et al. 2018).

Home-based care workers and domestic workers are typically even less protected than institution-based care workers. The vast majority of them lack social security coverage, which means no paid sick leave, access to health care, or unemployment insurance. As a result, containment measures restricting their ability to go to work have put nearly three quarters of domestic workers around the world at significant risk of losing their jobs and incomes (ILO 2020g). Figures for forty countries before and after the onset of the COVID-19 crisis reported in table 8.1 show that in lower-middle income countries and in upper-middle income countries, women domestic workers lost approximately 1 percentage point of employment in median terms. Those informally employed faced termination of employment or forced unpaid leave, and some who remained employed did not receive their salaries. Migrant domestic workers were particularly vulnerable, as they could not return to their home countries due to the lockdown measures, nor could they continue sending remittances when staying. In contrast, live-in domestic workers mostly continued to work in confinement with their employers. They faced longer working hours due to school closures and more housework chores as persons stayed at home. They also faced increased contagion risks because they continued to be in close contact with their employers (ILO 2020g).

Care Workers in Education

Care workers in education, including early childhood education, primary and secondary school and higher education teachers and professors, technical and vocational training personnel, as well as support personnel, accounted for 4.8 percent of global employment and 7.4 percent of women's employment before the onset of the COVID-19 pandemic. Approximately 60 percent of all education workers around the world are women (Addati et al. 2018). Virtually all of these 157 million education workers as well as 94 percent of the world's students were affected by school and educational facilities' closures, in what has been called the most severe disruption to global education systems in history (UNESCO 2020b).

Teachers had to adapt to the new context, including moving to online teaching. In developing countries, however, teachers lacked the skills and equipment to provide distance education effectively. When possible, they met the challenge facing increased workloads, including meeting their own increased care demands (ILO 2020a). Indeed, school closures made evident that children need to be taken care of in order for their parents to continue to work for pay, either in their workplace or in the new teleworking arrangements that emerged. In many places, schools remained open in order to care for the children of health care workers—a local form of "care chain."

Generally more protected than other care workers, most teachers were able to keep their jobs and livelihoods during the pandemic, particularly if they were in the public sector (UNESCO and ILO 2020). Indeed, table 8.1 shows that in upper-middle income and high-income countries, employment in education expanded markedly, especially among women. There is indication, at least for Organization for Economic Cooperation and Development countries, that this is the result of the recruitment of temporary teachers or other staff in 2021 to help minimize the impacts on students' learning outcomes (OECD 2021).

In low-income countries, however, where fee-paying schools dominate, teachers and support personnel lost their livelihoods, as parents could not continue to pay the fees, in particular if they were on temporary contracts (United Nations 2020).

In many places, schools reopened with the second-wave lockdowns to avoid further learning losses but also to allow parents to go back to paid work. Along with other care workers, teachers effectively became "essential workers," continuing working face-to-face during the pandemic. Health risks associated with schools' reopening are not clear, however, and measures to minimize them, like maintaining physical distancing, the use of masks, and frequent handwashing might not be feasible with poor infrastructure. Improving and expanding school infrastructure are key in this regard, adding to the urgent calls for investing in care (United Nations 2020).

A "Caring" Economic Recovery

Care workers found themselves in a paradoxical position: while their jobs were mostly on demand and deemed "essential," therefore facing relatively low dismissal risks (at least in the short term), their working conditions were further strained during the worst of the pandemic. The previous account showed that in each of the care sectors, the COVID-19 crisis exacerbated already deficient working conditions, plunging some care workers into unemployment and poverty, making others overwork, and exposing most of them to heightened health risks. The previous account also offers indication that the more deficient the working conditions of care workers, the less prepared care services were to cope with the crisis, given the close relationship between the qualifications, protection, and pay of care workers and the quality and resilience of the services they provide.

Such unpreparedness was the result of long-term underinvestment in care services, following expenditure cuts in health and education budgets, and in wages of public sector workers in the aftermath of the 2008 financial crisis. Expenditure cuts had a disproportionate effect on women and children at the time (Ortiz and Cummins 2013). As is now evident, they also entailed long-term costs for care workers and care recipients, as well as for unpaid carers, who had to cope with higher care demands in a context of high employment and income losses. The COVID-19 crisis exacerbated and concentrated these costs in such a way that it was, finally, impossible to turn a blind eye to them. The plight of care workers, whose contribution has been essential to overcoming the pandemic, became undisputable, bringing with it the opportunity to leverage better working conditions, wages, and representation for care workers. The "heroes" deserve better, and yet these improvements are failing to materialize.

The fragility of those in need of care—now anyone from prime ministers to street vendors, although the elder more than the young—coupled with pervasive inequalities in the access to the infrastructure needed to self-isolate, to safe working conditions, to quality care services, and, lately, to vaccines, calls for a different, more inclusive recovery. As opposed to the 2008 financial crisis, though, this time around high- and upper-middle-income countries have prioritized investments in health care services as part of the emergency response, ramping-up public expenditures toward strengthening the public health system. The least developed countries have had less fiscal space to run the same policies, while middle-income countries have also experienced limitations due to the collapse in international trade, domestic and foreign revenues, and the weakening of their external positions (ILO 2020i; Parisotto and Elsheikhi 2020). Moreover, efforts need to be sustained in time, to guarantee universal access to health care and avert future pandemics, and extend to other care services, in particular education, to counteract the deleterious effects of school closures.

Past the worse of the pandemic, however, investments in care services might come under pressure, as there is a risk (already evident in some quarters) of a return to austerity policies (Ortiz and Cummings 2022). Lessons learned from past crises indicate that expenditure cuts weaken care services' coverage and quality and negatively impact care recipients, care workers, and unpaid carers. In the current crisis at the crossroad of employment and care, there is growing consensus that health and education budgets need to be protected and that investments in care must be part of the COVID stimulus packages and the postpandemic recovery efforts (ILO 2021c; United Nations 2020; UN Women 2020b). Investments in care, including care-related infrastructure, are not superfluous costs to be spared. They are the only reassurance that next time around the world would be more prepared to respond to a pandemic. There is also ample evidence that investments in care services have the potential to generate decent jobs, particularly for women (and indirectly for men as well) (Addati et al. 2018), contributing to a job-rich, more inclusive, and more sustainable recovery. Funding for these investments, and avoiding quick fixes, including in creating care jobs with less than decent working conditions, is the challenge ahead.

NOTE

1. Estimations based on micro-datasets for forty countries, before and after the onset of the COVID-19 crisis.

9

Caring for Children and the Economy

The Uneven Effects of the Pandemic on Childcare Workers, Primary School Teachers, and Unpaid Caregivers

PILAR GONALONS-PONS AND JOHANNA S. QUINN

Every year in August and September, over 130,000 K–12 schools across the United States open their doors to start their semesters, welcoming over 55 million children. In 2020, most schools did not physically open. They went fully online due to the continuing health risks of COVID-19 and the lack of planning and resources devoted to ensuring the possibility for safe in-person return.[1] The decision to move to online education was controversial and contested, reviving well-worn tropes, pitting teachers against children and the economy. The federal government, for example, argued that closed schools "could damage our children's education for years to come and hinder our nation's economic comeback."[2] While business leaders and newspaper editorials described teachers as "incredibly selfish, putting their fears, largely unfounded, ahead of the needs of their students, their communities and their country."[3] Others expressed well-founded concerns about how shuttered schools and online-only instruction would deepen existing inequalities and put additional stress on families.[4]

The debates about schools reopening viscerally illustrate a point that feminists have long understood: the paid workforce depends on paid and unpaid care workers' crucial labor. In 2019, there were nearly 27 million U.S. households with at least one child under 12, and 55 percent of all the adults in the households were in the paid workforce. These households rely on the labor of nearly 5 million paid care workers who take care of their children, implying that paid care workers directly *enable* the employment of at least 14.6 million individuals. This equates to one in ten members of the workforce. Suppose we add into this estimate the size of the workforce that depends on *unpaid* caregivers' work. In that case, the estimate amounts to 22 million paid workers, or one in seven members of the workforce, depending daily on paid and unpaid care workers freeing their time for waged work.[5]

The pandemic has revealed our reliance on carework, making it impossible to ignore the economy's dependence on care workers. The continuity of care jointly provided by childcare workers, teachers, and unpaid caregivers has suffered an unprecedented interruption. We should seize this interruption to rethink how we organize the responsibilities and value of caregiving.

This chapter reviews the existing evidence about how the pandemic has affected paid and unpaid carework for children ages 0 to 11 in the United States. We synthesize findings from published research and reports supplemented with original descriptive analysis using data from the Current Population Survey (CPS) 2019–2020 (Flood et al. 2022). Our analysis shows that the pandemic has affected caregivers in ways that reflect the legacies of gendered, racialized, and classed social institutions and norms that structure and divide those who care for children. By integrating the analysis of the different groups of caregivers, we seek to highlight how interdependencies between these groups are structured in ways that reinforce and reproduce devaluation, invisibility, and stratification. We argue that an integrated analysis of paid and unpaid caregivers offers a new approach for building alliances to advocate for changes in how caregiving is organized in ways that benefit children, families, and care workers.

The Paid U.S. Workforce Caring for Children during COVID-19

In the United States, the paid workforce caring for children under 11 includes nearly 6 million nannies, childcare workers, and preschool and primary school teachers.[6] These jobs disproportionately employ women, but teachers are overwhelmingly white, and childcare workers are disproportionately Black and Latina (table 9.1). The distinctive racialization of the two occupations is related to the separate histories of these jobs and the racial stratification of carework among women (Duffy 2011; Glenn 1992; Roberts 1997). Emerging research on the pandemic shows a stark divide in the kinds and forms of hardship endured by care workers for children 0–5 and teachers working with children 6–11, which has deepened existing racial and class divides.

Childcare Workers during COVID-19

Nannies and childcare workers, disproportionately Black and Latina women, have experienced significant job losses and sharp increases in economic insecurity and hardship during the pandemic. The only exception to this pattern has been workers in public institutions, such as Head Start schools, which offer subsidized childcare to children from poor families, and pre-kindergarten teachers who work in public schools. Jobs and wages for both of these groups of public childcare workers have been more protected.

There have been several published reports and studies documenting the challenges that the childcare sector and childcare workers faced during the pandemic. Some of the early evidence came from an extensive survey of 3,355 New York early childhood educators conducted in May 2020 (Nagasawa and Tarrant 2020a, 2020b;

TABLE 9.1

Economic impact of the pandemic on paid child caregivers

	Teachers	Childcare workers	Preschool and pre-K
N (unweighted)[a]	1008	280	161
Women	81.1	92.9	99.4
Nonwhite	19.1	37.1	29.8
% Becoming unemployed	2.2	10.4	6.8
% Becoming non-employed[b]	7.2	26.4	18.0
% Experiencing:			
Declines in weekly earnings (among those employed)	44.5	47.9	42.1
Declines in weekly labor income	48.3	63.0	52.9
Declines in household labor income	46.9	57.1	52.6
Declines in hours of work	27.9	41.4	39.8
Average change in weekly labor income	−33.0	−71.7	−74.1
Average change in household weekly labor income	−35.0	−93.5	−49.0
Average change in hours of work	−2.1	−5.1	−6.2
Pre-pandemic job quality[c]			
% In a union:			
In 1990	65.5	7.6	24.9
In 2019	49.6	7.2	17.7
% With pension benefits:			
In 1980	81.7	7.6	41.2
In 2019	65.3	14.1	33.7

Source: CPS 2019–2021 (Flood et al. 2022).

[a] The CPS has a rotating panel structure and waves 4 and 8 include earnings data. Our analytical sample includes respondents who are in wave 4 between April 2019 and January 2020 and who are observed again in wave 8 between April 2020 and January 2021. The sample is restricted to respondents ages 15–55 whose occupation at wave 4 is either childcare worker, preschool teacher, or elementary school teacher.

[b] Becoming non-employed includes people who become unemployed as well as those who exit the labor force (i.e., become inactive or go back to study). The unemployed category refers only to people without a job who are actively looking for employment.

[c] Data on pre-pandemic job quality come from the CPS ACS files for 1980 and 2020 and the CPS MORG files for 1990 and 2019.

Tarrant and Nagasawa 2020). The findings show substantial increases in financial hardship and insecurity among all workers; for instance, that only 60 percent of program leaders report paying their staff in full. The survey also finds that many private programs have closed and laid off all staff members (Tarrant and Nagasawa 2020). Other studies have confirmed these patterns of childcare closures and financial hardships among childcare workers across the country (Barnett and Jung 2020; Barnett, Jung, and Nores 2020; Bassok et al. 2020, 2021; Burwick et al. 2020; Campbell, Patil, and McSwain 2020; Crawford et al. 2021; Daily and Kazi 2020; Ewing-Nelson 2020; Lee and Parolin 2021; Pardee, Schneider, and Lamb 2021; Smith and Granja 2021). Family childcare workers, the type of childcare most likely to stay open when allowed, report the highest levels of financial hardship, resulting from lost revenue during stay-at-home orders and lost clients after reopening. Pre-pandemic these workers were already the lowest paid among childcare workers, thus declines in income result in severe stress, a situation that pushed many to reopen as soon as possible despite the lack of personal protective equipment and support to deal with health risks (Bassok et al. 2020; Nagasawa and Tarrant 2020a). All types of childcare workers report challenges accessing welfare benefits and declines in mental health and emotional well-being. Many work in person at a center or in their own homes while their children, who would usually be at school, are also home. As a result, childcare workers often report experiencing increased work–family balance challenges (Bassok et al. 2020; Crawford et al., 2021; Nagasawa and Tarrant 2020b; Smith and Granja, 2021; Tarrant and Nagasawa 2020).

The only group of early childhood workers who have seen their financial status relatively protected are those tied to public programs like Head Start or pre-kindergarten, representing a small percentage of early childcare workers (Datta and Borton 2020). Head Start, a federally funded program, provides free family services and education programs for low-income and disabled children ages 3–5. Though a national program, Head Start programs are run by state and local non-profit organizations, community action agencies, and school districts. Some states additionally offer pre-kindergarten programs that provide free and low-cost education and childcare to children ages 3–5 during the school year and are often part of the public school system. Unlike fee-dependent childcare centers, workers in public programs like Head Start and pre-kindergarten have been eligible for their full payments based on the approved budgets. While job and wage protection have shielded this group from intense financial hardships, other stressors and challenges have been similar. Those who offer in-person care report concerns over managing health risks and work–family balance, while those who remain remote express worry about children and families' well-being (Bassok et al. 2020; Smith and Granja, 2021; Tarrant and Nagasawa 2020).

The descriptive analysis of CPS data reinforces these findings. Table 9.1 shows that childcare workers as well as workers in preschool and pre-K grades have experienced elevated rates of transitions to unemployment and nonemployment, as well as declines in work hours and labor income. Across all economic metrics, however, childcare workers have fared worse than workers in preschool and pre-K grades.

We argue that the intensified job and income insecurity experienced by child-care workers reflects the legacy of the privatized, classed, and racialized develop-ment of paid childcare services in the United States. For most of the twentieth century, paid care for young children has been conceptualized in relation to the race and class of the mother whose children childcare workers looked after and their own intersecting racial and class status. For white upper-class housewives, paid carework was depicted as "help," whereas for poor single mothers, it was pitched as a service to promote their employment (Glenn 2010; Hays 2003; Michel 1999). Public acceptance of these tropes hindered care workers and mothers; rich women were seen as not needing public investment and poor women as undeserv-ing of additional support (Glenn 2010; Hays 2003; Michel 1999; Swinth 2018). Nei-ther of these conceptions afforded status nor meaningful public investment in the childcare sector, leaving these workers in a situation of high vulnerability dur-ing the pandemic.

Another factor hindering the childcare workforce stems from racism and the devaluation of work performed by women of color (Branch 2011; Wooten and Branch 2012). During the first decades of the twentieth century, paid care workers were disproportionately Black, Asian, and Latina women working in private homes as nannies or domestic workers, reflecting racialization processes of domestic service and the legacies of slavery (Glenn 1992). Few communal facilities existed for children too young to attend school, and prevailing cultural norms relegated white women to the home (Michel 1999) and nonwhite women to positions of servitude (Glenn 1992). The out-of-home care sector for young children slowly developed over the second half of the twentieth century, mainly in the form of private small businesses with little public support, except for Head Start schools and pre-K grades. Thus nannies and domestic workers have been historically construed as low-skilled ser-vants deserving limited labor rights (Glenn 1992, 2010; Wooten and Branch 2012).

More recently, concerns over the importance of quality childcare have moti-vated a push to professionalize the sector and a stronger focus on educational goals, generating an upper layer of early-childhood educators that are relatively higher in status (Chaudry et al. 2017). On the whole, however, these jobs are still low paid and have few benefits, and all continue to disproportionately employ Black, Latina, and immigrant women (Duffy 2011). As shown in table 9.1, in 2019 only 14.1 percent of childcare workers and 33.7 percent pre-kindergarten teachers had pension ben-efits, and only 7.2 percent of childcare workers and 17.7 percent of pre-kindergarten teachers had unionized jobs.

Like nannies and domestic workers before them, the job of childcare workers today is often seen as being low-status and a good fit for "low-skilled" racialized women (Branch 2011). The effect of cultural legacies depicting these jobs as "help" for rich mothers and employment-enabling for poor ones, combined with the lack-ing sense of public responsibility for the care of young children, has resulted in a mostly privatized, "deregularized," and scattered network of paid care centers that have been vulnerable to the shock of the pandemic. The stark contrast between care workers' experiences in public settings like Head Start schools and pre-K grades versus the majority of the childcare workforce during the pandemic offers a strong testament to the relevance of public infrastructure. Had more of the care for young children looked like Head Start or pre-K jobs, much of the workers' financial stress could have been mitigated, and reopening efforts could have been better coordinated and better resourced.

Primary School Teachers during the Pandemic

In contrast to those who work with young children, the majority-white U.S. primary school workforce has suffered fewer job losses, and their salaries have remained relatively protected. Table 9.1 confirms that the economic impact of the pandemic has been less severe on teachers than on childcare and preschool workers; teachers have seen relatively smaller declines in employment, hours of work, and labor income. Despite faring relatively well economically, teachers have faced harsh public criticism, and their more defined role as public servants has meant that teachers experience significant hardships relating to the challenges of adopting remote learning and the stress and responsibility of maintaining quality education while simultaneously working to protect communities from the spread of the virus. The pressure and concern over teaching are reflected in the much higher volume of research and studies conducted on teachers' experiences during the pandemic than on childcare workers and the public debates about the need for teachers to return to in-person instruction.

Since the pandemic started, several studies have tracked the rollout of remote learning and teachers' experiences, challenges, and concerns in this process. The overall picture that emerges is that teachers have been working hard to make remote learning successful. Many of them report having increased work hours, increased stress involved in adjusting to remote learning, and increased burnout (Diliberti and Kaufman 2020; Hamilton et al. 2020). A Rand poll from October 2020 finds that 49 percent of teachers have a workweek of 48+ hours, up from 24 percent before the pandemic, and over 57 percent list feelings of burnout as a major concern (Hamilton et al. 2020). Teachers working in schools in high-poverty neighborhoods are navigating staggering deficits in access to technology and the internet. In a nationally representative survey of full-time public school teachers, over 50 percent of teachers in schools serving low-income students report serious concern about the lack of access to technological tools or high-speed internet. In contrast, in schools serving higher-income students, only 16 percent of the teachers report this concern (Educators for Excellence, 2020). Teachers report stress related to the responsibility of having remote learning work for all students and say they are concerned about keeping up with student learning outcomes in light of declines in students' attendance, engagement, and learning (CRPE 2020;

Educators for Excellence 2020). These concerns are well founded. The evidence demonstrates an exacerbation of inequalities in attendance, engagement, and learning between schools in middle-class and wealthy areas and schools in poorer ones (CRPE 2020; Educators for Excellence 2020; EdWeek 2020). In addition to the increased stressors at work, teachers also report experiencing increased work–family conflict. An Upbeat survey from Spring 2020 shows that 41 percent of teachers have caregiving responsibilities at home that interfere with their work (Kraft and Simon 2020). Teachers also report experiencing increased levels of financial stress related to members of the household losing jobs or seeing their incomes decline (CRPE 2020; Educators for Excellence 2020).

Those pressures have resulted in substantial declines in teacher morale (Hamilton et al. 2020; Kurtz 2020). Between May and August 2020, the percentage of teachers reporting that they were unlikely to leave the occupation before but are likely to leave it now more than doubled, from 12 to 32 percent (Kurtz 2020). While there is increasing support among teachers to return to in-person instruction, there is more support for this among white teachers than among their colleagues of color. An August 26–28 poll by EdWeek reports that only 49 percent of nonwhite teachers, principals, and district leaders say all instruction should be in-person, while 63 percent of white educators favor this. These disparities reflect racialized inequalities in exposure to COVID-19 and the types of schools and communities the teachers serve. Trust in the ability to safely reopen schools in impoverished school districts is low due to decades of underinvestment and cuts in public education resources (Morgan and Amerikaner 2018). Unlike childcare workers, the unionization among teachers allows existing teachers' unions to coordinate efforts and bargain for conditions that allow safe reopening, albeit with mixed results. During the 2020–2021 school year, large school districts with long-established collective bargaining agreements were better able to negotiate remote instruction and school closures, but districts with larger numbers of Trump voters were more likely to have in-person instruction. Partisan politics often outmatched teachers' and unions' preferences (Marianno et al. 2022). With increased pressures to reopen schools despite the persistently high community spread of the virus, negotiations between teachers and governments were tense with few indications that supports had been put in place to improve morale.

The way the pandemic has affected elementary school teachers also reflects gendered and racialized legacies tied to this occupation. Unlike care for younger children, elementary school education developed as a public institution over the twentieth century. This development began offering good teaching jobs to white women, as men were fleeing the occupation for better-paid jobs in other fields (Sedlak and Schlossman 1987). Until the 1970s teachers experienced improved pay and working conditions, owing largely to high levels of unionization in the sector. Teachers' salaries across the United States increased steadily, though workers in other occupations requiring similar training and credentials earned more (Sedlak and Schlossman 1987). However, in recent decades, teachers have witnessed growing credentialism that has not been met with better working conditions or pay. Teachers' work has intensified and become more stressful (Williamson and Myhill 2008), and pay and benefits have declined (Allegretto and Mishel 2018) (See also table 9.1 statistics on teachers' benefits and unionization.) This shift in work conditions is related to high-stakes accountability reforms like No Child Left Behind that increased and intensified teachers' work responsibilities and bureaucratic demands (Bartlett 2004; Valli and Buese 2007), and coincides with the greater racial diversification of the workforce (Ingersoll, May, and Collins 2017).

The legacy of teachers' relatively higher-status and unionized public sector jobs have offered important protections to elementary school teachers during the pandemic. However, the recent deterioration of working conditions in the profession has meant that teacher burnout was already high when the pandemic hit (Dworkin 2008). The environment of high-stakes accountability only accentuates the pressure and worry about the transition to remote learning. The legacy of high-unionization and the recent wave of teacher strikes in 2018 and 2019 means that teachers are better prepared for bargaining the conditions for safe reopening, at least in comparison to childcare workers. At the same time, however, the feminized perception of teachers as self-sacrificing caregivers and the villainizing of teachers' unions tend to lower teachers' bargaining power.

The Unpaid Workforce Caring for Children during COVID-19

The pandemic has increased unpaid childcare at work, and emerging research shows that this increase has been disproportionately shouldered by women, exacerbating work–family conflicts and existing economic inequalities (Calarco et al. 2020). Single parents who must report to work sites have had to find new paid or unpaid care arrangements for their children or been forced to quit or change jobs (Hertz, Mattes, and Shook 2020; Montenovo et al. 2020; Zhou et al. 2020). In households with more caregivers (i.e., dual-parent households), care arrangements depend on adults' employment, and in heterosexual couples, the intensified work–family conflict is exacerbating gender inequalities (Alon et al. 2020; Collins et al. 2021a, 2021b; Feng and Savani 2020; Landivar et al. 2020; Zamarro and Prados 2021).

Much of the research and media attention on this topic has focused on middle-class, two-parent, heterosexual couples with professional remote-work-friendly jobs. With children being full time at home, adult paid workers' ability to focus on their jobs is impaired and has potential long-term career consequences. Studies unambiguously show that mothers shoulder the lion's share of this work and the brunt of the negative impacts. Mothers have increased their time on unpaid care and housework, including helping children with remote learning, more than their male partners (Adams-Prassel et al. 2020; Alon et al. 2020; Lyttelton, Zang, and Musick 2020; Petts, Carlson, and Pepin 2021; Zhou et al. 2020; but see Carlson, Petts, and Pepin 2020; Craig 2020; Craig and Churchill 2021). An Oxfam-Promudo-U.S. survey shows that unpaid care responsibilities increased more dramatically for

Black, Latina, and Asian women than for white women (Dugarova 2020; Oxfam, Promundo-US, and MenCare 2020). Studies find that mothers in heterosexual couples are more likely than their partners to have cut and reduced paid work commitments (Collins et al. 2021a; Feng and Savani 2020; Myers et al. 2020). Studies also find declines in well-being that are more accentuated for mothers than for fathers (Calarco et al. 2020).

Research on unpaid childcare in other family formations is relatively sparser. Studies on single parents (mostly mothers) show intensified stress due to the inability to simultaneously attend to paid work obligations and children's care needs at home (Hertz, Mattes, and Shook 2020; Montenovo et al. 2020; Zhou et al. 2020). This situation has forced many to quit jobs or reduce hours, resulting in increased economic insecurity and financial stress, and finding a new job while children are at home is challenging. Since most single-parent households are mothers, these patterns further contribute to the gender disparity in adverse economic impacts of the pandemic (Mertehikian and Gonalons-Pons, 2022). There are only a few studies focusing explicitly on queer families. These studies document how queer families face both similar and distinct challenges during the pandemic. Manley and Goldberg (2021), for instance, highlight the barriers to maintaining relationships with non-cohabiting children among consensually nonmonogamous LGBTQ parents. Pre-pandemic patterns indicating that same-sex and single LGBTQ parents are more likely to live near poverty compared to non-LGBTQ counterparts (Moore and Stambolis-Ruhstorfer 2013; Whittington, Cadfield, and Calderón 2020) suggest that these families are likely to have experienced increased unemployment, economic insecurity, and work–family conflict as well.

Table 9.2 summarizes the economic impacts of the pandemic on households with children under 12 and shows substantial declines in the number of earners and increases in the prevalence of household unemployment. These changes have been generally more accentuated among nonwhite households and among households with two or more adults. Racialized economic inequality and differences in work–family trade-offs likely play a role in explaining these differences.

The way the pandemic has affected the unpaid caregiving in families similarly reflects the consequences of racialized, gendered, and classed understandings of unpaid care work. Because unpaid care work is seen as a status responsibility of mothers (Glenn 2010), increased demand for unpaid caregiving has disproportionately fallen on them, with intensive motherhood accentuating the pressure. Fathers have increased unpaid childcare as well, but the research shows that their contributions have increased less than those of mothers (Altintas and Sullivan 2017). The intensified work–family conflicts and economic insecurities associated with the pandemic also reflect the limited availability of paid leave and other supports for unpaid caregiving.

The patchwork system of care in the United States has long been expensive and difficult for families to navigate. From birth to age 4 or 5, with the exception of programs like Head Start, parents are left to pay for and manage childcare on

TABLE 9.2

Economic impacts of the pandemic on unpaid caregivers

	1 Adult nonwhite	2 Adults nonwhite	3+ Adults nonwhite	1 Adult white	2 Adults white	3+ Adults white
N (unweighted)	482	1505	653	569	4381	729
% Experiencing:						
Declines in number of earners in the household	15%	19%	36%	11%	14%	35%
All adults unemployed	26%	9%	8%	21%	4%	10%
Declines in household weekly labor income	42%	53%	55%	43%	49%	52%
Declines in households' weekly hours of work	27%	35%	47%	27%	36%	50%
Declines in women's weekly hours of work	24%	21%	32%	18%	23%	36%
Average change in household weekly labor income	22.1	–117.1	–275.4	–10.2	–84.3	–206.7
Average change in household weekly hours of work	0.1	–3.7	–9.4	–0.7	–2.4	–11.2
Average change in women's weekly hours of work	–1.4	–1.0	–4.1	–1.1	–0.8	–5.6
Average decline in household weekly labor income	–320.7	–607.9	–865.5	–421.4	–646.2	–834.0
Average decline in household weekly hours of work	–23.8	–29.0	–41.9	–21.9	–25.4	–38.7
Average decline in women's weekly hours of work	–23.9	–24.5	–33.1	–23.2	–19.4	–29.1

Source: CPS 2019–2021 (Flood et al. 2022).

Notes: The CPS has a rotating panel structure and waves 4 and 8 include earnings data. Our analytical sample includes households who are in wave 4 between April 2019 and January 2020 and who are observed again in wave 8 between April 2020 and January 2021. The sample is restricted to households with a child under age 12 in the household.

their own. Even when children reach school age, school days are shorter than typical workdays, leaving parents to cobble together care for those unaccounted hours. For example, Brown and colleagues (2016) estimate that pre-pandemic for families to pay care workers to cover the excess days and hours schools are closed while parents work would cost an average of $6,600 a year, well beyond what most families can afford (Brown et al. 2016). This notorious lack of work–family policy and public infrastructure for childcare has exacerbated the negative impact of the pandemic on families with children.

Concluding Remarks

The review of the evidence on the impacts of the pandemic on paid and unpaid caregiving for children under 12 illuminates the relevance of what Eggers, Grages, and Pfau-Effinger (chapter 15, this volume) refer to as "care arrangements," the combined cultural, institutional, and policy mechanisms that organize and structure essential carework in the U.S. context. The intersecting classed, gendered, and racialized notions about who needs childcare and who is best fit to provide it, combined with the notion of solely private and familial responsibility for the care of young children, powerfully shapes childcare policy. When paid care for young children is depicted as a luxury service for careerist women, or when it is depicted as a structural incentive to promote poor mothers' "economic independence," it reinforces arguments against the development of public childcare infrastructure and intensifies racial and class inequalities among women. In both cases, paid and unpaid care for young children is feminized and devalued. Pre-pandemic unpaid caregivers lacked government support, and paid childcare work was precarious and poorly remunerated. In the United States, the pandemic exacerbated inequalities structured through the care arrangements, but as we detail, it also exposed how these groups' interests are interconnected.

By integrating the study of childcare workers, primary teachers, and unpaid caregivers, we have sought to emphasize the underlying structure of their interdependence and how this structure can serve to reinforce devaluation, invisibility, and stratification, but also how it can, and should, be leveraged for potential coalitions among these groups. The stark contrast between the impact of the pandemic on childcare workers versus teachers shows how public institutions can protect essential workers and the vital services they provide. The intensified work–family conflict and financial distress among families with children demonstrates how privatized and familialized responsibility for children's care harms unpaid caregivers and families. These interconnected fates contrast with narratives that pit teachers against children, bringing renewed meaning to the slogan "teacher working conditions are student learning conditions."

The pandemic has exacerbated problems for families and care workers and revealed the need to address divisions between early childcare workers and teachers and provide support for families with young children. While there have been long-standing divides in pay, prestige, and working conditions between workers who provide care to children ages 0–5 and those working with kids 5–11, families are often reliant on care workers across sectors, and teachers and childcare workers are dependent on paid and unpaid caregivers to do their work. There are high-stakes collective benefits to challenging the gendered, racialized, classed institutions and tropes that serve to divide, devalue, stratify the essential work of paid and unpaid caregivers. Such benefits would improve the lives of caregivers and those who receive care. Building alliances across groups of caregivers is the way forward.

NOTES

1. Education Week research showed that 74 percent of the 100 largest school districts chose remote learning only, out of a sample of 907 districts 49 percent were fully online, 27 percent hybrid, and 24 percent full in-person: https://www.edweek.org/ew/section/multimedia/school-districts-reopening-plans-a-snapshot.html.

2. Source: https://www.whitehouse.gov/briefings-statements/president-donald-j-trump-supporting-americas-students-families-encouraging-safe-reopening-americas-schools/.

3. Joe Nocera, July 29, 2021, Crain's. Source: https://www.chicagobusiness.com/opinion/teachers-unions-are-putting-biden-bind.

4. There have been many opinion and expert pieces on this point. Here is one example written by sociologist Jessica Calarco: https://theconversation.com/online-learning-will-be-hard-for-kids-whose-schools-close-and-the-digital-divide-will-make-it-even-harder-for-some-of-them-133338.

5. Authors' calculations using data from the 2019 Current Population Survey Annual Social and Economic Supplement (CSP-ASEC). The quantities are defined as follows: number of households with one or more children under 12, number of households with all adults employed and one or more children under 12, and number of households with one or more children under 6 plus number of households with all adults employed and one or more children under 12 (but no children under 6). These calculations simplify many complexities. Families may rely on unpaid care of friends or relatives, parents may simultaneously work remotely and care for children at home (a not ideal but common situation in the pandemic), and paid care workers may themselves be parents and primary caregivers.

6. Authors' calculations using the 2019 Current Population Survey Annual Social and Economic Supplement (CSP-ASEC). The paid workforce caring for children under 6 is calculated as the sum of workers in the following categories (using the 1990 Census occupations classification): childcare workers (468), preschool and pre-kindergarten teachers (155), and primary school teachers (156).

10

COVID-19 and Care for the Elderly People in Africa

An Analysis of South Africa's Mitigation Measures

ZITHA MOKOMANE AND AMEETA JAGA

According to the United Nations, there were 31.9 million sub-Saharan Africans aged 65 years in 2019. This number is projected to increase more than threefold to reach over 101.4 million in 2050 (United Nations 2019b). Research evidence also shows that life expectancy in North Africa increased from 48.7 years in 1965 to 74.5 years in 2015 and is projected to reach 76.9 years by 2045–2050. As a result of these trends, the proportion of older people aged 60 years and above in Africa is projected to reach 19 percent (approximately 50 million in absolute terms) in 2050, a significant increase from the 6.7 percent reported in 2015 (Sibai et al. 2017). The United Nations (2019b, 3) posits that such trends in population aging may reflect a reduction in the risk of premature death due to improved public health and socio-economic development. In the context of sub-Saharan Africa, however, service providers' and families' efforts to meet older persons' needs and demands (Mokomane 2013) are often hampered by low social protection and social security coverage, public health, and social infrastructures that are ill-equipped to care for older persons' needs (Cohen and Menken 2006, 23; Kronfol, Rizk, and Sibai 2015, 839). According to the International Labour Organization (2017), for example, only 29.6 percent of older people in Africa have effective social protection coverage. This is much lower than the global average of 67.9 percent. By the same token, only 9.0 percent of sub-Saharan Africans in the labor force are active contributors to old age pension schemes.

Against this background, the extended family continues—as it did in the traditional setting—to be the main source of instrumental and effective care and support for older people. Indeed, the United Nations (2019a) has shown that Africa is one of the world regions where it is most common for older people to live in multigenerational households. In these households, older people typically receive various forms of care and support from their children and/or grandchildren. The older people, on the other hand, are a major source of assistance for childcare and socialization in the households (Kalomo and Besthorn 2018; Mokomane 2013; Wusu and Isiugo-Abanihe 2006). Given the constant social contacts and daily interactions that characterize these reciprocal caregiving relations, multigenerational households are often seen as potential sources of disease spread, particularly during covariate public health shocks (Stokes and Patterson 2020). During the 2013 West African Ebola epidemic, for example, grandparents' traditional role of caring for children placed the elderly among those at a heightened risk of contracting the virus (Abramowitz et al. 2015).

Public health shocks also tend to increase the care burden of older people. For example, during the peak of the HIV and AIDS epidemic in East and South Africa in the 2000–2010 decade, high levels of AIDS-related morbidity and mortality "altered the contours of living arrangements and traditional roles among the African family" (Kalomo and Besthorn 2018, 35). For the most part, as many young adults of working age—the traditional caregivers for the elderly—became sick or succumbed to AIDS, older parents typically became the main caregivers of their infected children and orphaned grandchildren. In 2000, the World Health Organization reported that female caregivers aged 50 years and over cared for more than 80 percent of HIV-infected family members in Africa (WHO 2000). In essence, therefore, at a time when they themselves should be taken care of, older people often take up the responsibility of caring for sick and dying family members during health shocks (Chazan 2015; Mokomane 2013).

This increased double burden of care creates an array of financial, health, and psychological challenges for older people. Typically, with young adults' morbidity and lost capacity to earn an income, older parents find themselves without the income transfers from the middle generations. Furthermore, with most of the attention directed at the prospects of those in their care (Marais 2005), older people often endure significant financial care obligations to a multigenerational household (Button 2017). As a coping strategy, older caregivers often have to sell their assets (such as land or property), use large portions of their meager monthly social pensions, or work precarious jobs (such as domestic workers or informal sector workers) to support those in their care (Kalomo and Besthorn 2018; Mokomane 2013). In cases of covariate public health shocks, therefore, it is common for net resource flows to be from, rather than to, older parents (Merli and Palloni 2006). Increased household chores and care duties also often prevent older caregivers from working full time or earning their previous level of income (Kidman and Heymann 2009). The overall resultant financial constraints, along with the physical demands of caregiving, often lead to a range of psychosocial vulnerabilities and distress among older people (Kuo et al. 2012; Oburu and Palmerus 2005; Ssengonzi 2009). This chapter uses evidence from South Africa, the country with the highest COVID-19 cases in Africa, to illustrate how public health shocks can have significant implications for the care needs of older people. There is particular focus on the implications of some of the main COVID-19 mitigation measures, such as restrictions on regular movements and suspended economic activities of family members.

COVID-19 and Elder Care

The first case of COVID-19 was confirmed in South Africa in March 2020 and, as part of the national government's efforts to mitigate the spread and impact of the virus, a nationwide 21-day lockdown was announced 9 days after detection of the first locally transmitted case (Magongo et al. 2020). This lockdown, which was eventually extended beyond the initial 3 weeks with various amendments, generally focused on public health and behavioral interventions as well as various community mitigation strategies. The latter are described as measures that people and communities can take to slow the spread of infection during a period when vaccines and medical treatments are not available (Anderson et al. 2020). In South Africa, these measures included containment strategies, such as home isolation of ill or potentially ill persons, restriction of consumption and production to essential services, restriction of public gatherings, closure of schools, social distancing of at least 1.5 meters between people, closing of international travel, and bans on nonessential domestic travel. The latter mitigation measures posed several challenges for caregiving roles in multigenerational households. The implications for older people, in particular, are succinctly discussed in the following sections, in no particular order of importance.

Focus on Essential Services

With consumption and production restricted to essential services, only about a third of the employed were able to continue working, while some employees adopted "work from home" approaches (Kerr and Thornton 2020). Data from the National Income Dynamics Study—Coronavirus Rapid Mobile Survey conducted to establish the impact of COVID-19, showed that between February and June 2020, about 15 percent of the workforce lost their jobs (2.8 million jobs) and one-third of the workforce lost their earnings from temporary layoffs during the lockdown period (Visagie and Turok 2021). This economic disruption brought several critical outcomes for the vulnerable elderly. For example, working-age children who became unemployed or who could no longer earn an income were suddenly unable to continue supporting their older parents as in the pre-COVID-19 era. Many older parents also experienced additional financial care burdens as more dependents became reliant on their meager income from their old age grants or from low-income work if it was deemed essential.

Social Distancing

At least 15 percent of the South African population lives in densely populated, informal urban settlements, often with communal taps and toilets. Anecdotal evidence suggests that when the lockdown was announced, expectations of economic hardships (such as rising cost of and limited access to food) propelled many extended families to move in together to share food and other resources. This move aggravated the already overcrowded living conditions in many areas of the country. To the extent that "extreme social distancing is a luxury that low-income populations struggle to afford" (Magongo et al. 2020, 5), this mitigation measure placed family members, especially the older persons—who are more susceptible to infectious diseases—at heightened risk of contracting the virus (A. Smith et al. 2020). Furthermore, it is the case that many informal settlements have a high prevalence of comorbidity factors, such as tuberculosis and HIV (Magongo et al. 2020).

Bans on Nonessential Travel

Temporary circular labor migration to urban areas continues to be an integral feature of the South African economy and is often characterized by migrants who retain membership in the rural households (Posel, Fairburn, and Lund 2004). Many of these migrants typically return to the rural areas on a regular basis: weekly, fortnight, monthly, quarterly, or yearly (Smit 2001) to provide affective and material care to family members, typically older parents and children left behind. With the restricted population mobility brought about by the travel bans of the national lockdown, many older people were unable to receive their usual care from their nonresident migrant children who, pre-COVID-19, visited on a more regular basis.

School Closures

COVID-19-related closure of schools and childcare facilities has been linked to, among other things, emotional exhaustion as well as high rates of depression and anxiety among caregivers (Spaull and Van Der Berg 2020). Thus, where parents worked in essential services or from home, many older family members, particularly grandmothers, became primary caretakers for school-age children. While this was the case in many families even before COVID-19, school closures heightened practical care demands during the lockdown. Accordingly, the increased care burdens associated with elevated time demands have implications for low-income grandmothers in South Africa managing the competing demands of care and income generation, and limiting their choice or agency (Hall and Posel 2019). These implications include emotional and psychological stress (Button 2017).

Existing Opportunities for Lasting Change

Given the devastating socioeconomic impact of COVID-19, there are calls for strategies in disease prevention and control that can shape current and future responses by all stakeholders (Shi et al. 2020; UNHCR and IOM 2020). In essence, there is a need to know how to better prepare, now that we "know that future epidemics can be so quickly and widely spread from almost anywhere" (Shi et al. 2020, 2). Also important is the need for an improved understanding of how health resources and care services should be more accessible for vulnerable persons, such as the elderly.

Evidence from past epidemics in many parts of Africa has demonstrated that focusing solely on the medical and epidemiological responses to covariate disease

outbreaks is often insufficient, particularly in contexts of poor health care infrastructures (Abramowitz et al. 2015). This is because the factors outlying these outbreaks are often structural and operate at multiple levels of influence. In the
context of HIV and AIDS, for example, these factors included inadequate access to
health care, poor-quality education, drug and substance abuse, unemployment,
poverty, gender inequality, and exposure to violence (Eaton, Flisher, and Aarø 2003;
Ellsberg and Betron 2010; Mbonu, van den Borne, and De Vries 2009; Vermund,
Sheldon, and Sidat 2015). For this reason, the development, implementation, and
expansion of social protection measures, such as unconditional cash transfers
and in-kind food distribution, are often being emphasized as they have been
shown to be effective in maintaining food security and supporting local economies during humanitarian crises and epidemics (Magongo et al. 2020).

Largely against the foregoing, during COVID-19 a number of countries across
the world, including South Africa, amended preexisting social protection programs. These included increasing coverage and benefit levels, making advance
payments, simplifying administrative requirements, plugging COVID-19 response
schemes into existing delivery platforms, and providing innovative design solutions, such as school feeding programs delivering food directly to children's
homes or nearby distribution points (Magongo et al. 2020, 12). However, given the
low social protection coverage in Africa as well as the "problems and formidable
financial and administrative hurdles of expanding formal social security [and
social protection] schemes" in the region (Cohen and Menken 2006, 37), the social
protection route may not be an option or feasible for many countries of the conti-
nent. We argue, therefore, that there is a need to focus on new models that incorporate Indigenous and local knowledge into policies to simultaneously meet the
care needs of older people and contain costs. These should typically be culture-
specific modalities of interventions that "shift the ideology of family care from
being a family responsibility to a societal one" (Sibai et al. 2017, 81). Indeed, according to Abramowitz and colleagues (2015, 4), "a key lesson from the West African
Ebola epidemic is that local community engagement is crucial for response, and
may have played a role in the decline in transmission rates." Abramowitz and colleagues report that communities particularly demonstrated resilience, innovation,
and rapid response to the Ebola crisis and that culture proved to be flexible and
supple in response to new public health messages. To this end, they argued, traditional or cultural caregiving practices can be effectively altered to protect uninfected individuals (Abramowitz et al. 2015, 4).

Against the foregoing, we argue that instead of solely relying on kin caregivers, reaching out to community-based organizations with the right capabilities and
knowledge of particular communities and broad distribution networks or close
community ties, is one way of supplementing the government's protection of vulnerable older people. An example of a plausible model is that of community-based
support and services (CBSS), which is designed to provide (and act as a link to)
specific resources for older adults and their caregivers. Such models often entail

wellness programs, nutritional support, educational programs about health and other aspects of aging, counseling services for caregivers, as well as general assistance with access to social services (Siegler et al. 2015). Using data from over 200 helplines in the United States, Brewster and colleagues (2020) noted the critical role of CBSS in complementing the intense and sustained effort of many health care and social care providers to meet the interrelated health and social needs of older adults, including alleviating experiences of social isolation and stress. Anecdotal evidence from Ethiopia also reveals that community-based organizations played a major role in the administration and implementation of the country's Community Based Health Insurance as well as other treatment and care services. For example, volunteers associated with NEP+ (a network of People Living with HIV in Ethiopia) made home deliveries to those on antiretroviral therapy, to ensure that they adhered to treatment during the COVID-19 travel restrictions. Table 10.1 shows aspects of the CBSS model that could be relevant for elder care in future epidemics in Africa, particularly where measures such as restricted movements or decreased employment of kin caregivers are put in place or where hospitals and other care facilities reach capacity.

Rather than being prescriptive, the support and services shown in the table are meant to illustrate the range of interventions that can complementarily enhance the health, care, and social welfare of older people during covariate public health shocks, such as COVID-19. Meals provision and nutritional information services, for example, can go a long way toward ensuring food security and nutrition, which are an important aspect in any compromised health situation. Personal care and adult care services can provide companionship and affective care that can reduce social isolation, while information and legal assistance can increase older people and their carers' awareness of other supporting services for which they may be eligible. Together with case management and outreach services, they can also be important referral resources to other available support services. The provision of chore services, on the other hand, can greatly reduce the burden of domestic tasks for older people as well as being a source of respite for family members who provide care.

Conclusion

In contexts of high poverty and inequality, as in many African countries, circumstances that challenge caregiving include precarious employment, low pay, inability to work from home, reliance on family networks for child and elder care, and cases where family members have underlying health problems related to cumulative disadvantage. Despite these being largely structural, in many parts of Africa, the care of family members is still dominantly seen as a private, individual responsibility, leaving gaps in care needs (Stokes and Patterson 2020). Using COVID-19 as an example, this chapter shows that intergenerational relationships, family structure, and public health are inseparable in many African societies, and the most

TABLE 10.1

Examples of community-based supports and services

Services	Description
Home delivered meals	Meals delivered to the home of those who cannot prepare or obtain adequate nutrition
Congregate meals	Meals served in a community setting to those who cannot prepare or obtain adequate nutrition
Personal care	Hands-on or cueing to assist individuals with activities of daily living (ADLs) or instrumental activities of daily living (IADLs)
Homemaker services	Services designed to maintain a healthy home environment, such as housekeeping, meal preparation, laundry, and shopping
Information and assistance	Used to help older people or their carers identify, access, and use support services (exclusive of case management)
Nutrition education and counseling	Assessment of and assistance in meeting an individual's nutritional needs by a licensed nutritionist or dietician
Adult day care	Community-based program offering social, recreational, and health-related services in a congregate setting
Case management	Professional management of an individual's health care; identification and assessment of biopsychosocial needs; monitoring use of services to ensure positive outcomes
Outreach	Informing and educating the public of the availability of services, benefits, and programs
Chore services	Household tasks, such as heavy cleaning and yard work
Legal assistance	Consultation and representation for social protection benefits

Source: Amended from Siegler et al. (2015, 3).

effective public health regimes and interventions will be those that recognize these intersections and design interventions accordingly. Our main thesis is that at the forefront of policy development and action should be a collaboration between the public health sector, families, and community-based organizations. In addition to reducing health inequities (Stokes and Patterson, 2020), this approach can ensure that older people continue to receive basic services, such as food provision as well as a range of information assistance, while family members focus on their caregiving responsibilities. In Africa, such an approach is particularly feasible given the broad absence of institutional facilities. Even where such facilities may be available, the adoption of the CBSS model can be an important pathway for averting some of the main factors that often hamper or limit continuity in care in such institutions. As Pat Armstrong and Janna Klostermann illustrate (chapter 6, this volume), factors such as inadequate or lack of formal training of staff, low staff morale, and insufficient infrastructure in care facilities can have profound implications for the right to care and also put pressure on families to continue providing care. We thus reiterate, in conclusion, that different locational complexities, such as resource-constrained southern realities, require a focus on new models that incorporate local knowledge and an intersectional analysis of gender, age, and social class for policy development and innovative responses grounded in the context. Furthermore, for a sustainable and equitable COVID-19 recovery, decisions on care and elderly people in the African context should involve engaging diverse people on what is practical and implementable to fine-tune relevant responses that support these populations, thereby preventing a one-size-fits-all approach (Jaga and Ollier-Malaterre 2022). Finally, a reconceptualization of work that values care work and the care needs of older people that acknowledges diverse family forms and kin obligations is needed to foster greater well-being and economic empowerment for older women.

11

Transnational Family Caregiving during a Global Pandemic

KEN CHIH-YAN SUN

Since early 2020, the coronavirus has continued to ravage the world. Like many other vulnerable populations, the lives of migrants and their families are also deeply affected by this large-scale pandemic (Bernstein et al. 2020). Many migrant workers, especially those who are low income, have trouble social distancing at work or in their own personal space. In Germany, slaughterhouses that rely heavily on Polish, Romanian, and Bulgarian migrant workers have become epicenters of the COVID-19 pandemic (Ruxandra 2020). In Singapore and Brazil, low-wage migrant workers living in the favelas and crowded dormitories are more susceptible to the virus, in turn affecting nonmigrant populations (Bengali and Jennings 2020; Stack 2020). These phenomena have reignited the debate on the interplay between migration, inequalities, and risk management, provoking further discussion of the resources that migrants need to protect their families and themselves.

This chapter takes the analysis of inequalities and immigration to a transnational level, examining the impact of a global pandemic on caregiving in the context of long-distance family dispersal. The global outbreak of COVID-19 brings changes and challenges to geographically dispersed family members, setting significant limits on the basic premise of migrant transnationalism. This chapter explores the impact of the coronavirus pandemic on three types of resources that are frequently exchanged through cross-border family networks: hands-on care, economic remittances, and emotional support. The highly contagious nature of COVID-19 not only precluded at-home families from traveling internationally but also made it virtually impossible for emigrants to return home and manage family crises. The financial recession in the context of a global pandemic restrains the ability of migrants to protect and provide for family members in the homeland. The "care circulation" that was well documented in the transnational family research has been significantly disrupted under the circumstances of this global pandemic (Ito Peng, chapter 3, this volume).

This chapter also raises questions about the circulation of emotions, information, and advice between globally dispersed families as the pandemic strikes many parts of the world. How dispersed family members represent themselves to each other likely becomes more complicated and has significant implications for intimate relations. Despite these limitations, some transnational family members still make efforts to support one another materially and emotionally. Living a transnational life also allows migrants to rethink the cross-border resources that it would take to anchor their families in these unsettling and anxiety-producing contexts. At the core of this chapter are the myriad and complex ways in which social inequalities mediate the family life of immigrants both nationally and transnationally.

The Circulation of Care across Borders

Economic and cultural globalization have pushed millions of people to move across borders, thereby resulting in the geographic separation of families (Horn and Schweppe 2015; Walsh and Näre 2016). The phenomenon of "transnational families"—which typically refers to family members from a household who are divided by national borders—has attracted the attention of both family and migration scholars over the past decade (Berckmoes and Mazzucato 2018; King et al. 2014; Sun 2020). Researchers have been particularly attentive to the negotiation of caregiving responsibility among families in which migrant parents work overseas and leave their children in the homeland (Hoang and Yeoh 2015; Paul 2017; Sun 2014, 191).

This research clearly demonstrates how the intersection of class disadvantage and gendered notions of parenthood affects and operates in the lives of members of transnational households. While migrant men can rationalize their absence by regularly sending money home, most migrant women who provide economically for their families are still expected to be emotionally and socially available to their children left back home (Dreby 2010). In addition to their contribution to the household budget, many migrant women who work as domestic workers in the receiving contexts regularly mail letters, send text messages, have expensive gifts delivered, make phone calls, plan family menus, and supervise their children's daily activities (Lan 2006). These migrant mothers believe that such gestures allow them to be a palpable presence in their children's everyday lives and to sustain emotional connections to the next generation in the homeland (Peng and Wang 2013). However, studies have found that children left behind, especially young children and teenagers, are more inclined to blame migrant mothers than fathers for not "being there" in daily life (Parreñas 2005; Yarris 2017).

Just as many migrant women and men have left their underage children behind, many also have parents living in their home societies and feel obligated to perform elder care from afar (Baldassar 2016; Guo et al. 2016; King et al. 2017).

Many elderly parents decide to stay behind, or are left behind, because they face various structural and cultural constraints (Leinaweaver 2010; Sun 2012; Zhou 2012). A growing number of studies on migrants and their stay-behind or left-behind parents affirm the continued significance of these relationships for all those involved. Despite the spatial distance, many migrant adult children seek to financially, emotionally, and symbolically support their aging parents back home (Baldassar 2014). Much of the global care chain literature documents the circulation of material and symbolic resources—regular visits, short-term hands-on care, and financial, emotional, and moral support—between migrants and their parents back home (Amin and Ingman 2014; King et al. 2014; Zechner 2017). Some migrant adult children send economic remittances to their parents in the homeland (Horst et al. 2014; Mazzucato 2007), and some take "the lead in coordinating and delegating the care their parents need" (Ciobanu, Fokkema, and Nedelcu 2017, 176). In addition, through modern information and communication technologies, many migrant children seek to create visibility, presence, and a sense of involvement in the everyday lives of their parents (Baldassar et al. 2016).

Likewise, while some parents feel a sense of ambivalence or even abandonment due to long-distance family dispersal (King and Vullnetari 2006), many seek to provide their children with critical and much needed support in the form of money and assistance with the care of grandchildren, either in the homeland or during extended visits to their children abroad (Da 2003; Karl and Torres 2015; Marchetti-Mercer 2012). Overall, this body of literature contradicts the preoccupation and assumptions in the gerontology literature that caregiving requires proximity "by highlighting how migrant children and their parents in the homeland can continue to help each other in the context of long-distance family dispersal" (Baldassar 2007, 276). Family intimacy, in many aspects, is sustained in transformative ways, rather than thwarted, by national borders (Lamb 2009; Sun 2021).

Changes and Challenges in the Context of the Coronavirus

However, COVID-19 challenges several premises that are foundational to the scholarship on transnational family caregiving. The global pandemic precludes many immigrants and their family members from traveling between their home and host societies, making it increasingly challenging, or even impossible, for transnational family members to exchange care resources across borders (Baldassar 2016). In a time when many international flights are canceled and many countries are enforcing strict border controls, it has become increasingly difficult for migrants to return home to visit children or care for older generations during a family crisis. It also becomes harder for families to stay with their children through extended visits in the host societies. International travel would be particularly risky for older generations since they are at greater risk of COVID-19 than the younger generations; if infected, they would be less likely to recover and would have a stronger need for personal and medical care (Li and Huynh 2020; Mahase 2020). These changes and challenges arising from the pandemic suggest that the circulation of care that migration scholars uncovered earlier could be severely thwarted.

To illustrate, transnational contexts significantly limit the options that mainland Chinese immigrants in the United States have regarding transnational family caregiving. On January 31, 2020, the White House (2021) set a number of restrictions on the entrance of people from China. As a result, Chinese immigrants and their parents may face extended separation. Therefore, immigrants from mainland China might be forced to be separated for an extended period of time. Concurrently, China does not recognize dual nationality. Once a Chinese citizen is naturalized overseas, they automatically lose not only citizenship in the People's Republic of China but also local *hukou* (a household registration system in China) and its corresponding rights (e.g., public health insurance and children's access to school education) (Lui 2016). This means that mainland Chinese immigrants who are naturalized as U.S. citizens have a harder time returning home, partly because they have limited access to local public services and partly because they would face barriers to bringing their families back to the homeland during a pandemic (e.g., enrolling their U.S. citizen children in local schools when many American schools offer limited in-person classes).

The large-scale outbreak of COVID-19 in many countries has also significantly limited migrants' ability to support their family members in the homeland through economic remittances. The World Bank (2020) estimates that due to the impact of COVID-19, the economic remittances from migrants' receiving to sending countries has declined about 20 percent (around U.S. $445 billion) in 2020. The money sent by migrants working in better developed societies is essential to whether families back home can satisfy the basic and medical needs of younger and older generations (e.g., food, housing, accommodation, schooling, and health care) (Cohen 2011; Hoang and Yeoh 2015; Thai 2014). This money also constitutes an important way in which transnational family members could sustain a sense of mutuality and reciprocity with each other (Abrego and LaRossa 2009). However, the global pandemic has made many migrants' employment situations precarious (Ruxandra 2020). Some of them may have lost their steady income, and others may face a significant salary cut. Some may be worried about the prospects of their work and career. These financial worries may not only affect the amount of economic remittances they send but may also have significant implications for younger and older generations who depend on this money.

Furthermore, the global pandemic may complicate the ways in which migrants and their family members in the home societies communicate with one another. Information and communication technologies certainly increase the possibility that transnational family members will understand each other's situation immediately (Baldassar et al. 2016; Levitt and Jaworsky 2007; Nedelcu 2017). Yet this intimate knowledge of each other's lives also has the potential to exacerbate the worries and concerns that the different generations have about each other. Therefore, some avoid communicating from afar, and others downplay or hide their challenging circumstances to protect their families from feeling overwhelmed (Bryceson and Vuorela 2002; Peng and Wang 2013). As COVID-19 sweeps the United States and other parts of the world, how would migrants and their families back home contact one another? In this deeply unsettling context, how do they feel about each other's virtual presence in each other's lives? Do they candidly talk about the difficulties they face? Or, do they selectively present their lives to their families back home?

Transnational Family Resources during COVID-19

Long-distance family dispersal is certainly challenging during a global pandemic. Yet for some immigrants, cross-border kin ties could be mobilized to cope with moments of crisis. Here, I draw on newspaper articles and my ongoing research on immigration from mainland China and Taiwan to illustrate how migrants use transnational family resources to construct or tighten their safety net in such unsettling contexts. Central to these examples are the ways in which social inequalities, such as family resources, class disparities, and citizenship status, are negotiated during renewed waves of COVID-19.

Some migrants shift their familial roles from "economic provider" to care recipient, relying on their kinfolk in the homeland to cope with the risks and uncertainties they face in the receiving contexts. Flavius Tudo—whose story was reported in the *New York Times* on July 27, 2020—was a telling example (Goodman 2020). Flavius was originally from Romania and worked at a nursing facility in England. Working abroad allowed him to send money to support his family, especially his mother, back home.

However, at the age of 53, Flavius encountered unexpected challenges brought about by the outbreak of the global pandemic. As COVID-19 struck the United Kingdom, he lost his job. Suffering from a high fever and persistent cough at the peak of the pandemic, Flavius was prohibited from entering the facility where he worked. As a result, he lost his income. This financial loss took an emotional toll on him. Working abroad to support his family back home had given his life purpose, but now he could no longer do so. Rather, Flavius relied on his mother to wire him money from Romania, which is one of the most underresourced countries in Europe. Living on his mother's retirement pension, Flavius felt both defeated and lost. Yet his experiences were definitely not unique in these unsettling and anxiety-provoking times, since many migrants were no longer able to send economic remittances to their homeland. Instead, they had to borrow money from their families who were also struggling financially.

In contrast to disadvantaged migrants like Flavius, those whose families have greater resources are more secure and better protected. These migrants knew that they could turn to their at-home families for help without becoming a financial burden to them. Ruby Chu—a Chinese immigrant whom we interviewed during the pandemic—worked for a nonprofit organization in New York City. She was aware of the potential impact of COVID-19 on her job, but she understood that she would have economic support from her family in China if the worst-case scenario happened. This, according to her, convinced her that she would be fine during moments of crisis: "There are many people who get sick and laid off here [in the United States]. Some of my friends lost their jobs, and some companies in my field started to fire people. I do not know whether the same thing will happen to me and whether I would end up being sick or unemployed. But my families said to me: if anything happens, or if you are too stressed out, just come back. We will take care of you. So, in a way, I know I am protected and thus feel safe."

Different from many blue-collar migrant workers, Ruby did not have to send economic remittances to support her family in the homeland. As her words show, she was even given the option to return home if she faced any trouble. Indeed, having a reliable family in the homeland made it easier for some immigrants to return to their homeland during the pandemic. While Ruby chose to stay in the United States at the time of the interview, Jacob Lin—a Taiwanese immigrant I interviewed—decided to move his entire family to Taiwan to escape the continued surges of COVID cases in the United States. In many ways, COVID-19 woke Jacob up from his American Dream. He had never seriously noticed that the United States has so many problems—especially the flawed health care system, loopholes in the social safety net (e.g., paid sick leave), and the lack of coordination between federal and state governments—let alone considered how these problems could turn the COVID-19 pandemic into a national crisis. He was also worried about how the uncertain future—such as risks associated with reopening school or online learning—might affect his children's education.

After consulting with his parents and siblings in the homeland, Jacob and his wife decided to leave the United States for Taiwan—at least for a couple of years—in summer 2020. His parents found him a conveniently located apartment in downtown Taipei soon after learning of his decision to return home. In addition, his siblings back home helped Jacob figure out the school district and enroll his children in the local school. Without such transnational support, moving his entire family internationally in the middle of the COVID-19 crisis would have been much more difficult, if not entirely impossible. Concurrently, his Taiwanese citizenship grants him and his immediate family members not only the option to live there, but also provides access to public health care at low cost. Jacob complained about staying up late every day in order to work in New York's time zone, but he appreciated the fact that his children could go to school, receive an education, and interact with peers in ways that he deems essential to human development (Aspinwall 2020; Ruiz, Horowitz, and Tamir 2020, 198). Jacob had an awakening moment in the context of COVID-19. That is, he realized his intimate life is deeply embedded in institutional and structural contexts. Although both he and his wife had good jobs and have respectable incomes, his family life—especially when it comes to child rearing—could still fall apart if the society could not operate normally. Jacob's ability to relocate somewhere safer than the United States during a global pandemic was a privilege, which stems from the combination of his family resources, dual citizenship status, and class advantage (e.g., the fact that he could work remotely).

Conclusion

Using successive global waves of the coronavirus pandemic as an example, this chapter explores the impact of a global pandemic on the transnational life of migrants. Specifically, I focus on their responses to three aspects of transnational parental caregiving. First, the global outbreak of COVID-19 set significant limits on the "care circulation" between home and host societies (Baldassar 2016). Second, their ability to financially support families back home under the circumstances of a global pandemic could be severely thwarted as well. Third, while some immigrants are able to secure transnational support from their family afar, some could intentionally hide their problems from or selectively disclose their problems to their loved ones in this deeply anxiety-producing context.

The care circulation literature emphasizes the ability of transnational family members to exchange resources such as money, information, advice, and emotional as well as moral support (Baldassar 2016). This chapter highlights the importance of studying how this transnational family support could be undermined in the times of global crisis; it is my hope that future research can continue to examine these issues. At the same time, this chapter also challenges the conventional understanding of the divide between the Global South and the Global North. Many migrants might mobilize resources in their home societies to cope with crises in their host societies—which are often assumed to be wealthier and offer stronger social protection than migrants' homeland—in such contexts as the global pandemic.

The transnational resources that migrant families could access also affect their strategies for coping with a pandemic. To cope with the perceived or actual inadequacy of the resources available in a national context, some immigrants strategized by using their family ties to secure myriad forms of protection across borders. Future research should further explore the ways and extent to which globally dispersed family members are able to protect and provide for their loved ones as a catastrophic disaster affects the transnational social field that they and their families inhabit.

Policymakers should consider and incorporate transnational family responsibilities and the obligations of labor migrants—especially those in an economically precarious situation—when drafting proposals for relief packages and even immigration reform. If migrants could access resources (e.g., money) in the receiving contexts, they would be better able to construct a stronger transnational safety net for themselves and their at-home family members. If migrants could bring their families to their host societies, they could avoid extended family separation during COVID-19.

Considering these issues is important not only because many migrants work abroad to protect and provide for their families who remain back home but also because many receiving countries benefit from the continued flow of immigrants, the labor force that these countries did not cultivate from scratch. As Douglas Massey and his colleagues (1998, 36) explain, "Because developing nations covered the costs of feeding, clothing, educating and maintaining the emigrants until they reached productive age," the transnational circulation of labor migrants creates "a subsidy of wealthy nations by the poor." This externalization of social reproduction becomes even more salient in the context of a global pandemic since many migrants have family—children, spouses, or parents—who remain in the homeland. These transnational family responsibilities are often handled at an individual level and through personal means (e.g., money, kinship, and market forces) in "normal" times, but many migrants might no longer be able to do so in the context of COVID-19. Resolving such thorny issues requires us to think about policy solutions beyond national borders. The well-being of globally dispersed family members depends on coordination between governments, market forces, the third sector, and individuals in bi- or multinational contexts (Levitt et al. 2017; also see Marchetti and Mesiäislehto, chapter 13, this volume).

PART THREE

Aftermath

After the immediate response of lockdowns across the globe, many governments followed up with additional policy efforts to mitigate the economic and social harm brought on by the pandemic. In this section, authors explore these early policy responses: What do they teach us about the value of care? Are they meaningful steps to change or replications of the same historical inadequacies and inequalities?

In the early days of the pandemic, we did see new emphasis on the importance of care and care workers. An economic and social crisis brought on by a worldwide pandemic necessarily involved discussions about health care workers and systems. As Franziska Dorn and colleagues note, the elevation of health care workers at all levels as "essential workers" brought many care workers into the public eye and paved the way for symbolic valuing of care. At the same time, however, fewer policy responses backed up this symbolic effort with material assistance.

One form of material assistance was supplemental pay provided to these essential workers. Dorn et al. describe the range of temporary wage bonuses offered in the United States, Germany, and Canada. While Canada and Germany provided more generous supplemental pay than the United States in the early days of the pandemic, these efforts were inconsistently implemented, and the bonuses were not substantial or long-lasting. Sabrina Marchetti and Merita Mesiäislehto similarly point to the symbolic value of extensions to migration policy for care workers during the pandemic but note that these policies did little to mitigate the larger context of long-term precarity for these workers.

The inadequacy of these policy responses is certainly foretold by the ideological and policy trends that preceded the pandemic. The dominance of the economic and cultural ideology that Tronto calls wealth-care is clearly seen in these early responses, as economic factors continue to take precedence, limiting the view of "need" to business interests and silencing care needs, as described in Orly Benjamin's analysis of the Israeli response. Benjamin also points to the role of the "experts' committee"—a group of thirty military and economic leaders, almost all men—in the shaping of this discourse, emphasizing the importance of who sits at the decision table.

These early policy responses are nested in a political environment that is both care-blind and gender-blind. As such, instead of governments responding to care needs directly, these authors describe efforts that fall back into the ill-fitting categories of labor policy, immigration policy, and health policy. These policy solutions fall short in addressing the complex relationships of health, care, and labor. These siloed responses are most visible in Marchetti and Mesiäislehto's analysis of European policy responses for migrant and domestic workers. Migration policy in some countries worked to facilitate labor supply, allowing more care workers to travel into the country, or extending immigration status. Labor policies, however, often worked to keep these migrants in more vulnerable position (like tying permits to first employer, or preventing domestic workers from applying for resident permits). Some hope appears, however, in evidence that pressure from domestic worker organizations resulted in more responsive policy efforts as the pandemic continued.

Of course, policy does not function independently of culture, as Thurid Eggers, Christopher Grages, and Birgit Pfau-Effinger highlight. In their examination of childcare policy responses early in the pandemic, Eggers and colleagues analyze the ways that cultural ideologies shape policy responses, and even limit the impact of these policies. They find that Denmark, which has consistent ideological support for nonfamilial childcare, was able to marshal resources to reopen nonfamilial childcare quickly and safely. In Germany and England, however, where cultural orientations are more supportive of familial care, measures supported retraditionalism of care arrangements, with Germany providing extended family leave, and England doing little to support either paid or unpaid carers, with additional burdens largely taken on by women.

Overall, the chapters in this section demonstrate that there are some glimmers of hope in attention to care during the early policy responses to the pandemic. However, lacking a solid foundation in stronger political and economic ideologies, and lacking a position of power for those who might advocate for care, these efforts fall short of meeting the substantial needs of families and workers in the pandemic. These efforts also fall short of creating long-term transformative change.

12

Cheap Praise

Supplemental Pay for Essential Workers in the 2020 COVID-19 Pandemic

FRANZISKA DORN, NANCY FOLBRE, LEILA GAUTHAM, AND MARTHA MACDONALD

Beginning in March 2020, policies implemented to respond to the COVID-19 pandemic shocked labor markets in the United States, Canada, and Germany, as elsewhere. Some workers were thrown out of work or forced to reduce their hours. Others shifted to working from home. However, those loosely defined as "essential" workers faced increased demands on their time and, often, heightened risks of infection as they continued to provide crucial services. Their commitment was widely appreciated. Health care workers, in particular, were often publicly applauded. Yet efforts to compensate them with bonuses or hazard pay have proved uneven, inconsistent, and short-lived.

Pandemic-related pay policies deserve close consideration for several reasons. They affect the well-being of essential workers and are likely to influence the supply of paid labor in long-term adaptation to pandemic threats. The care services—health care, education, and social services—brought into sharp focus during the pandemic constitute an important part of essential paid work. Moreover, noncare essential services during the pandemic resemble carework in terms of the social benefits they create, and the normative commitments they require. The public goods aspects of care imply that, in the absence of public policy, care workers and other essential workers are likely to be underremunerated and underprotected, especially given the risks of COVID-19 infection that many of them face on the job.

Comparative analysis of private and public-sector strategies across countries confirm this suspicion. Our analysis of supplemental pay policies implemented in the first half of 2020 in three countries with federal structures allowing variation in public policy across provinces and states—United States, Canada, and Germany—highlights two key problems: (1) inconsistencies in the definition of essential work and attendant risks of infection and (2) erratic and inadequate levels of compensation. It also shows that the United States lagged far behind two comparable countries in its public provision of supplemental pay.

Risks, Rewards, and Essential Workers

While the experience of health care workers during the pandemic encapsulates many of the questions of health risks, bargaining power, and pay that are central to this chapter, many of the supplemental pay policies that we analyze also cover other, noncare, essential workers. The broader category of essential work in the pandemic has close parallels to carework, including spillover effects, the overrepresentation of women and/or minorities, and significant health risks. We therefore consider all essential workers (defined differently across settings, but usually including employees in health care, energy, utilities, information and communication technologies, food, water, transportation, safety, government, and some manufacturing) in our analysis, while narrowing our focus to the subset of essential care workers where appropriate.

It is difficult to imagine a better illustration of spillover effects than measures aimed at minimizing the transmission of contagious disease—measures ranging from social distancing and mask-wearing to vaccination. It follows that *all* workers who expose themselves to contagion in order to prevent and treat it also create positive spillovers—diffuse benefits for those not directly involved in any market transaction. Limited bargaining power helps explain why essential workers in general (and care workers in particular) were often unable to demand adequate compensation for their services during the pandemic, despite serious shortages of protective equipment and high risks of infection. While some larger companies offered bonuses as a goodwill gesture, government intervention was a far more important source of hazard pay in Canada and Germany than in the United States.

Worker bargaining power is influenced by many factors, including the unemployment rate, union membership, and workers' race/ethnicity, gender, and citizenship (Mishel et al. 2012). Also relevant are the type of services that workers provide. The positive spillovers associated with care services help explain why markets undervalue care provision, and also why workers in care industries—even those in relatively unskilled occupations—are strongly bound by moral and social obligations to care. Research shows that workers in essential care jobs in the United States are paid less than would be expected based on their education and other characteristics (Folbre, Gautham, and Smith 2021).

In the United States, Europe, and Canada, women, racial and ethnic minorities, and immigrants are heavily overrepresented among low-wage essential workers (Peng, chapter 3, this volume; Estabrooks et al. 2020; Rho, Brown, and Fremstad 2020). According to the United Kingdom's Office for National Statistics, men in low-skilled jobs are four times more likely to die from the virus than men in professional occupations, while women working in low-paid care jobs are twice as likely to die as those in professional and technical roles (Office for National Statistics 2020a). Comparable statistics are not available for the United States, but similar patterns of occupational exposure help explain why low-wage workers, especially

Blacks and Hispanics, have suffered far higher mortality than high-wage workers (Kinder and Ross 2020). Black women's overrepresentation in health care jobs was critical to understanding their higher risk during the pandemic (Akosionu et al., chapter 4, this volume).

Even prior to the pandemic, carework was associated with significant risks: for instance, job-related injury rates for direct care workers were often greater than for construction workers (Kurowski, Boyer, and Punnett 2015). These hazards were often made invisible by relational commitments; care workers, prioritizing the well-being of those they cared for, often dismissed workplace-related risks as "part of the job" (Zelnick 2015). The COVID-19 pandemic further heightened risks, while the structural factors limiting worker bargaining power remained in place.

Supplemental Pay Policy in Canada, Germany, and the United States

Political jurisdictions offered different rationales for supplemental pay, which took many different forms. Pandemic-related bonus pay is often described as hazard pay, a concept with origins in the military, where soldiers typically receive a bonus for combat duty. Indeed, in Canada, military troops who provided assistance in several nursing homes with severe COVID-19 outbreaks received the bonus associated with deployment (Armstrong and Klostermann, chapter 6, this volume). The U.S. Department of Labor defines hazard pay as "additional money for work that causes extreme physical discomfort and distress not adequately alleviated by protective devices and deemed to impose a physical hardship."[1] Large numbers of essential workers, health care workers among them, have been exposed to unsafe working conditions with little or no hazard pay.

The hazard pay policies implemented in the United States, Canada, and Germany in 2020 differed substantially in their scope, eligibility, and rationale. Our analysis of the policies described in table 12.1 reveals important cross-country similarities, but also documents the comparative weakness of the U.S. response.

Sources of the Initiatives

In contrast to Germany and Canada, hazard pay in the United States was characterized by the absence of policy at the federal level. While the proposed U.S. Heroes Act included a provision for $13/hour "pandemic premium pay," it stalled for lack of congressional approval. Only a few states opted to use general federal relief funds to implement their own programs. By contrast, both Canada and Germany enacted hazard pay at the federal level, with different levels of flexibility at the provincial or state level. Canada provided federal funding for each province to design its own program, whereas the German central government provided a bonus for a specific set of occupations. Two German states implemented separate policies in addition to the federal provisions. Across all three countries, private hazard pay was largely confined to a handful of large retail corporations, especially those selling groceries.

TABLE 12.1

COVID-19 supplemental public pay policies in the United States, Canada, and Germany in 2020 (expenditures in national currency; note distinction between $US and $CAN)

Source	Eligibility	Means-testing	Size and source of compensation	Timing
U.S.				
Federal government	Essential workers		No federal hazard pay but CARES Act made funds available for state governments	
State governments				
Pennsylvania	Employees in seven critical industries	Full-time and part-time employees earning less than $20 per hour	COVID-19 PA Hazard Pay Grant funded by CARES Act: one-time payment up to $1200 per worker	August 16, 2020, through October 24, 2020
Vermont	Public and private employees in essential services that deal with the public	Employees earning $25 per hour or less and working in a job with an "elevated risk"	Frontline Employee Hazard Pay Grant Program funded by CARES Act: one-time payment of $1200–$2000 per worker	March 13 through May 15, 2020
Louisiana	Public and private employees in critical industries	Adjusted gross income of $50,000 or less	Louisiana Frontline Worker Rebate Program funded by CARES Act: one-time $250 payment	March 22–May 14, 2020

TABLE 12.1 (continued)

COVID-19 supplemental public pay policies in the United States, Canada, and Germany in 2020 (expenditures in national currency; note distinction between $US and $CAN)

Source	Eligibility	Means-testing	Size and source of compensation	Timing
Maryland	Public employees in "24/7 jobs," e.g., law enforcement, corrections, hospitals		COVID-19 Response Pay: $3.13 per hour pay raise	April 1–September 10, 2020
Virginia	Home health care workers serving Medicaid members		Hazard Pay for Home Health Workers funded by CARES Act: one-time $1500 payment	March 12 and June 30, 2020
Michigan	First responders and direct care workers providing Medicaid-funded care		First Responder Hazard Pay Premiums Program funded by CARES Act: one-time $1000 for first responders; $2 per hour increase for direct care workers	First responders, July 26–September 30, 2020; direct care workers, July 1–December 31, 2020
New Hampshire	First responders and frontline workers at Medicaid-funded care facilities		Long Term Care Stabilization Program funded by CARES Act: $300 weekly payments	April 16–June 30, 2020; reactivated November 16–December 30, 2020

(continued)

TABLE 12.1 (continued)

COVID-19 supplemental public pay policies in the United States, Canada, and Germany in 2020 (expenditures in national currency; note distinction between $US and $CAN)

Source	Eligibility	Means-testing	Size and source of compensation	Timing
Canada				
Federal government	Workers in essential sectors		Up to $3 billion to increase the wages of low-income essential workers, eligibility and amount of support determined by province or territory. Provinces to contribute $1 billion in cost-sharing agreements.	
Provincial governments				
Newfoundland and Labrador	Providers of essential services in accordance with Public Safety Canada guidelines	Gross monthly income <$3000 (later increased to $3500) and more than 190 hours worked over eligibility period (March 15– July 4, 2020)	Essential Worker Support Program (EWSP). Lump sum scale: $600–$1500 based on hours and earnings over 16 weeks	Ended on July 4, 2020

TABLE 12.1 (continued)

COVID-19 supplemental public pay policies in the United States, Canada, and Germany in 2020 (expenditures in national currency; note distinction between $US and $CAN)

Source	Eligibility	Means-testing	Size and source of compensation	Timing
Nova Scotia	Health care employees, including long-term care	Worked March 13–July 13	Essential Health Care Workers Program. Max. $2000 bonus	March 13–July 13, 2020
Prince Edward Island	Providers of essential services	Gross monthly income <$3000, hourly wage $18.75 or less, and worked a minimum of 60 hours April 6–May 3, 2020	$1000 bonus	April 6–July 26, 2020
New Brunswick	Direct care employees in care services	Hourly wage $18 or less; worked >10 hours per week	Up to $500/month	March 19–July 9, 2020
Quebec	Employees in essential services, focus on long-term care and COVID-19 hospital units	Weekly income $550 or less, annual income $5000–$28,600	$100/week (all); further $600 per 4 weeks for full-time workers in facility with active COVID-19 case	March 15–July 4, 2020

(continued)

TABLE 12.1 (continued)

COVID-19 supplemental public pay policies in the United States, Canada, and Germany in 2020 (expenditures in national currency; note distinction between $US and $CAN)

Source	Eligibility	Means-testing	Size and source of compensation	Timing
Ontario	Phase 1 employees in health care, long-term care, social services, corrections Phase 2 limited to personal and direct care workers in publicly funded care	Only direct care workers, hours per month >100, excluding management and doctors	Phase 1 $4/hour bonus; plus $250 lump sum/month Phase 2 $3 or $2/hour depending on sector	April 24–August 15, 2020 October 1, 2020–August 23, 2021
Manitoba	Phase 1, employees in essential services; Phase 2, direct care providers in these services	Earns $5000/month or less and worked >200 hours; Phase 2 wage < $25	One-time lump sum of $1530 or $5/hour wage supplement	March 20–May 29, 2020; November 1, 2020–January 10, 2021
Saskatchewan	Workers in essential care facilities, emergency and transition shelters, integrated health care facilities, or providing care to seniors in their own home	Excludes care services contracted out; must earn a wage less than $24/hour and have gross earnings less than $2500 over the 4-week period; no income cutoff in Phase 2	$400 every 4 weeks for up to 4 months	March 15–July 4, 2020; November 19–December 16; December 17, 2020–January 13, 2021

TABLE 12.1 (continued)

COVID-19 supplemental public pay policies in the United States, Canada, and Germany in 2020 (expenditures in national currency; note distinction between $US and $CAN)

Source	Eligibility	Means-testing	Size and source of compensation	Timing
Alberta (no program in first wave)	Workers in health, social services, and education	Excluded doctors, teachers	Lump sum of $12,000	October 12, 2020–January 31, 2021
British Columbia	Health, social services, corrections employees		Lump sum, about $4/hour	March 15–July 4, 2020
Yukon	All those providing essential services	Earning $20/hour or less	$4/hour wage increase for up to 40 hours a week OR an amount to bring pay up to $20/hour for up to 40 hours a week	Phase 1, March 15–October 3; Phase 2, October 15, 2020–February 15, 2021
Germany[a]				
Federal government[b]	Public employees, states and municipalities		3.2% to 4.5% increase in hourly wage, depending on salary grade, plus one-time bonus of €300–600	Stepwise increase until December 2022

(continued)

TABLE 12.1 (continued)

COVID-19 supplemental public pay policies in the United States, Canada, and Germany in 2020 (expenditures in national currency; note distinction between $US and $CAN)

Source	Eligibility	Means-testing	Size and source of compensation	Timing
	Nurses	Nurses explicitly exposed to COVID-19 in hospitals; all nurses in elder care	8.7% increase in hourly wage for nurses, 10% increase for nurses in intensive care, plus lump sum up to €1500, depending on weekly working hours; up to €1500 for all elder care nurses	Same as above
	Doctors in public health departments		€300 monthly allowance	Permanent increase after March 2021
Berlin	Hospital staff at Charité and Vivantes, two state-owned hospital groups		€450 bonuses to all their workers	€150 added to monthly wage April–June 2020
	Public employees	Those particularly exposed to changing conditions due to COVID-19	Up to €1000 paid by the state	No fixed dates, eligibility and payment varied by department

TABLE 12.1 (continued)

COVID-19 supplemental public pay policies in the United States, Canada, and Germany in 2020 (expenditures in national currency; note distinction between $US and $CAN)

Source	Eligibility	Means-testing	Size and source of compensation	Timing
Bavaria	Nurses in hospitals Public employees		€500 bonus	For the year 2020

Sources: See appendix at the end of this chapter.

[a] The German Ministry of Finance allowed special payments due to the COVID-19 crisis to be tax-free up to €1500. Voluntary for any industry; any employee could benefit, from March 1, 2020, to December 31, 2020.

[b] General wage negotiations took place in Germany at the end of 2020, making it unclear whether the wage increases were pandemic-specific.

Eligibility

Federal agencies in Canada, Germany, and the United States provided loose definitions of essential work as jobs in certain critical sectors: health care, energy,
utilities, information and communication technologies, finance, food, water,
transportation, safety, government, and some manufacturing. These definitions
were operationalized in a variety of ways (based on industry, occupation, or a combination thereof) that influenced lockdown policies. Supplementary pay in Germany focused mainly on a few health care occupations and public employees. Often
as a result of budget constraints, provincial and state governments in the United
States and Canada narrowed eligibility to specific groups, such as first responders
(Michigan, Maryland, New Hampshire), health care (Nova Scotia, Quebec), or long-
term care and social service employees (Manitoba Phase 2, Saskatchewan).

Targeting and Means-Testing

Across most Canadian provinces and some U.S. states, eligibility was further
restricted to low-wage/income workers. In lieu of an income cutoff, targeting also
took the form of excluding certain highly paid occupations like doctors and hospital management (such as in Ontario and British Columbia in Canada). While
means-testing was often driven by limited funding (e.g., in Pennsylvania in the
United States) and the need to make low-paid essential work attractive relative to
offered income security benefits (Canada), it was also rationalized as a means of
raising the wages of workers who were poorly paid to begin with.

   Other kinds of targeting included exposure to COVID-19 risk. For instance,
Germany provided extra compensation for health care workers only in hospitals
with a certain threshold of COVID-19 cases. Requirements that eligible workers be
full-time or directly employed were also common, excluding workers in services
that were contracted out (a common practice in hospital and long-term care settings) or those working multiple part-time jobs. Some programs restricted eligibility to only direct care workers (New Brunswick, Ontario, Manitoba Phase 2),
leaving out workers such as cleaners and dietary staff. Overall, the implementation of supplemental pay targeting was inconsistent and frequently excluded workers who experienced significant risks of contagion.

Size and Source of Compensation

Given the lack of systematic accounting on public expenditures on hazard pay, we
attempt an approximate estimate of the scale of funding. Our back-of-the-envelope
calculations of government expenses on supplemental pay for essential workers
show that while the United States spent about $0.8 billion, Canada and Germany
spent about $3 billion and $0.4 billion dollars, respectively (all currencies con-
verted to $U.S. using average nominal exchange rates for 2020).[2] When scaled by
the size of the paid labor force (as given by the Organization for Economic Cooperation and Development 2020 Indicators), Germany spent roughly twice as much

as the United States per employed worker, whereas Canada spent thirty times as much.[3] Conditional on eligibility, payments to individual workers were not particularly large: in the United States, even the most generous payments to health care workers (such as in Pennsylvania) were equivalent to raising wages for a full-time employee by about $3 per hour for 2 months. In Germany, the best-case payment (to a full-time eldercare nurse or a nurse in a hospital with high exposure to COVID-19) would amount to a 3.13 euro (or 3.6 U.S. dollar) increase in hourly wages for 3 months. In Canada, the best-case scenario was 5 Canadian dollars (or 6.7 U.S. dollars) per hour (Manitoba Phase 2), while three jurisdictions paid 4 Canadian dollars (or 5.4 U.S. dollars) per hour for 4 months (most provinces paid essential workers an increase of about 2.67 Canadian dollars [2 U.S. dollars] per hour for about 4 months). The top-ups offered by private employers in the United States and Canada were typically $2 per hour, with some companies also providing a one-time bonus.

Timing

Payments in the United States and Canada generally took the form of a one-time bonus or a temporary wage increase, ending by July–September 2020. The programs offered by private companies in Canada and the United States were even shorter-lived, with most ending in the late spring of 2020. During the second wave (autumn 2020) only four Canadian jurisdictions reintroduced programs, two of which were more tightly targeted to essential care facilities than in the first round. Permanent wage increases were confined to continuing care assistants in nursing homes and home care in Nova Scotia, Canada, and to a few essential workers in Germany, but these were an exception to the rule. The fact that the timing of supplemental pay rarely coincided with the duration—or severity—of the pandemic suggests that the pay raises were largely symbolic in nature, and not intended as a substantive compensation for workplace hazard.

Rationales

Neither governments nor private employers embraced the term "hazard pay," preferring to frame payments as driven either by gratitude or the need to retain workers rather than by employer obligations for fair compensation. Words such as "bonus" or "supplemental" convey generosity. The names of many specific programs are revealing in this respect: Incentive Program to Retain Essential Workers (Quebec), Temporary Pandemic Pay (Ontario, British Columbia), the Corona Bonus in Germany, the Thank-You Bonus in Berlin, and the Heroes Act and pandemic premium pay in the United States.

Conclusion

Lack of compensation for exposure to dangerous working conditions dovetails with other issues of economic justice raised by the pandemic (Tronto, chapter 1, this volume). It also connects to principles of pay equity that often conflict with market-driven outcomes. In the absence of consistent and equitable pay policies and greater protections for worker safety, essential workers are likely to experience burnout, employers are likely to suffer high staff turnover, and all of us will find it harder to obtain the care services we need. Many essential workers have expressed concern and anger over their lack of remuneration, as illustrated in the following sample of comments from the United States:

> In America, a hero is something you label somebody when they do something you don't want to fairly compensate them for.

> Got a letter that says I'm an essential worker and a paycheck that says I'm not.[4]

Employer liability for worker exposure to COVID-19 is difficult to define or enforce. For many workers, supplemental pay matters less than their own health and that of their families and friends. Indeed, paying workers a risk premium can be a way of sidestepping costly health and safety protections. On the other hand, placing responsibility for hazard pay on employers rather than the public sector could strengthen private incentives for improvement of workplace safety. These policy options are not necessarily inconsistent: public and private responsibility could go hand-in-hand, combining modest subsidies with strict regulations and legal liability guidelines for private firms.

The inadequacy of hazard pay and workplace safety provisions in the private sector demonstrates the inability of market forces to adjust to big, external health shocks. Our analysis shows that U.S. policies could have been much more generous. It also highlights the lack of any coordinated attempt to fairly compensate essential workers. Definitions of eligibility were inconsistent and ad hoc, particularly in the health care sector. Workers who faced significant work-related health risks, from contract or part-time workers to hospital cleaning and administrative staff to relatively well-paid physicians, were often excluded from consideration.

Dangerous and stressful working conditions during the pandemic—including lack of consistent hazard pay—have likely contributed to high rates of attrition among essential workers. A recent national survey of U.S. health care workers found that approximately one in five physicians and two in five nurses intend to leave their current practices (Sinsky et al. 2021). A pre-pandemic global shortage of nurses has intensified (ICNM 2022; WHO 2020d). The depletion of the health care workforce threatens the quality of patient care. Although compensatory pay in most jurisdictions has ended, the pandemic has not.

APPENDIX: SOURCES FOR TABLE 12.1

Background Sources

UNITED STATES

City of Portland. 2020. "Minimum Wage Ordinance." Accessed January 21, 2021. https://www
.portlandmaine.gov/1671/Minimum-Wage#:~:text=Effective%20January%201%2C%20
2021%2C%20employers,be%20paid%20to%20tipped%20workers.

Governor of New Hampshire. n.d. "Establishment of the COVID-19 Long Term Care Stabilization Program." Accessed January 21, 2021. https://www.nhes.nh.gov/services/employers
/documents/emergency-order31-ltcs-program.pdf.

Governor of New Hampshire. n.d. "New Hampshire Reactivates Long Term Care Stabilization
Program." Accessed January 21, 2021. https://www.governor.nh.gov/news-and-media/new
-hampshire-reactivates-long-term-care-stabilization-program.

Governor of Virginia. 2020. "Governor Northam Authorizes Hazard Pay for Home Health Workers." Accessed January 21, 2021. https://www.governor.virginia.gov/newsroom/all-releases
/2020/october/headline-860858-en.html.

Kinder, Molly, Laura Stateler, and Julia Du. 2020a. "The COVID-19 Hazard Continues, but the
Hazard Pay Does Not: Why America's Essential Workers Need a Raise." Accessed January 21, 2021. https://www.brookings.edu/research/the-covid-19-hazard-continues-but-the
-hazard-pay-does-not-why-americas-frontline-workers-need-a-raise/.

Kinder, Molly, Laura Stateler, and Julia Du. 2020b. "Windfall Profits and Deadly Risks." Accessed
January 21, 2021. https://www.brookings.edu/essay/windfall-profits-and-deadly-risks/.

Michigan Dept. of Health and Human Services. n.d. "Skilled Nursing Facility COVID-19
Response: Direct Care Worker Wage Increase; Frequently Asked Questions." Accessed
January 21, 2021. www.michigan.gov/documents/mdhhs/MDHHS_SNF_COVID19_DCW
_FAQs_v4_07.30.20_697986_7.pdf.

Michigan Dept. of Treasury. n.d. "First Responder Hazard Pay Premiums Program (FRHPPP)."
Accessed January 21, 2021. https://www.michigan.gov/treasury/0,4679,7-121-1751_2197
-532758—,00.html#:~:text=Premiums%20Program%20(FRHPPP),2020%20to%20Decem-
ber%2029%2C%202020.

Pennsylvania Department of Community and Economic Development. 2020. "COVID-19 PA
Hazard Pay Grant." Accessed January 21, 2021. https://dced.pa.gov/programs/covid-19-pa
-hazard-pay-grant/.

State of Louisiana. 2020. "Louisiana Frontline Worker Rebate Program." Accessed January 21,
2021. https://frontlineworkers.la.gov/.

State of Vermont. 2020. "Governor Phil Scott Announces Expansion of Frontline Employee
Hazard Pay Grant Program." Accessed January 21, 2021. https://governor.vermont.gov
/press-release/governor-phil-scott-announces-expansion-frontline-employee-hazard
-pay-grant-program.

Wood, Pamela. 2020. "Maryland to Bump Salaries of Frontline Workers in Coronavirus Crisis;
Rates Still Below Double Pay Received Earlier." Accessed January 21, 2021. https://www
.baltimoresun.com/coronavirus/bs-md-pol-state-worker-pay-20200401-yuxwqngljvck
nev5z5w7k5ga4y-story.html.

CANADA

Note: Unfortunately many of the documents used for the table have disappeared
from the provincial government websites. In those cases less detailed press releases
or media articles have been included.

Alberta: Accessed October 17, 2022. https://www.theglobeandmail.com/canada/alberta/article
-alberta-requested-far-less-in-federal-wage-top-up-for-essential/.
          Accessed October 17, 2022. https://www.alberta.ca/critical-worker-benefit.aspx.
British Columbia: Accessed October 17, 2022. https://globalnews.ca/news/7523601/bc-hospital
-workers-pandemic-pay-delay/.
Manitoba: "Manitoba Risk Recognition Program." Accessed October 17, 2022. https://manitoba
.ca/covid19/infomanitobans/mrrp_eligible.html.
          Accessed October 17, 2022. https://manitoba.ca/covid19/restartmb/mrrp.html#overview.
New Brunswick: Accessed October 17, 2022. https://www2.gnb.ca/content/gnb/en/news/news
_release.2020.05.0290.html.
Newfoundland and Labrador: "Essential Worker Support Program." Accessed October 17, 2022
.https://www.gov.nl.ca/releases/2020/exec/0615n04/.
Nova Scotia: "Essential Health Care Workers Program." Accessed October 17, 2022.https://
novascotia.ca/news/release/?id=20200507004.
Ontario: "COVID-19 Temporary Pandemic Pay." https://www.ontario.ca/page/covid-19-tem
porary-pandemic-pay.
          Government of Ontario. 2020. *Eligible Workplaces and Workers for Pandemic Pay.* May 29.
                    Accessed October 17, 2022. https://www.ontario.ca/page/eligible-workplaces-and
                    -workers-pandemic-pay#section-1.
          Accessed October 17, 2022. https://news.ontario.ca/en/release/60798/ontario-extending
                    -temporary-wage-enhancement-for-personal-support-workers.
          Accessed October 17, 2022. https://news.ontario.ca/en/release/1000284/ontario-extending
                    -temporary-wage-increase-for-personal-support-workers.
Prime Minister. 2020. "Prime Minister Announces Agreements to Boost Wages for Essential
Workers." May 7. Accessed October 17, 2022. https://pm.gc.ca/en/news/news-releases
/2020/05/07/prime-minister-announces-agreements-boost-wages-essential-workers.
Prince Edward Island: "COVID-19 Support for Essential Workers." Accessed October 17, 2022.
https://www.princeedwardisland.ca/en/news/province-announces-support-for-essen
tial-workers-small-business-and-fisheries.
"Public Safety Canada's Guidance on Essential Services and Functions in Canada during the
COVID-19 Pandemic." Accessed October 17, 2022. https://www.publicsafety.gc.ca/cnt/ntnl
-scrt/crtcl-nfrstrctr/esf-sfe-en.aspx.
Quebec: Accessed October 17, 2022. https://www.cbc.ca/news/canada/montreal/covid-19-health
-care-bonuses-quebec-1.5560287.
          "Quebec Government COVID-19 Measures." Accessed October 17, 2022. https://mrcbm
.qc.ca/covid19/QuebecGovernmentCoronavirus_RelatedMeasures_8May2020.pdf.
Saskatchewan: Accessed October 17, 2022. https://regina.ctvnews.ca/temporary-wage-sup
plement-applications-open-for-low-income-essential-workers-1.4941604.
          Accessed October 17, 2022. https://www.saskatchewan.ca/government/news-and-media
                    /2020/november/18/new-phase-of-temporary-wage-supplement-program-intro
                    duced-to-support-those-caring-for-seniors,
Yukon: Accessed October 17, 2022. https://globalnews.ca/news/6977373/yukon-coronavirus
-essential-workers/.
          Yukon Update: https://yukon.ca/en/health-and-wellness/covid-19-information/economic
                    -and-social-supports-covid-19/yukon-essential.

GERMANY
Bonus for public employees: Accessed October 17, 2022. https://oeffentlicher-dienst-news.de
/corona-sonderzahlung-im-oeffentlichen-dienst-anspruch-hoehe-auszahlung/.

Bundesfinanzministerium. 2021. "Sonderzahlungen jetzt steuerfrei: Anerkennung für Beschäftigte in der Corona-Krise". Accessed January 30, 2021. https://www.bundesfinanzministerium.de/Content/DE/Pressemitteilungen/Finanzpolitik/2020/04/2020-04-03-GPM-Bonuszahlungen.html.

Bundesministerium für Gesundheit (BfG). 2020. "Pflegebonus." *Bundesministerium für Gesundheit.* Accessed September 17, 2020. https://www.bundesgesundheitsministerium.de/pflegebonus.html.

Federal payment regulations: Accessed October 17, 2022. https://www.bundesfinanzministerium.de/Content/DE/Pressemitteilungen/Finanzpolitik/2020/04/2020-04-03-GPM-Bonuszahlungen.html.

Accessed October 17, 2022. https://www.tagesschau.de/wirtschaft/tarifeinigung-oeffentlicher-dienst-111.html.

Accessed October 17, 2022. https://www.verdi.de/presse/pressemitteilungen/++co++df6f2fd0-16ad-11eb-bacd-001a4a160129.

Berlin

Berlin Bonus/Alltagshelden: Accessed October 17, 2022. https://www.bz-berlin.de/berlin/corona-praemie-fuer-berliner-alltagshelden-wird-ausgezahlt.

Berlin.de. 2020. "Prämie für «Corona-Helden» soll bald fließen." Berlin.de. Das offizielle Hauptstadtportal. Accessed September 17, 2020. https://www.berlin.de/aktuelles/berlin/6178306-958092-praemie-fuer-coronahelden-soll-bald-flie.html.

Bonus Charité and Vivantes: Accessed October 17, 2022. https://www.aerzteblatt.de/nachrichten/111772/450-Euro-extra-fuer-Pfleger-und-Aerzte-bei-Vivantes-und-Charite.

Total Care Bonus (Pflegebonus): Accessed October 17, 2022. https://www.bundesgesundheitsministerium.de/pflegebonus.html.

Bavaria

Bayrisches Staatsministerium für Gesundheit und Pflege (BSGP). 2020. "Maßnahmen." *Bayrisches Staatsministerium für Gesundheit und Pflege.* Accessed September 9, 2020. https://www.stmgp.bayern.de/coronavirus/massnahmen/#Anerkennung-des-Personal.

Additional Sources/Updates

UNITED STATES: BLOG POSTS AND POPULAR PRESS

Associated Press. 2021. "Who's a Hero? Some US States, Cities Still Debating COVID Hazard Pay." September 25. https://www.voanews.com/a/who-s-a-hero-some-us-states-cities-still-debating-covid-hazard-pay/6328647.html.

Kamper, Dave, Jaimie Worker, and Jennifer Sherer, Economic Policy Institute. 2021. "Few Midwestern States Are Providing Premium Pay to Essential Workers, Despite American Rescue Plan Funding." October 13. https://www.epi.org/blog/few-midwestern-states-are-providing-premium-pay-to-essential-workers-despite-american-rescue-plan-funding/.

Karla Walter. 2021. "Higher Pay for Caregivers." Center for American Progress, June 28. https://www.americanprogress.org/article/higher-pay-caregivers/.

Kinder, Molly. 2021. "With Federal Aid on the Way, It's Time for State and Local Governments to Boost Pay for Frontline Essential Workers." April 6. https://www.brookings.edu/blog/the-avenue/2021/04/06/with-federal-aid-on-the-way-its-time-for-state-and-local-governments-to-boost-pay-for-frontline-essential-workers/.

Kinder, Molly, Laura Stateler, and Julia Du. 2020. "The COVID-19 Hazard Continues, but the Hazard Pay Does Not: Why America's Essential Workers Need a Raise." October 29.

https://www.brookings.edu/research/the-covid-19-hazard-continues-but-the-hazard
-pay-does-not-why-americas-frontline-workers-need-a-raise/.

Lieb, David A. 2021. "Bonus Pay for Essential Workers Varied Widely across States," AP News,
July 11. https://apnews.com/article/joe-biden-business-health-government-and-politics
-coronavirus-pandemic-8cbdd37a71cf34c812150b93f0e3da17.

UNITED STATES: ACADEMIC RESEARCH

McConnell, Doug, and Dominic Wilkinson. 2021. "Compensation and Hazard Pay for Key
Workers during an Epidemic: An Argument from Analogy." *Journal of Medical Ethics* 47,
no. 12: 784–787.

Ng, Matthew A., Anthony Naranjo, Ann E. Schlotzhauer, Mindy K. Shoss, Nika Kartvelishvili,
Matthew Bartek, Kenneth Ingraham et al. 2021. "Has the COVID-19 Pandemic Accelerated
the Future of Work or Changed Its Course? Implications for Research and Practice."
International Journal of Environmental Research and Public Health 18, no. 19: 10199.

Orleck, Annelise. 2021. "And the Virus Rages On: "Contingent" and "Essential" Workers in the
Time of COVID-19." *International Labor and Working-Class History* 99: 1–14.

Romer, Christina D., and David H. Romer. 2021. *A Social Insurance Perspective on Pandemic Fiscal
Policy: Implications for Unemployment Insurance and Hazard Pay.* National Bureau of Economic Research Working Paper 29419 (forthcoming in *Journal of Economic Perspectives*).

GERMANY: BLOG POSTS AND POPULAR PRESS

Bundesministerium der Finanzen. 2022. "Entlastungen für Bürgerinnen und Bürger sowie
Unternehmen: Weitere steuerliche Erleichterungen zur Bekämpfung der Corona-
Pandemie." February 16. https://www.bundesfinanzministerium.de/Content/DE/Pressemit-
teilungen/Finanzpolitik/2022/02/2022-02-16-weitere-steuerliche-erleichterungen-corona
-pandemie.html.

Öffentlicher Dienst News. 2022. "Pflegebonus 2022: Wer bekommt bis zu 3000 Euro Corona-
Prämie?" February 20. https://oeffentlicher-dienst-news.de/corona-bonus-1500-euro
-sonderpraemie-fuer-beschaeftigte-in-der-stationaeren-langzeitpflege-und-der
-ambulanten-pflege/.

Tagesschau. 2022. "Corona-Prämie—Wo bleibt der Pflegebonus?" February 21. https://www
.tagesschau.de/inland/innenpolitik/pflegepersonal-bonus-101.html.

Tagesschau. 2022. "Geplante Corona-Prämie Bis zu 550 Euro Bonus für Altenpflegekräfte." February 22. https://www.tagesschau.de/inland/pflegebonus-corona-eckpunkte-101.html.

Ver.di. 2021. "Tarif- und Besoldungsrunde 2021 für die Beschäftigten der Länder Spürbare
Einkommensverbesserungen im Gesundheitswesen." November 11. https://unverzichtbar
.verdi.de/++co++b3ea091a-50fa-11ec-9593-001a4a16012a.

CANADA: BLOG POSTS AND POPULAR PRESS

Bundale, Brent. 2022. "Grocers Pressured to Bring Back 'Hero Pay' amid Omicron Surge. January 7. https://www.cbc.ca/news/business/grocers-hero-pay-unifor-1.6307698.

Canadian Union of Public Employees. 2022. A Permanent Wage Top-Up Is Required in Community Care. January 19. https://cupe.ca/permanent-wage-top-required-community-care.

Gorman, Matt. 2022. "CCA Raise Should 'Make Life Easier' for Other Health Workers, Says N.S.
Minister." February 10. https://www.cbc.ca/news/canada/nova-scotia/long-term-care
-ccas-wage-increase-1.6347001.

Proudfoot, Shannon. 2021. "The Working Class Has Had Enough." *MacLeans Magazine*, September 13. https://www.macleans.ca/longforms/the-working-class-has-had-enough/.

Thomson, Aly. 2022. "Continuing Care Assistants in N.S. Getting 23% Wage Increase." February 7. https://www.cbc.ca/news/canada/nova-scotia/nova-scotia-continuing-care-assistants-25-per-cent-wage-increase-1.6345604.

CANADA: ACADEMIC RESEARCH

Gaitens, J., M. Condon, E. Fernandes, and M. McDiarmid. 2021. "COVID-19 and Essential Workers: A Narrative Review of Health Outcomes and Moral Injury." *International Journal of Environmental Research and Public Health* 18, no. 4: 1446. https://doi.org/10.3390/ijerph18041446.

Lamb, D., R. Gomez, and M. Moghaddas. 2021. "Unions and Hazard Pay for COVID-19: Evidence from the Canadian Labour Force Survey." *British Journal of Industrial Relations* (November 1): 1–29. doi: 10.1111/bjir.12649.

Rao, A., H. Ma, G. Moloney, J. Kwong, P. Jüni, B. Sander, R. Kustra, S. Baral, and S. Mishra. 2021. A Disproportionate Epidemic: COVID-19 Cases and Deaths among Essential Workers in Toronto, Canada. *Annals of Epidemiology* 63: 63–67. https://doi.org/10.1016/j.annepidem.2021.07.010.

NOTES

1. See U.S Department of Labor, accessed February 6, 2021, https://www.dol.gov/general/topic/wages/hazardpay.

2. These estimates include both federal and state-level spending. The U.S. estimate includes spending from Virginia ($50 million), Vermont ($50.5 million), Louisiana ($50 million), New Hampshire ($100 million), Maryland ($33.3 million), Virginia ($73 million), and Michigan ($420 million). The estimate for Canada includes federal spending of $3 billion Canadian dollars and $1 billion from the provinces, converted at an exchange rate of 1.34 Canadian dollar/U.S. dollar. German federal spending was €100 million at the federal level, €131.6 million, and €41 million on the part of Bavaria and Berlin, respectively, and approximately €50 million from the other fourteen states that provided a €500 bonus to eligible nurses, converted at 0.877 €/U.S. dollar.

3. Estimates on the size of the labor force in 2020 are taken from the OECD 2020 Indicators, accessed February 9, 2020, https://data.oecd.org/emp/labour-force.htm.

4. "30 Hilarious Essential Worker Memes," at www.boredpanda.com, accessed July 10, 2020, https://www.boredpanda.com/essential-workers-jokes/?utm_source=google&utm_medium=organic&utm_campaign=organic.

13

Migrants in Europe's Domestic and Care Sector

The Institutional Response

SABRINA MARCHETTI AND MERITA MESIÄISLEHTO

The COVID-19 pandemic shattered the globe in spring 2020. Worldwide, countries took policy measures to prevent the spread of disease and support their citizens against the distress it caused (Gentilini et al. 2020). In Europe, the needs of migrant workers evoked a range of policy interventions, with different strategies for protection. Internationally, migrant care workers and domestic workers constituted a category most affected by the pandemic (ILO 2020g; Marchetti and Boris 2020). Because of their status as migrants and often also as informal workers, these workers often lack labor market protection. In each European country, their conditions during the pandemic were the result of the intersection of migration and labor market policies.

In Europe, care workers and domestic workers, in particular undocumented migrants, were especially vulnerable. As Maria Nieves Rico and Laura Pautassi (chapter 7, this volume) suggest, the "social impact" of the COVID-19 epidemic was stronger for those whose socioeconomic status rendered them already disadvantaged, and for temporary and undocumented migrants, lack of full citizenship rights exacerbated vulnerabilities. Care workers and domestic workers are "essential workers" and, as Joan Tronto (chapter 1, this volume) explains, they are often from the most disadvantaged backgrounds and so were forced to risk their lives while others could avoid the worst dangers of the pandemic (Fasani and Mazza 2020). The case of migrant care workers and domestic workers thus confirms Tronto's view that the health and socioeconomic crises wrought by COVID-19 will have the strongest impact on racialized groups who provide "basic care." Current policies, she argues, neglect the most vulnerable.

In Europe, the COVID-19 pandemic turned migrant care into a "showcase of precarious EU labor market arrangements" (Kuhlmann et al. 2020). Europe's dependence on a migrant workforce, particularly in elder care, led some governments to take rather drastic measures to ensure the inflow of circulating migrants. For example, in Romania, during the lockdown in the first weeks of the pandemic, nearly 200 chartered flights left for other European countries at a time when scheduled flights had been canceled (Mutler 2020). With trains departing from Timişoara to Vienna, transportation was also organized for care workers serving the elderly (Creţan and Light 2020).

Our focus is on migrant care workers and domestic workers because they are more likely than other workers to face precarious labor conditions. Indeed, a migrant background increases the risk of precarious labor, including both low wages and informal and irregular work arrangements (Jokela 2019; Lightman 2017). Institutions, however, play a crucial role. For example, state policies simultaneously shape both migrants' citizenship status and their employment status (Hellgren 2015; Jokela 2017; Williams and Gavanas 2008). Governments may either enhance migrants' conditions of employment through regulation or promote precariousness through informal and irregular work or through incentives for households (e.g., vouchers) that weaken workers' positions (Jokela 2017; Morel 2015). Also important are policy approaches to the care needs of households with elderly members or young children (Marchetti and Farris, 2017).

Regional and global efforts are thus important to ensure that the COVID-19 crisis does not reinforce existing inequalities (Ito Peng, chapter 3, this volume). Policy measures include the ratification (and implementation) of ILO Convention number 189 of 2011, which demands that domestic workers be treated equally to other workers.[1] In addition, the 2016 European Parliament Resolution, "Women Domestic Workers and Carers in the EU," emphasizes the importance of protecting workers in this sector against abuse and lack of social and legal recognition.[2] More recently, the European Economic and Social Committee published a report on live-in care workers in selected EU countries (the UK, Germany, Italy, and Poland), supporting the request for more protection and labor rights (Rogalewski and Florek 2020).

The status of domestic workers differs across Europe. For example, Germany, Denmark, Poland, the UK, Sweden, Hungary, and Greece lack specific laws on domestic work, but general labor law applies. Ireland, the Netherlands, and Spain lack specific collective agreements for this sector (Triandafyllidou and Marchetti 2014, 2017). The specifics of work in this sector, especially for live-in workers, can then leave workers vulnerable, as their working conditions differ from those of other jobs. Yet most national laws on domestic workers fail to grant these workers the rights afforded other workers (Marchetti and Triandafyllidou 2014, 2017). A telling example is the absence of paid sick leave, which, given the high risk of domestic workers' contracting the disease, assumed paramount importance in the COVID-19 pandemic.

For migrant care workers and domestic workers, precarity concerns not only working conditions but also a lack of full citizenship rights. These limitations include restrictions on the duration of residence permits, the right to family reunification, access to goods and services (property, health care, education, financial credit, etc.), and more generally the scarce opportunities these workers have for labor and social mobility. Such limitations also apply to the many EU migrants moving from eastern countries to the West, including most of those employed in the domestic and care sector, especially women. All these factors contribute to the position of migrant care workers and domestic workers as "partial citizens" (Marchetti, 2016; Parreñas 2001).

Most non-EU migrants working in this sector are forced, through a range of policies, to assume undocumented status (Triandafyllidou and Marchetti 2014, 2017). In Denmark, Germany, Ireland, and the Netherlands, workers in this sector are prevented from applying for residence permits. In Belgium and the UK, permits are tied to a worker's first employer and are lost when that worker changes jobs. In Italy and Greece, quotas limit the numbers and nationalities of workers in this sector who can apply for residence permits each year. In Denmark, Belgium, Finland, the Netherlands, Sweden, and the UK, the au-pair program is often abused to facilitate the arrival of migrant workers. Undocumented status in Europe is therefore common among care workers and domestic workers, putting them in a highly precarious position. The pandemic amplified these vulnerabilities.

The Impact of the Pandemic on the Care and Domestic Sector

In the European Union, carework and domestic work are together categorized as a critical sector. In March 2020, the European Commission published guidelines to ensure the continued free movement of workers in critical occupations during the COVID-19 outbreak.[3] These occupations, also referred to as essential work, included jobs often performed in private households, such as cleaners, helpers, and personal care workers. Estimates based on the European Labour Force Survey suggest that non-EU citizens accounted for 25 percent of cleaners and helpers and 14 percent of personal care workers in Europe (Fasani and Mazza 2020). According to the same estimates, these are also the largest groups among migrant essential workers (figure 13.1). The estimates suggest that one-third of EU-mobile workers (i.e., migrant workers from other EU countries) and around 45 percent of non-EU workers were employed as cleaners, helpers, and personal care workers.

In June 2020, the ILO estimated that 55 million domestic workers were at risk for significant effects of COVID-19 (ILO 2020g). According to estimates, 50 percent of domestic workers in northern, western, and southern Europe had been "significantly impacted" by job losses, reduction in earnings, or reduction in the number of hours of work. The EU Labour Force Survey provided more detail by using the most recent data from the Eurostat database, which does not provide disaggregated information by occupation. Domestic workers were therefore defined as persons employed by private households, or those in a category defined as "activities of households as employers of domestic personnel," in a statistical classification of economic activities in the European community referred to as NACE (ILO 2011). The numbers thus left out domestic workers who were self-employed or employees of companies. As official statistics, the data also left out undocumented migrants, whose invisibility in data charting the pandemic is an important issue in need of consideration (Pelizza, Milan, and Lausberg 2021).

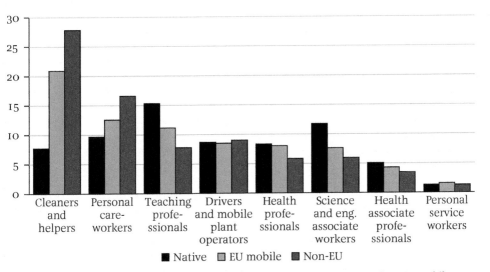

FIGURE 13.1 Proportion of workers in selected occupations among native, EU-mobile, and non-EU workers.

Source: Fasani and Mazza (2020).

Figure 13.2 depicts changes in domestic workers' employment in fifteen countries between the first quarter of 2018 and the third quarter of 2020. During spring 2020, employment in paid domestic work dropped dramatically in some countries, particularly in Spain, where the sector employed 90,000 fewer persons after the first quarter, and in Italy, where employment fell by 73,000 persons. In Romania, the sector employed around 40,000 persons at the beginning of 2020 but only half that number after the COVID-19 outbreak. In Austria, Switzerland, Finland, and Portugal, however, the employment rate of domestic workers evidenced no notable change. These stable numbers may have several explanations. First, protection of care workers and domestic workers, as with workers generally, differed significantly across countries. Another explanation may be the impact of the crisis on women, with high unemployment in the service and travel industries and an increased care burden due to the closing of schools and kindergartens. Households may thus have been better able to employ care workers and domestic workers in some countries than in others. The numbers do indicate, however, that after June 2020, employment in the care and domestic sector was close to prepandemic levels in most countries.

Recent research and reports on migrant care workers suggest that the social and economic consequences of the COVID-19 crisis have been particularly difficult for circulating migrants. Because of travel restrictions, these workers either had to extend their stays in the countries where they worked or remain in their home countries without income (Leiblfinger et al. 2020; Leichsenring et al. 2020). Those who extended their stays often worked for weeks without days off. Thus, while some care workers and domestic workers experienced job loss, others

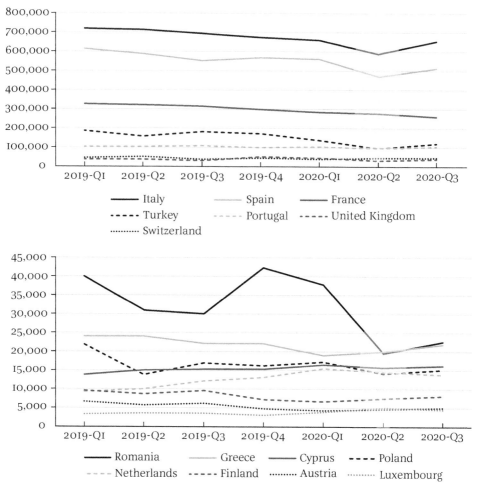

FIGURE 13.2 Number of domestic workers employed in selected countries in 2019–2020.
Source: European Labour Force Survey, https://ec.europa.eu/eurostat/web/lfs.

struggled with increased workload. The uncertainty was also a mental and emotional strain, especially for personal care workers who spent weeks in isolation with those who were sick (Leichsenring et al. 2020).

Home-Based Care Workers and State Policies during the Pandemic

Throughout the pandemic, countries in the European Union took different approaches in supporting their citizens. Gentilini and colleagues (2020) offer an overview of these measures in a "living paper" that the World Bank regularly updated after the breakout of the pandemic.[4] The report delves into the social protection measures taken by states and distinguishes among the following types of policies:

- Social assistance: utility waivers, cash-based transfers (including childcare support), and in-kind transfers (food, vouchers, etc.)
- Social insurance: pensions, paid sick leave, unemployment benefits, health insurance for workers, and social security contributions
- Labor markets interventions: reduced work time, wage subsidies, labor market regulations, and activation measures

As the authors of the report emphasize, regions in the world have combined these initiatives differently. In Europe (and Central Asia), 47 percent of measures focused on social assistance, 35 percent on social insurance, and 18 percent on labor market interventions (Gentilini et al. 2020, 9). The combination of measures adopted strongly depended on the organization of social services and benefits and on the labor market institutions that existed before the pandemic. The great variation in this respect between European countries explains how it is possible that Denmark enacted only one intervention (on wage subsidies), while Italy enacted nine initiatives of different types.

Some European countries supported migrants. Given the limited functioning of the institutional and bureaucratic infrastructure, these measures targeted migrants whose status was pending—for example, those with expiring visas or those waiting for the outcomes of procedures (including expulsions). In France, for example, all migrants' residence permits due to expire during the lockdown were extended for 6 months.[5] In Spain, all expiring residence permits were deemed valid for the duration of the emergency.[6] Detention centers for undocumented migrants were also closed and detained people released.[7] In Portugal, an important measure allowed all undocumented migrants and asylum seekers with pending applications to regularize their status and have "access to the national health service, welfare benefits, bank accounts, and work and rental contracts."[8]

These categories do not always correspond to the profile of migrant care workers and domestic workers. These workers often remain undocumented for many years without opportunities to apply for regularization because in most EU countries visa applications are closed to migrants considered to be low skilled. For them, only Ireland instituted an applicable measure. There, after the outbreak of the pandemic, all undocumented migrants were allowed to apply for several one-off cash-transfer provisions, such as the "COVID-19 pandemic unemployment payment," the "exceptional needs payment," or the "urgent needs payment." Guidelines made clear, however, that applications would be evaluated without assurance that every applicant would be granted payment.[9]

Measures taken by governments to protect workers more generally rarely made explicit mention of domestic workers and home-based caregivers. In countries where they are included in the general labor law, the protection that applies to other workers presumably applies to them as well. Less clear, however, is whether they are included in measures targeting self-employed and general workers because the specifics of their status vary across countries. In Italy and Austria, for example, families could apply for financial support to pay for childcare during the period of school closure, but both the modalities for payment and the degree to which these cash transfers benefited the nannies working for these families remained unclear.

Michael Leiblfinger and colleagues (2020) explain that, in Austria, self-employed migrant care workers were unable to access COVID-19 support because they lacked Austrian tax numbers and bank accounts. In Germany, migrant care workers were excluded from benefits because, under the EU directive, they are usually posted workers or are self-employed and paying taxes in their home countries. These two cases exemplify the conditions of the many care workers and domestic workers who have residence and work permits and yet remain "partial citizens," not entitled to the social and health rights available to the country's citizens.

In a few cases, governments explicitly targeted care workers and domestic workers. In several countries, the government asked these workers to stay home to avoid the risk of contagion for themselves and their employers' families. In Belgium, for instance, "corona unemployment" subsidies covered payment for lost hours when care workers and domestic workers had to reduce their hours or stop working entirely. The subsidy, however, was very low for these low-wage workers, many of whom complained of feeling obliged to return to their jobs too soon.[10] The French government adopted an ad hoc compensation mechanism for domestic and care workers, giving employers an 80 percent reimbursement of the hours not worked during the lockdowns, on the condition that they kept the employees in place.

In Spain, after an open letter by several domestic workers' organizations, the government extended the "COVID-19 unemployment benefit" to this sector.[11] This was the first time Spanish domestic workers were included in provisions for unemployment benefits.[12] In Italy, we assisted a grassroots mobilization to draw attention to the vulnerability of care workers and domestic workers during the lockdown.[13] Even the Italian International Labour Organization headquarters mobilized for workers in this category with a special policy brief (ILO 2020g). As a result of this pressure, the Italian government extended a monthly cash transfer called emergency income to care workers and domestic workers, although the amount was lower than for other workers. The Italian government also launched a regularization of informal workers, including undocumented migrants, in the home-based care sector. Because of the costs and bureaucratic procedures, however, the number of applicants was not very high.[14]

Conclusion

An assessment of the impact of COVID-19 pandemic on the employment of care workers and domestic workers and the policy responses in European countries reveals a severe impact in many countries. Among domestic workers employed by households, a large proportion lost jobs during the spring lockdown because many could not work or had employers who were afraid of contagion. In some countries, however, policy measures, such as temporary layoffs instead of unemployment insurance and subsidies for households employing these workers, made the immediate effect less visible. Knowing how many migrants left for their home countries would be interesting, but data are difficult to find.

Policy measures taken by European governments to support migrants included both general migration policies and specifically targeted measures. A number of initiatives were designed to support the employment of migrant workers. For example, chartered flights and trains moved migrant care workers between Romania and Austria, ensuring care for the elderly and disabled in the host country even when borders were closed for everyone else. Residence permits were extended in several countries to allow migrant workers to stay and continue working. A closer look at the policies protecting workers from job loss and poverty, however, shows that these measures were not particularly favorable to migrant care workers and domestic workers, especially those who worked informally or who were undocumented. As "partial citizens," these workers could not take full advantage of government support. Many were live-in workers and dependent on their employers' families, with little opportunity to isolate and avoid contagion. During lockdowns, they had to renounce free days and personal lives to stay "at home." A crucial question then becomes who is entitled to help and who is left outside the scope of protection.

In many countries, the fast spread of the COVID-19 virus, together with its social and economic consequences for individuals and families, led governments to introduce new policies or extend existing policies to new socioeconomic groups. In some countries, these changes extended unemployment insurance for domestic and care workers for the first time or offered subsidies for households employing them. These benefits may be temporary, but they do demonstrate the possibility of change for the better in the wake of the pandemic. To effect long-term change enhancing the rights of care workers and domestic workers, however, political pressure will be essential.

For migrant care workers and domestic workers, the situation remains most problematic. The International Domestic Workers' Federation seemed to have welcomed successful campaigns, such as those in Spain and Italy.[15] We agree with Statewatch, which stated that "caution must prevail when celebrating the recent measures in the field of migration under the state of emergency."[16] Although these initiatives do have great value at the symbolic level, as they emphasize that care workers and domestic workers are indeed like other workers, they generally have little practical impact. Rather, the precarity of these workers continues to render them vulnerable.

Even in European countries where COVID-19 support initiatives were the most generous, the conditions of work and life for migrant workers and providers of basic care prevented them from fully enjoying opportunities to access rights and benefits. Their experiences throughout the pandemic magnify the chronic inequalities that continue to determine their social, economic, and citizenship positionality in European societies. These structural inequities in systems of care provision dominate in Europe, where countries rely on the temporary, precarious, and invisible work of migrant women from both distant and neighboring countries and on their marginalization.

NOTES

1. As of October 2020, C189 had been ratified by Belgium, Finland, Germany, Ireland, Italy, Portugal, Sweden, and Switzerland. The updated list of European countries that have ratified the ILO convention can be found at https://www.ilo.org/dyn/normlex/en/f?p=NORM LEXPUB:11300:0::NO::P11300_INSTRUMENT_ID:2551460, accessed October 25, 2020.

2. The full text of the resolution is available here: https://www.europarl.europa.eu/doceo /document/TA-8-2016-0203_EN.html, accessed October 25, 2020.

3. "Communication from the Commission: Guidelines Concerning the Exercise of the Free Movement of Workers during COVID-19 Outbreak," EUR-Lex, March 30, 2020, https://eur -lex.europa.eu/legal-content/EN/TXT/?uri=CELEX:52020XC0330(03).

4. We are here considering the version of this paper published on June 12, 2020, which included policies initiated between February and May 2020, a period of generalized lockdown in Europe (Gentilini et al. 2020).

5. "France—Prolongation exceptionnelle des titres de séjour en raison de COVID-19," European Commission, May 15, 2020, https://ec.europa.eu/migrant-integration/news/france -prolongation-exceptionnelle-des-titres-de-sejour-en-raison-de-covid-19.

6. "Spain Introduces Special COVID-19 Integration Measures," European Commission, April 14, 2020, https://ec.europa.eu/migrant-integration/news/spain-introduces-special -covid-19-integration-measures.

7. "Spain/Portugal/Italy: Partial Relief: Migrant Regularisations during the COVID-19 Pandemic," Statewatch, June 8, 2020, https://www.statewatch.org/analyses/2020/spain -portugal-italy-partial-relief-migrant-regularisations-during-the-covid-19-pandemic/.

8. "Portugal to Treat Migrants as Residents during Coronavirus Crisis," *Reuters*, March 28, 2020, https://www.reuters.com/article/us-health-coronavirus-portugal-idUSKBN21F0N7.

9. "Rights of Undocumented Workers to Access Social Welfare Supports during COVID-19," MRCI, April 22, 2020, https://www.mrci.ie/2020/04/22/rights-of-undocumented-workers -to-access-social-welfare-supports-during-covid-19/.

10. Amandine Cloot, "Coronavirus: Les aides ménagères reprennent le travail sans garantie," *Le Soir*, April 23, 2020, https://www.lesoir.be/296225/article/2020-04-23/coronavirus -les-aides-menageres-reprennent-le-travail-sans-garantie.

11. http://www.nadiesinfuturo.org/IMG/pdf/NdeP_Territorio_domestico_24M.pdf, accessed October 24, 2020.

12. Sophie Davies, "Spain Starts Subsidy for Domestic Workers Hit by Coronavirus," *Reuters*, March 31, 2020, https://www.reuters.com/article/us-health-coronavirus-domestic-workers -idUSKBN21I2Q9.

13. "Towards a Caring Democracy," *European Law and Gender*, April 9, 2020, https://elan.jus .unipi.it/blog/towards-a-caring-democracy/.

14. Applications to regularize, amounting to 176,848 applications, were received between June and July 2020. See https://www.interno.gov.it/sites/default/files/2020-08/dlci_- _analisi_dati_emersione_15082020_ore_24.pdf, accessed October 25, 2020.

15. "International Domestic Workers Federation (IDWF): The Impacts of COVID-19 on Domestic Workers and Policy Responses," May 1, 2020, https://idwfed.org/en/resources/idwf -policy-brief-the-impacts-of-covid-19-on-domestic-workers-and-policy-responses/@@ display-file/attachment_1.

16. "Spain/Portugal/Italy."

14

Budgeting Care Services during the COVID-19 Crisis

ORLY BENJAMIN

On the first day of the COVID-19 lockdown, all social workers employed by Israel were deemed "nonessential workers" and sent home on unpaid leave. Rates of food insecurity and violence against women increased immediately. Nonetheless, the emergency was defined as military and scientific, not a matter for those providing care. How was this temporary halt to caring services constituted as rational? I examine changes in the meaning of "care" and in related policy decisions made by Israel's Ministry of Welfare, by the Bank of Israel, and by the country's Ministry of Finance. Applying feminist critical discourse analysis, I find that the rationale for ignoring care was constituted in two ways: by deploying distinct silencing mechanisms and by appropriating the concept "categories of need." Consistent with earlier analyses of the disproportionately high cost to women of policies dealing with the COVID-19 crisis, this rhetoric ignored the crisis in care by detaching government assistance from need. Discursive framing thus undermined any radical feminist response to the crisis and to greater provision for formal and informal care.

A feminist tradition in philosophy, psychology, sociology, and economics has identified a labor process for carework embedded in relationships and emotional connection. Care thus represents an orientation distinct from neoliberal principles of competition, individualism, and rationality (Duffy, Albelda, and Hammonds 2013). Welfare services, which provide formal assistance for those in need, are a common site of contestation between an orientation to care and a neoliberal, managerialist orientation that limits formal care (Benjamin 2016). In the neoliberal state, economic crises and policy reforms have been opportunities to limit welfare services, and hence carework, often through deskilling and reduced professionalization (Klenk and Pavolini 2015; Trappenburg and van Beek 2019). In Israel, the COVID-19 pandemic also coincided with a power struggle between advocates for care and those seeking to underfund health care, welfare services, and education. How, then, was the pandemic used to further a neoliberal, managerialist orientation rather than greater budget allocation to the urgent crisis of care?

One visible step that marginalized advocacy for care in Israel was the convening of an experts' committee. The committee was commissioned to chart a path toward exiting the lockdown, during which social services facilities had been closed. The committee's thirty members, however, were mostly men, principally scientists and military personnel, with only two women serving as research assistants. Therefore, as in Canada (Cranford, chapter 16, this volume), the country's planning ignored both the need for care and the service employees who provide it and who continued to rely on hourly pay and lack of regulatory protection. For example, employees who lacked a sufficient number of paid sick days had to prioritize economic survival over both their own health and the health of those they cared for.

Particularly problematic during the lockdown was the closure of childcare facilities, followed by the partial operation of the school system. Employed parents became isolated, without even the practical support of grandparents, whose family support remained unacknowledged. Decisions instead reflected taken-for-granted attitudes that families, including dual-earner families, could scrape by, even as parents struggled to maintain their work status at a time of high unemployment. As a result, women assumed the burden of unpaid care; food insecurity rose dramatically; and incidents of domestic violence spiked while shelters lacked adequate space or suitable alternatives. The impact was especially harsh for Israeli Palestinian women, immigrants from Ethiopia and the former Soviet Union, and refugees from Sudan and elsewhere. Many women in these groups live at the intersection of poverty and ultrapatriarchal masculinity and thus lack material and emotional support.

In Israel, as elsewhere, care workers in the long-term elderly care sector were deemed essential workers. Yet, in Israeli hospitals, only those working directly with coronavirus cases were supplied with equipment needed for protection from the hazardous working conditions. Other workers were expected to work without protection or to acquire what they could at their own expense and without additional pay, despite their very low incomes. After teachers were furloughed, the teachers' unions did force the Ministry of Finance to fund online teaching, but the ministry eliminated this provision at the earliest opportunity. Many precariously employed teachers were thus made redundant. Budgeting policy changed in later stages, still excluding most aspects of carework, failing to fund increases in care workers' income, not dealing with the care crisis, leaving the intensified workload untackled. At the beginning of 2022, the finance minister fiercely refuted the public campaign for an increase in the minimum wage affecting the paycheck of thousands of care workers.

Methodology: Silencing, Power, and Rationality

This chapter considers the rhetorical measures that allowed the described marginalization of care to constitute rational decision making. The COVID-19 crisis required the reallocation of resources and so created an opportunity to consider the position of care and caring services in relation to other funding issues. To understand the alternative logic that led to budget cuts at a time of urgent need, I consider the language that announced relevant policies. I focus on a sequence of decisions at the Ministry of Welfare and on two announcements concerning the allocation of funding at the Bank of Israel and at the Ministry of Finance. Importantly, the analyzed materials do not represent the overall COVID-19 budgeting policy. Rather, they represent the approach taken by policymakers during the first month of the crisis. To analyze these announcements, I followed Lazar's (2005) approach to feminist critical discourse, together with the perspective on silencing proposed by Clair (1998) and Deetz (1992). Both posit silencing mechanisms that facilitate "not hearing" power-related content in rational forms of speech.

Bringing together these approaches, I first asked how the category "citizen in need of support" was discursively disconnected from issues related to carework. I then identified text that deals with "needs" and highlighted specific silencing mechanisms, typically a combination of neutralization and topic avoidance. As Deetz (1992) notes, such instances occur when speech presents a benefit for all, with no injured parties. Using Lazar's (2005) understanding of the appropriation of feminist categories by hegemonic discourse, I show how the category "need" was manipulated; stripped of its gendered, care-related significance; and imbued only with considerations of finance and resource management.

The Ministry of Welfare

Social workers experienced silencing at the onset of the pandemic. Israeli democracy is exceptional in that it retains a legal arrangement dating back to the British Mandate that, in effect, maintains an operational state of emergency. Since independence in 1948, any minister can impose emergency regulations when the measures are deemed justified for defending the state, public security, and the maintenance of supplies and essential services. On March 15, 2020, the Israeli government exercised this option, designating some state employees essential.[1] The designation, however, included very few social workers. Most were required to take unpaid leaves of absence.

Crucial to any understanding of the significance of this act is that a week later, on March 22, the Ministry of the Interior called on all social workers employed by local municipalities to return to work and perform all aspects of their regular jobs. The call was not enforced. On March 29, human rights NGOs wrote a protest letter to the chair of the women's status committee of the Israeli Parliament demanding that she should interfere in ensuring that all care workers were back.[2] Instead, many local municipalities downsized their workforces of social workers, recalling some only after the social workers' trade union intervened. While the union's success remained limited, the downsizing persisted until the end of March. Only on April 8 did the government define all social workers as essential. For an entire month of intense need in the care sector, therefore, a broad range of services was disrupted.

The Ministry of Welfare was also quick to slash payments routinely transferred to local municipalities for "operational budgets." Although funded by the Ministry, these disbursements are not counted as part of its budget. They cover outsourced welfare services for diverse "special" interventions, including work with adolescent girls, young adults without family support, and families living in poverty. Slashing these payments pushed local municipalities into mothballing many services and placing the relevant employees on unpaid leave. On March 31, the ministry did attempt to reactivate payments, but many services (e.g., for people with disabilities) remained unfunded and some (e.g., for the LGBT community and for holocaust survivors) were only partially funded. Social workers in these areas remained on unpaid leave.

Silencing Care at the Central Bank of Israel

Between 2013 and 2018, the Bank of Israel had a female governor. At the beginning of the COVID-19 crisis, she gave an interview about the required policy steps and stated, "Israel has a debt/GDP relation that could allow for extensive government activity, even at the price of a temporary rise in the financial deficit." She said nothing, however, about the specific conditions women faced in the crisis and instead recommended government support for small businesses. Analyzing the Bank of Israel's policy during the beginning of the crisis, I reviewed a statement made on March 24 by the bank's current governor:

> As the regulator of the banking system, we act systematically with the banks in order to support business and households during this time. We entered the pandemic with a strong banking system, with a quality credit file and proven resilience in harsh conditions. . . . We have guided the banks in increasing credit for business and households, and we have advertised the regulations that would support this. I'm pleased to see that the banking system is willingly supporting businesses and households to deal with the crisis. We have devised quite a few steps for assisting the public and weak populations in managing their relationship with the banking system. . . . Let me emphasize: I stand in close connection and full collaboration, around the clock, with the Prime Minister and the Finance Minister, in order to set forth a fiscal program that will shortly be introduced by them. Whoever knows me knows that already, in my inaugural speech I emphasized the necessity of reducing our budgetary deficit and to stabilize the relationship between debt and GDP during ordinary times. But these are no ordinary times—we therefore need today to shake older conventions which were right for different periods. In these times, we need to support businesses and citizens, so that

the crisis won't intensify, and businesses will recover quickly once the health limitations are dropped. We need to assist those in society that were hurt, and those whose business income was cut, and they have to manage their expenses. Likewise, we need to assist those who were made redundant, as well as those who were sent on unpaid leave and are left with no income. This is what governments around the world are doing, in huge sums.[3]

The statement repeatedly expressed three notions guiding policy: "business," "assistance," and "the world." I examined the use of these words to identify the ways in which carework and feminine knowledge of formal and informal care were downplayed, as well as the ways those in need were isolated. The notion of "business," conveying reference to the market, was repeated six times. Underlining commitment to the market constituted marginalization, not only of hospitals but also a range of health care and nongovernmental organizations involved in the provision of social and health care services. Hospitals in Israel have since the early 1990s conducted significant commercial activity, and over 90 percent of welfare services, particularly in the area of food insecurity, are provided by nongovernmental bodies. Yet the central bank's notion of "business" marginalized these businesses.

Possible alternatives—"service providers," "corporations," "civil society organizations," "nongovernmental organizations"—might have implied inclusion of these economic entities. Instead, the announcement of financial support offered rhetorical exclusion. In this respect it resembled the U.S. Senate's decision to drop proposed legislation supporting hazard pay for essential workers likely to be employed by hospitals and health care services (Dorn et al., chapter 12, this volume). In Israel, hospitals and health care services encountered huge financial difficulties from the onset of the crisis but remained outside the announcement's ambit. Further, repetition of the phrase "businesses and households" promoted a spirit of individualism, with "household" implying a small-scale survival struggle with no connection between isolated household members and sources of formal support already excluded from the category "businesses."

Instead, the central bank's governor promoted banking activity as a form of assistance. Management of debts and loans is important, of course, but banking assistance is primarily concerned with commercial loans, offered with interest and related terms. During the crisis, these approximated the terms of loans common in normal times. This assistance, then, turned the ethic of care on its head, irresponsibly offering loans while ignoring both their risks and the meaning of debt for families. Notably too, contemporary feminist analysis finds links between debt and economic abuse (Adams, Littwin, and Javorka 2020). For example, a documented practice among owners of small businesses in Israel reflects gendered power relations: men force women to take loans in their names, freeing the men to disappear and leave their partners shouldering the debts (Krumer-Nevo, Gorodzeisky, and Saar-Heiman 2017).

Equating assistance with bank loans excluded people in several categories: the unemployed, those on unpaid leave, and anyone else left without income. By presenting banking as a form of "assistance" to "business"—a concern separate from those in need—the central bank's scope for assistance also rendered care workers irrelevant. Avoiding mention of financial support for social and health care services, the rhetoric silenced discussion of the employment these services offer. Language thus performed social action. Any assistance to support care, employment, or responsible assessment of "need" fell outside the boundaries of a financialized definition consistent with a neoliberal orientation to care.

The notion of "the world" operated in tandem with this silencing. Maman and Rosenhek (2011) exposed a necessity logic as typical to the Bank of Israel: each neoliberalization step has been introduced as following allegedly best practices applied by the U.S. and the UK economies. Moreover, these researchers showed that a common threat being used to frame any alternative as irrational, contained the phrase "international markets will punish us." In the analyzed statement, "The world" seems to stand for a similar purpose, providing a major source of legitimation for deviating from "ordinary days" and ordinary forms of action. The bank's rhetorical deployment of "the world," however, limited its scope and mobilized a deceit. For example, the definition of "world" denied the Israeli public access to information about Germany and the UK, both of which applied a different policy: funding salaries to keep redundancies to a minimum. Other governments, including Spain and (to a certain extent) the United States, embraced policies providing universal income. Justifying loans as responses common to "the world" was thus deceitful.

This limited notion of "the world" had broader effects. It served to legitimize the exclusion of a feminist ethic of care based on human need, and it blocked a responsible, skillful response to observed needs. Notable for feminists committed to an ethic of care, "the world" is an important signpost in campaigns to address human need. An inclusive definition of "the world" can enhance both global principles and the carework required for health care, welfare, and education. These efforts, however, must be a transnational project closely aligned with transnational organizations committed to generous funding of education, health care, and welfare services. Without such a broad notion of "the world," local change is hard to imagine.

Care-Free Rhetoric at the Ministry of Finance

Economists at Israel's Ministry of Finance and the Bank of Israel are professionally homogeneous. Why then analyze their respective rhetoric separately? In Israel, the law regulating the central bank prohibits its interference in government action and specifically prohibits the bank from printing money according to government needs. This regulation is a remnant of Israel's severe inflation crisis in the early 1980s, when Israel implemented its "new economic plan," a set of policies consistent with the "Washington consensus" in the United States (Maman and Rosenhek 2007). Analyzing the rhetoric of the Ministry of Finance, however, reveals a framing of economic policy consistent with the central bank's, as the ministry discursively avoided mention of care or care workers. This announcement was delivered at the end of March, three weeks into the crisis:

> The Prime Minister and the Minister of Finance are extending the relief pack guarding the stability of the economy: the total sum devoted so far to managing the crisis stands at 80 billion shekels (about $23.5 billion). The plan allocates 41 billion (51%OB) to the business sector, 11 billion (14%OB) to strengthening the healthcare system including civil actions for facing the pandemic, 20 billion (25%OB) for extending the social security net, banking assistance for households and the regulation of liberalization plans. In addition, a sum of 8 billion (10%OB) has been allocated for accelerating the economy.
>
> Seeking to support the citizens of Israel who had been affected by the Corona Virus pandemic, the Ministry of Finance put together an economic relief plan for the coming months. The plan seeks to respond to the crisis on four levels: the Healthcare and civil response, aiming to provide the healthcare system with all instruments required for facing the virus and its ramifications; extending the social security net, aiming at a response to employees, small business owners and freelancers during the coming months; supporting businesses, allowing them to traverse the crisis; and an acceleration plan and investment in growth engines that aims to provide the support for a rapid recovery at a future time in which the pandemic will be over. Overall, the plan is divided between 50 billion for budget, grants and allowances, and 30 billion for credit and monetary flows.[4]

The announcement was followed by details for each area. Recruitment of additional labor is mentioned only for the health care system and is counted with other significant expenses, leaving very little for salaries. The section directing a plan for extending the social security net mentions loans for nongovernmental organizations providing welfare, health care, and education services, together with some small grants to philanthropies. In practice, however, loans for health, welfare, and education meant no support because these operations depend on contracts with the state, and cancellation of existing contracts means no income available to cover the loans.

In the plan, "business support" refers to a range of steps, none relating to salaries. The plan's details describe directing money to "citizens," but without allocation for any of the services that provide formal support to populations in need. Moreover, nothing was allocated to cover the costs of online teaching or to addressing huge disparities in access to child care, mental health services, and a range of other social needs. Indeed, no action was taken to support working women or to protect existing arrangements and interventions. Instead, in the crisis budget of 90 billion shekels ($30 billion USD), none of the listed items had any relevance for working women or for systems of education and welfare services. The 9 billion shekels allocated to the health care system was entirely allocated to equipment purchases and additional positions for doctors.

Conclusion

Peck (2020) proposed that the COVD-19 crisis be termed a "she-cession" or a "fem-cession," a designation clearly applicable to Israeli policies that avoided funding care services and care workers during the first months of the epidemic. Beyond the disproportionate costs for women—particularly working-class women and women from ethno-national-racial minorities, Israel excluded both formal and informal care during decision-making processes. The silencing of care as a category of concern occurred through two mechanisms. First, topic avoidance allowed formal institutional texts to ignore issues relating to care and carework and to focus instead on "business." Second, emergency regulations neutralized any concern for care, as though the urgency of defending the country from disease rendered formal care services unnecessary.

A second rhetorical instrument was the presentation of "categories of need" that failed to include care and carework. Formal announcements regarded only the need for loans and banking services, implying no relevance for responsive care in addressing the crisis. Consequently, defined categories of need became dissociated from both formal and informal care. A major achievement of neoliberal policies during the COVID-19 crisis has thus been the exclusion of carework, accomplished by silencing all mention of care-related need. Shifting the focus to financial need, to be served by loans, established an environment in which banking services overrode all other concerns. Policies developed during the first month of the crisis thus suggested that Israeli society can rationally manage without carework and without caring services.

NOTES

1. Government decision on March 20, 2020, https://www.gov.il/he/departments/policies /dec4910_2020.

2. Opinion paper sent by women's organizations to the chair of the Israeli Parliament on women's status, on March 29, 2020, protesting the harsh disruption of social services, https://fs.knesset.gov.il/23/Committees/23_cs_bg_568131.pdf.

3. Speech of the head of the Israel National Bank, March 24, 2020, https://www.boi.org.il /he/NewsAndPublications/PressReleases/Pages/24-3-2020.aspx.

4. News release by the Finance Ministry on steps guarding markets stability, March 30, 2020, https://www.gov.il/he/departments/news/press_30032020_b.

15

Policy, Culture, and COVID-19

European Childcare Policies during the Pandemic

THURID EGGERS, CHRISTOPHER GRAGES, AND
BIRGIT PFAU-EFFINGER

This chapter analyzes and seeks to understand the various childcare policies of European welfare states during the COVID-19 pandemic. For the first wave of the pandemic, in the spring of 2020, European governments implemented a lockdown of the extrafamilial daycare centers for children as an important intervention against the spread of COVID-19. Consequently, in most countries, children had to stay home for several weeks. This situation was particularly challenging for dual-earner parents, many of whom had to balance their jobs and childcare. This affected countries as a whole because many children had been cared for in extrafamilial daycare facilities.

Employed parents had to choose between two stressful options. They could work in home offices and combine their employment with parental childcare, which is linked to a high risk of work–family conflicts (Andrew et al. 2020). If they could not work at home, the second option was for them to take a temporary leave or quit. This was predominantly applied to parents in low-skilled jobs who could not access emergency care for "system-relevant" workers. This option was in part connected to substantial financial risks for the caregiving parent (Andrew et al. 2020; Bujard et al. 2020). Studies on the first wave of the COVID-19 pandemic showed that in most countries, mothers provided the main portion of necessary childcare at home (Andrew et al. 2020; Czymara, Langenkamp, and Cano 2020). This triggered a sociological debate about "retraditionalizing" gender roles and family relations (Carli 2020; Hipp and Bünning 2021; Kulic et al. 2021).

To cushion this challenge for parents, especially mothers, European welfare states introduced several family policy measures. However, their policy responses clearly differed about childcare. This chapter argues that the policy responses of different countries not only depended on the preexisting family policy but were significantly influenced by the dominant cultural ideas about work–family relations, care provision, and women's employment. We define "culture" as a system of collective ideas relating to the "good" society, the "ideal" way of living, and (morally) "good" behavior. The main cultural ideas of a society can be contradictory; they can be contested among actors and are changeable (Pfau-Effinger 2005a). Furthermore, we briefly discuss the consequences of gender equality in the work–care relationship, as associated with different family policy responses to contain the COVID-19 pandemic.

The Interplay of Culture and Family Policies in the Context of Care Arrangements

To understand the leeway that different governments had for tackling the care-related challenges of parents during the first wave of the COVID-19 pandemic, it is necessary to consider the welfare state's various political, structural, and cultural points of departure. To analyze the complex interrelation between these factors, we use the theoretical "care arrangement" approach of Pfau-Effinger (2005b). The approach assumes that the work–welfare behavior of women and men, as well as the structures of the work–welfare relationship, can be understood based on predominant cultural ideals, particularly on ideas about the "best" form of childcare and parental work–welfare behavior, and how they interact with family policies, bearing some socioeconomic factors. This means that family policies do not determine work–family behavior, since cultural ideas can modify their influence in an inconsistent care arrangement.

We usually expect that in welfare states, which offer a generous family policy for extrafamilial childcare, that the population would also consider it the "best" form of care and make significant use of it. For example, in several Nordic welfare states, the main cultural ideas within the population and family policy institutions support women's full-time employment, while women's labor force participation rate, and the proportion of children in a formal daycare, are relatively high (Pfau-Effinger 2012, 2014; Jensen et al. 2017). Nevertheless, it is also possible that a welfare state could introduce a generous policy in extrafamilial childcare, while traditional cultural ideas of motherhood and childcare still dominate the population, and where a "good childhood" entails that mothers (and perhaps, to some degree, fathers) provide childcare at home. In such an inconsistent care arrangement, it is possible that mothers have relatively low labor market participation rates, or work part time, because their more traditional cultural orientation may limit their choices. This inconsistent relationship between progressive family policies and traditional cultural ideas offers an explanation for the traditional labor market behaviors of these mothers within the care arrangement of certain conservative European welfare states (Pfau-Effinger 2012). It is also likely that the family policy has low generosity because the welfare state takes little responsibility for financing daycare, although cultural ideas and labor market behavior shows that this is relatively valued in the population, which is the case of the care arrangement of several southern European countries (Pfau-Effinger 2014).

TABLE 15.1

Employment of women with children under 3 in different types of "care arrangements"—Denmark, England, and Germany

		Denmark	England	Germany
Main features of the "care arrangement" (according to Pfau-Effinger 2005b)	Generosity of policies toward women's employment and extrafamilial care for children under school age (institutional level)	Relatively high	Relatively low	Relatively high
	Cultural support for extrafamilial childcare for children under school age	Relatively high	Relatively low	Relatively low
Employment of mothers	Extent of mothers' employment with children under school age (on the basis of employment rate, part-time rate)	Relatively high	Relatively low	Relatively low

Denmark, England, and Germany represent different types of care arrangements and hence provide interesting examples for our comparative analysis of European countries' responses to family policies during the first wave of the COVID-19 pandemic.

The Danish care arrangement is rather coherent and is based on a high degree of gender equality (see table 15.1). Family policy generously supports extrafamilial childcare and the employment of mothers, since it offers comprehensive and affordable, publicly funded daycare for children aged from 26 weeks to school age (Rostgaard and Ejrnæs 2020). This corresponds with the main cultural ideas in the Danish population: most people believe that extrafamilial daycare is the "best" form of childcare for babies over 1 year old and that mothers, like fathers, should be fully employed (Jensen et al. 2017). Accordingly, the majority of children under 3 years old and almost all children age 3 to school age are in formal daycare in Denmark (Eurostat 2020b). In addition, having children does not affect mothers' employment, since their employment rate is nearly identical with that of women without children. Moreover, less than one-third among employed mothers of children less than school age work part time (Eurostat 2020a).

Since the "Nordic turn" in German family policies in the mid-2000s, the German childcare policy has had a level of generosity similar to that of the Danish system (see table 15.1). Children from 1 year old to school age have an individual right to affordable, publicly funded, full-time daycare (Schober et al. 2020). However, in Germany, most people adhere to traditional cultural ideals, where home childcare should be provided by parents and mainly mothers when children are under 3 years old, while two-thirds of mothers only work part time until the child starts school (Eurostat 2020a). This is why having young children can negatively affect women's employment rate, which is significantly lower than for women without children (Eurostat 2020a). The relatively traditional cultural orientation of Germans helps explain why numbers of children in formal daycare are relatively low for children under 3 years old, at less than one-third. It is considerably higher for 3- to 6-year-old children, since almost all of them are in formal daycare, but a third only receive part-time care (Eurostat 2020b). Accordingly, the German care arrangement shows an inconsistency; even if Germany has a generous childcare policy that supports full-time extrafamilial childcare, most mothers of young children show a more traditional employment pattern, based on longer leave and part-time work. This is why gender inequality remains relatively high in Germany.

The English care arrangement is somewhat less inconsistent. Both the family policy and the dominant cultural ideas of the population offer a relatively low degree of support for the employment of mothers and extrafamilial childcare (see table 15.1). Parents can get funding for short part-time care of children, from 3 years old to school age, while full-time care and care for 2-year-old children are offered only for low-income families (Lewis and West 2017). The cost of childcare for parents in England is among the highest in Europe (OECD 2020a). Additionally, formal daycare for children is not popular. Two-thirds of the population regards family care as the "best" care for children under age 3, while less than a third considers formal daycare preferable (Pfau-Effinger and Euler 2014). In this context, the negative employment effect for women with children under school age is also significant, and more than half of them work part time (Eurostat 2020a). In line with the low generosity of policies toward extrafamilial childcare, the number of children in daycare facilities is slightly more than one-third, which is relatively low for those under 3 years old and is almost exclusively based on part-time care. More than two-thirds of children from 3 years old to school age receive care in daycare facilities, but for more than one-third it is only part time (Eurostat 2020b). In all three countries, fathers of children under school age have a higher employment rate than fathers without children.

For welfare states like Germany and England, where care by family members is still regarded as the "best" method of childcare, a generous family policy for parental leave could support mothers in their decision to provide most of the care themselves and ensure social rights and financial support. England has a maternity leave program of 52 weeks (11 weeks before birth, 41 weeks after birth) for employed women. After childbirth, mothers can stay at home with their child for 28 weeks based on paid leave, which is paid with 90 percent of the average gross weekly earnings or a flat-rate payment of £604 (about $772) (whichever is lower), and an additional 13 unpaid weeks (Atkinson, O'Brien, and Koslowski 2020). The pay is generous for western European standards, but a generous duration of paid leave would last about 1 year (Yerkes et al. 2022). Women can transfer 50 weeks of the leave to the child's father. In addition, parents can take up to 4 weeks of unpaid leave annually per child. This means that most mothers can take lengthy leave only if they receive financial support from their husband. In contrast, in Germany, the program for paid parental leave with job protection is relatively generous, as it offers 12 months of paid parental leave or 14 months if both parents share it, with an income substitute of 65 to 67 percent or 100 percent for low-income earners. Parents can extend their leave for up to 36 months, but this is not very attractive, since it is unpaid. Employed parents can also take fully paid family responsibility leave to care for sick children for 10 days per annum (Schober et al. 2020). Even though the Danish population does not consider family care to be the "best" form of childcare, the family policy offers the most generous parental leave among all three countries: parents can take paid parental leave for 11.5 months, with 100 percent income compensation and job protection, and both parents can share this. They also have the option to extend this to an unpaid leave of 36 months and can get fully paid family responsibility leave to care for sick children of 12 to 24 days per annum (Rostgaard and Ejrnæs 2020).

Overall, this section shows that all three countries differ in their care arrangements regarding the relationship between family policies and cultural ideas, and regarding the work–family relationships that have developed in this context. Accordingly, the countries had different points of departure when the first wave of the COVID-19 pandemic began.

Policy Responses for Childcare during the First Wave Of the COVID-19 Pandemic

Regarding the accelerating COVID-19 pandemic in the spring of 2020, European welfare states were forced to adjust their family policies to deal with the care-related challenges resulting from the temporary closure of daycare facilities. Against the background of the aforementioned differences in care arrangements, we expect that the Danish government would focus on a fast reopening of daycare facilities for children under school age, due to the dominant cultural ideal and policy orientation toward extrafamilial care. Due to the traditional cultural orientation of the German population, we further assume that the German government would rely on parental childcare, based on preexisting policy instruments. We expect that the English government would provide little support for parents for childcare, essentially leaving the responsibility to the market and families, following the existing targeted family policy and cultural ideals.

Our analysis shows that the Danish government's family policy response focused strongly on extrafamilial childcare. Accordingly, all childcare facilities were only closed for around 4 weeks (March 16–April 15) (Andersen, Schröder, and Svarer 2020), except for parents working in "essential jobs," although only a few families used these (Rostgaard and Ejrnæs 2020). The possibility of a quick reopening was strongly supported by the relatively short duration of higher infection rates in Denmark, due to a low degree of community transmission (Stage et al. 2020). Nevertheless, this was based on large-scale financial and organizational efforts in a very short period, to meet strict regulations regarding hygiene and social distancing, such as small groups and higher staff ratios, more rooms, divided playgrounds, and rules for dropping off and picking up children (Guthrie et al. 2020). Due to rapid reopening, the Family Ministry did not offer a particular leave program for parents. Instead, they asked employers to offer parents the opportunity to take their remaining or nonstatutory holidays with their paid leave (Greve et al. 2021). The childcare policy response of the Danish government corresponds to the main characteristics of the Danish care arrangement, as extrafamilial childcare for children over 1 year old plays a particularly relevant role in Danish culture and families. People give priority to formal daycare, which they consider the "best" form of childcare. This point of departure created a comparably strong pressure on the Danish government to rapidly reopen the daycare facilities, to support the work–family reconciliation of the prevalent dual-earner couples, and to meet their childcare ideals. Therefore, the policy successfully prevented prolonged risks for working women, who would otherwise have been forced to provide care at home instead of (or in addition to) keeping their jobs (Blum and Dobrotić 2021).

Unlike many other European countries, Germany never issued a strict curfew because the duration with higher infection rates was moderate (Wieler, Rexroth, and Gottschalk 2020). Nevertheless, together with the general lockdown on March 22, the German government closed all childcare facilities until the end of May (10 weeks later). While children of the so-called key workers (i.e., health, care, food supply, public safety; later on education, government, single parents) were entitled to "emergency childcare," most parents had to provide childcare at home, based on reductions in work time or on working from home. To support parents in providing childcare at home, the government could have easily adapted the already available family policy instruments to suit the conditions of the pandemic. The main instrument was a variant of the existing parental leave program: parents of children under 12, and of disabled children who reduced or interrupted their employment for childcare reasons, could take extra leave of up to 10 weeks per parent, with an income compensation of 67 percent of their regular net wage (20 weeks for single parents) (Bujard et al. 2020). However, since the COVID-19–related parental leave offered only a 67 percent income substitute for all parents, women with lower wages who stayed at home for childcare incurred high financial risks. In addition, to care for their own children, parents of healthy children could take family responsibility leave for up to 25 days, with an income compensation of

70–90 percent (Schober et al. 2020). In conclusion, the German government's policy response was built on the preexisting family policies and provided relatively generous support for parents who stayed at home. A quick reopening of childcare facilities was not the top priority in Germany, even though preexisting policies also generously support extrafamilial care. The main reason for this is that the government was able to link its policy responses to the prevalent, traditional, cultural ideal of parental childcare, which also sets the cultural foundation for the female workforce who, to a large scale, could combine gainful employment and childcare work with part-time work, even before the pandemic started. The relatively strong support regarding time and finances for parental childcare at home ensured the financial autonomy of the (predominantly female) caregivers. However, such a policy tends to replicate the traditional gender division of labor, and, as a consequence, mothers tended to take over most childcare tasks during the pandemic and spent significantly more time on childcare than fathers (Bujard et al. 2020; Hank and Steinbach 2021).

The childcare policy of the English government during the initial months of the pandemic was based on the closure of all daycare facilities for about 10 weeks (March 20–June 1), while "key workers" were still eligible for extrafamilial childcare (Blum and Dobrotić 2021). Overall, the government's support for childcare was relatively low, as it offered relatively little support for parents to combine work and childcare or to receive compensation while reducing working time. The main instruments were the "job retention scheme," which is a temporary full-time, or part-time leave, and unpaid part-time or full-time parental leave, for which parents have no legal right because they require their employer's consent (Andrew et al. 2020; Office for National Statistics 2020b). The government's policies during the COVID-19 pandemic correspond to the dominant cultural ideas of childcare in England, which are largely based on the responsibility of parents to provide or finance childcare themselves, and with a more traditional gender division of labor that is based on lower female full-time employment and lower use of extrafamilial care. Against this background, the government did not significantly intervene in childcare provisions during the lockdown and continued to rely on families to organize care provisions for themselves. Apart from the "job retention scheme" and unpaid parental leave, no new instruments were introduced to help parents combine work with childcare. This reflects the low generosity of paid parental leave. Shifting the predominant responsibility for childcare to the family household, without any noteworthy support, strongly disadvantaged mothers who often shoulder childcare, without the possibility of acting as financially autonomous caregivers. Therefore, the English policy response not only promoted a traditional division of labor but also increased female dependency on male breadwinners (Andrew et al. 2020).

In summary, the study shows that, for all three countries, the preexisting family policy and dominant cultural ideals about work–family relations significantly contributed to our understanding of differences between welfare states' policies in childcare during the COVID-19 pandemic. Furthermore, it can be concluded that those countries which had already placed a stronger focus on gender equality in their family policies before the pandemic, also chose strategies that supported gender equality during the pandemic, even if this was associated with higher additional costs.

Discussion and Conclusion

What can we learn from the findings on family policies that support parents during a pandemic? In our opinion, the following issues are particularly important: First, the focus on family policy alone is not sufficient to explain cross-national differences in women's work–family behavior and the structures of childcare and female employment. The integration of cultural ideals of childcare and parenting should be added into the explanatory framework, and how such cultural ideals and family policy institutions interact in the context of the respective care arrangement of society offers a more adequate approach toward understanding these differences. Second, regarding family policies, it seems that generous policies in extrafamilial childcare *and* familial care offer important preconditions for the support of parents during a pandemic. The extent to which governments use each of these family policy instruments to support parents during a pandemic seems to differ substantially among various care arrangements. Accordingly, a care arrangement with generous political and cultural support of extrafamilial care offers an adequate basis for a pandemic policy that keeps a short-term lockdown of formal daycare, thus reducing financial risk for parents. Third, in societies with care arrangements in which most of the population thinks that parental childcare is best, governments can introduce lengthier lockdowns more easily. The reason is that they can rely on more parents, especially mothers, who have already worked for shorter hours or stayed at home prior to the pandemic. If these countries already have generous parental leave programs, governments can easily adapt these instruments to the new conditions, which can help reduce the financial risks of parents who must interrupt their employment to provide home childcare during the closure of formal daycares. Nevertheless, there is a risk that traditional labor structures with gender divisions are maintained, and women bear more financial and career-change risks. If generous parental leave systems do not exist, these risks are much higher. In summary, the findings indicate that welfare states who offer generous family policies to extrafamilial daycare and parental childcare have higher sustainability than others for the conditions they offer in support of parents during a pandemic.

Acknowledgment

We would like to thank Editage (www.editage.com) for English language editing.

PART FOUR

Transformation

The COVID-19 pandemic exposed and exacerbated the gaps and inequalities in care infrastructure around the world. But does this moment of catastrophe also hold within it the possibilities to catalyze a transformative change in care systems? Immediate policy responses had both progressive and regressive elements, and in many ways reflected and reinforced the existing devaluation of care and those who do it. In this section, the authors explore the potential to use this tragic historic moment to create truly transformative social, political, economic, and cultural change.

One of the key themes that emerges from these chapters is the central role that ethics and ethical decision making must play in creating the care systems of the future. Cindy L. Cain urges us to use the pandemic moment to consider how to incorporate lessons from hospice and palliative care about the ethics of balancing quantity and quality of life in care decisions. Helen Dickinson and Catherine Smith argue that ethical considerations of the needs of care workers and those being cared for must be taken into consideration as technological changes in care that were accelerated by the pandemic further advance. Cynthia J. Cranford and Katherine Ravenswood challenge us to envision care structures that are not only efficient and effective but also fair. And Julie Kashen lays out a plan for the creation of a care infrastructure in the United States that would transform all aspects of our current system, building a just system on ethical principles.

These arguments about the primacy of ethical decision making hearken back to Joan Tronto's call in chapter 1 of this book to move beyond a value system that prioritizes the accumulation of wealth above all else. Tronto argues for the creation of a caring democracy, a term that makes visible the critical interface between the values that a society stands for and the citizens who have power. The authors in this section also emphasize that the voices of unpaid caregivers, paid care workers, and those receiving care must play a central role in the transformation of care at the macro-, meso-, and microlevels.

Ravenswood and Cranford both offer analyses that demonstrate the potential for the collective voice to change the nature of care in a qualitatively different way than can be achieved by individuals acting alone. The examples described by Cain and Cranford provide models for including the voices of care workers, those cared for, and family members in decision making at the microlevel of daily living, at the organizational level, and at the policy level. Dickinson and Smith note the absence of input from these very voices into the development of new technologies in the care arena, and that proceeding ethically means creating mechanisms for care workers and care recipients to help design technology with their needs at the fore. And Kashen reminds us to center the perspectives that have been most excluded—the women of color and migrant women who have been pushed to the margins of care.

What emerges from listening to these voices, according to our authors in this section, is in part a call to expand our understanding of the nature of care beyond a medically centered model and to conceptualize care as a set of humans in relationship and not simply a set of services provided. Cain argues that the pandemic has demonstrated more than ever that the holistic approach to care practiced by end-of-life providers needs to be expanded to other arenas of care. And Cranford shows that we will transform care only when all aspects—social and emotional as well as medically defined—are made visible and recognized rhetorically and financially. In a similar vein, Dickinson and Smith caution that if we think of care as a set of services or a set of tasks separate from the relational component we risk developing technology that further degrades carework rather than supports it. Kashen echoes this argument in her call for policymakers to recognize that "services" means "people who provide care" and that policy needs to be built around the needs of caregivers, paid and unpaid, as well as those who receive care.

Taken as a whole, these chapters weave together many of the threads that emerged in earlier sections of the book to paint a powerful picture of some of the central elements of a path to truly transforming care in the wake of COVID-19.

16

Exposing Fault Lines, Flaring Tensions, and the Need for New Alliances

Home Care in the Time of COVID-19 in Ontario, Canada

CYNTHIA J. CRANFORD

Joyce Balaz both receives home care services, thanks to a wound inflicted by a persistent ulcer, and provides them to a man at risk of fatal seizures—the man is Joyce's employer, but he also lives with Joyce and her family. Such a particular nexus of gendered intimate care and employment arrangements is not understood or attended to by the public, the state, or even some arms of the labor movement, which reinforces interlocking inequalities. Lack of understanding of the particularity of home care; insufficient action; and intersecting inequalities of race, citizenship, class, gender, age, and disability that flow from them, have been exacerbated by COVID-19. Joyce, for example, took up tending to her own wound when the visiting nurse was exposed to COVID-19 at another care job (Baxter 2020). Joyce's experience is only one of many unique, but similarly complex, assemblies of care and employment in private homes (Cranford 2020). Home care includes skilled nursing, but, as Joyce's story illustrates, this skill is frequently overlooked and turned into unpaid work (Armstrong and Armstrong 2005). The move of much care from hospital to home has facilitated deskilling so that the majority of home care workers are personal support workers. Personal care and support (e.g., paid help with daily activities like bathing and eating) provided to people who need such help due to age, disability, or chronic illness is at the bottom of a health care hierarchy and hidden in the home, which became more apparent during COVID-19. This reflects the devaluation of life for those with chronic illnesses and disabilities and for older people whose long-term needs are at odds with a medical model (Mauldin, chapter 5, this volume). It also signals the racialized labor market that funnels immigrant women and women of color into the most precarious care sectors (Akosionu et al., chapter 4, this volume; Cranford 2020; Peng, chapter 3, this volume). Racialized workers are not only concentrated in the care jobs with the least protections but also face racism in the health care system (Allen 2020). Thus, as in other types of care in other places, within home care we are seeing a crisis of gendered, racialized, ableist injustices (Tronto, chapter 1, this volume).

This chapter focuses on state-funded, privately provided home care in Ontario, Canada's most populated province, where roughly 35,000 home care workers provide services to 650,000 people (Lorinc 2020). Opposition parties, physicians, and employers have called for increased funding so seniors could leave, or avoid, long-term residential care (LTRC) (Jeffords 2020; Zinchuk 2020), or to take the strain off hospitals (Benner 2020; Casey 2021). Notwithstanding the dire situation in LTRC (Armstrong and Klosterman, chapter 6, this volume) and the importance for hospitals to address surgery backlogs, lack of attention to the specificities of home care reflects its marginalized position within the health care system. As a result, COVID-19 exacerbated the devastating impact of inadequate funding, reinforced gendered and racialized labor market inequalities, and flared tensions in home workplaces within Ontario home care.

The unique, and varied, qualities of homecare beg the question of *how* we can use this pandemic-induced immediacy to rethink ways to challenge long-standing, intersecting inequalities in home care. I argue that we must theorize new alliances between home care workers, receivers, and allies to push for multilevel changes in how we organize home care. At the heart of this argument is a call to listen to collectives of home care workers and receivers in line with what Tronto (2013; chapter 1, this volume) calls "democratic caring." What would home care look like if it were designed by workers like Joyce and the man who both receives Joyce's care and employs her? I suggest an intimate community unionism could help conceptualize new alliances to challenge the long-standing (home) care crisis exacerbated by COVID-19.

Multilevel Inequalities in Home Care

Inequalities in home care are multilevel. Inequalities are structured by inadequate state funding, which both reflects and reinforces gendered and racialized labor markets that define who does what kinds of home care work under which conditions. Structural fault lines driven by inadequate funding and labor market inequities contour more intimate tensions in home workplaces (Cranford 2020).

Inequalities are generated in part by insufficient funding reflecting the trend toward wealth-care (Tronto, chapter 1, this volume), as in the United States, but the case of Ontario also illuminates the problems with narrowly medical funding. In home care, there are two dynamics to consider; the first is the place of home care within the health care system. Health care systems are based on a medical model—the notion that different bodies must be cured or made to match a "normal" body or otherwise contained and managed in institutions (Garland-Thompson 2002; Mauldin, chapter 5, this volume). Yet much home care is long-term care to support daily activities, what is often called social care (Twigg 2000). Social care includes LTRC, but the location of care in the home makes it even more invisible and ideologically connected to women's unpaid family work (Grant et al. 2004). The Federal Canada Health Act mandates socialized hospital care, but home care is left up to the provinces (Bourgeault 2015). Ontario home care is not means tested, but priority is given to people recovering from acute illnesses while long-term support hours have been cut, so home care clients have long felt merely "fed and watered" (Aronson 2004). This medical bias results in poorer-quality care for seniors and worse conditions for workers (Cranford 2020).

A second dynamic is marketization. To reduce cost, the Ontario government contracted out delivery, mostly to for-profits, echoing trends in other Anglo, (neo) liberal countries (Anderson and Shutes 2014; Charlesworth and Malone 2017; Nazareno et al. 2022; Williams and Brennan 2012), and new forms of privatization were pushed through during COVID-19 (Zalev 2020). Marketization has augmented labor market precariousness.

Home care labor markets are precarious in Ontario as elsewhere. Workers earn low wages and have few benefits, and this coupled with part-time or temporary contracts results in high turnover (Akosionu et al., chapter 4, this volume; Martin-Matthews, Sims-Gould, and Naslund 2010; Price-Glynn and Rakovski 2015). The mostly nonunionized for-profit home care companies classify workers as casual, resulting in employment insecurity. Given people's intermittent needs and limited hours of work offered, combining jobs in LTRC and home care is widespread (Cranford 2020).

Home care precarity reflects continuity with gendered and racialized labor markets that have long organized domestic service, supported by ideologies of gender, race, and class inferiority that posit women of color as suited for the most devalued, dirty work (Chun et al. forthcoming; Duffy 2011; Glenn 2010; Parreñas 2015). In Ontario, as in other Anglo (neo)liberal countries, insufficient funding and poor working conditions mean employers rely on immigrants, often with precarious citizenship status (Bourgeault 2015; Nazareno et al. 2022). Justifications of recruitment of immigrant and racialized women into devalued home care are conveyed by employers in Ontario as elsewhere (Cranford 2020; Guevarra 2014; Schwiter, Strauss, and England 2018). Home care receivers also sometimes hold racialized preferences and for-profit, nonunion companies are more likely to appease them than nonprofit, unionized ones (Cranford 2020). This racialized and citizen-based division of labor shapes tensions in the daily labor process.

Studies emphasize the rewards of home care intrinsic to the job, yet given inadequate and narrowly medical funding, and gendered and racialized labor markets, there are also tensions in the labor process. Home care workers value "relational autonomy," operating in and through relationships with home care receivers and their families (Parks 2003). But this relational aspect is a double-edged sword, requiring workers to manage boundaries between getting too close or too distant and can result in self-exploitation (Cain 2015; Price-Glynn and Rakovski 2015; Stacey 2011). For workers of color working with white clients, this boundary work is part of ensuring that the work does not morph into servitude (Cranford and Chun forthcoming). Some American studies find that workers employed by agencies feel agencies help them set boundaries with clients (Cain 2015; Price-Glynn and

Rakovski 2015). In Ontario, however, workers are critical of agencies' unrealistic "depersonalizing" policies (Aronson and Neysmith 1996), and many agencies only contingently respond to workers' and clients' concerns (Cranford and Miller 2013). Where funding is narrowly medical and care is organized through racialized, gendered labor markets, tensions ignite over what is done and how (Cranford 2020).

How Has the COVID-19 Crisis Exacerbated Inequalities?

COVID-19 exacerbated the impact of inadequate home care funding. Exposing the position of long-term care in a health care system defined by the medical model, in Ontario home care funding was shifted to LTRC to get elderly patients out of hospital beds in the early days of COVID-19 (Picard 2020). In July 2020, a Health Ministry spokesperson said Public Health Ontario could not even distinguish home care workers from other health care workers in the data they collect (Baxter 2020), also reflecting the marginal status of home care within the system. It took efforts by journalists to disaggregate the data, and subsequent reports of lower COVID-19 cases in home care compared to LTRC (Star Staff 2020) were cited by employers, physicians, and others in calls for increased home care funding (Jeffords 2020). However, specific funding for the sector was not included in the 2021 budget (Ontario 2022a) so home care continued to receive less than 5 percent of health care funding (Payne 2021).

COVID-19 reinforced gendered and racialized inequalities that structure home care labor markets. Unions, receivers' advocates, and employers' associations called for government funding to help recruit and retain home care workers early in the pandemic (Contenta 2020; Star Staff 2020). In October 2020 the Ontario government introduced a Temporary Wage Enhancement of $3.00/hour (approximately $2.00 USD) for workers who deliver publicly funded personal support services, including home care workers (Ontario 2020). This raise was extended several times and is now permanent (Ontario 2022b). Even with the increase, however, earnings are low since the vast majority of home care workers work part time without guaranteed hours (Cranford 2020). By 2021, upon losing home care workers to better-paid sectors, employers were adding their voices to worker and receiver advocates' critiques of the wage gap between home and institutional care (Ketchen 2021; Thompson 2022).

The mismatch between hours of work paid and workers' need to make a living that drives multiple job holding across LTRC and home care was also intensified by COVID-19. In April 2020, the Ontario government banned workers from working in more than one LTRC home, after significant criticism, but only issued guidance for home care, leaving it up to employers (Baxter 2020; Grant and Anderssen 2020). A Ministry of Health spokesperson justified this, and normalized insufficient funding, arguing that "limiting their work location to one setting means many clients would go without publicly funded care and many home and community care providers would be limited in their working hours" (Baxter 2020). One employer who provided both home care and supportive housing services in Toronto explained that since a good number of their staff work in other locations, if the single workplace directive was applied to the sector it would have been, according to journalist Baxter (2020), "chaotic." By April 2021, fully vaccinated workers were permitted to work in more than one health care setting to ensure appropriate levels of care, yet again home care was not the focus (Canadian Press 2021). Given the labor shortage, and indicative of a general move to temporary migrant labor, the federal government launched the Home Support Worker Pilot June 2019, which admits up to 2,750 primary applications a year under temporary contracts (Canada n.d.). Thus the gendered deskilling evident in Joyce's story was increasingly racialized and tied to citizenship during COVID-19 (Alhmidi 2020). This pilot allows for a permanent residence pathway after 24 months of work experience, providing that education and language standards are met (Canada n.d.). Importantly, it allows family to accompany the temporary migrant and apply for work or study permits, and makes it easier for workers to change employers (Immigration, Refugees and Citizenship Canada 2021). These changes reflect long-standing critiques by migrant workers and advocates, suggesting more openness to such demands under COVID-19. However, the program does not provide the (permanent) "landed status now" called for by advocates (Caregivers' Action Centre et al. 2020). Thus it reflects continuity with racialized gendered servitude (Glenn 2010).

Finally, there is evidence of heightened tensions in home workplaces. Some families with extensive needs continued to have certain home care workers come, although they were fearful. One Ontario home care employer reported that a client sprayed the home care worker with Lysol (Lorinc 2020). Several media reports highlighted concerns from home care receivers or families who knew the nurse or personal support worker coming was also likely to work in residential settings (Baxter 2020; Contenta 2020). Such tensions are fueled by minimal health and safety requirements on employers. At the height of the first COVID-19 wave, the Ontario Ministry of Health guidelines and industry association protocol based on it only required full personal protective equipment if a home care client reported COVID-19 symptoms (Lorinc 2020) with devastating effects on workers and receivers (Allen 2020). Employers said they could not get enough protective equipment (Paikin 2020). In April 2021, the Ontario government, which cut paid sick leave pre-COVID-19, implemented 3 paid sick days for COVID-related illness, after pressure from health experts, workers' advocates, and the general public (Crawly 2021). This temporary program expires March 31, 2023 (Levy and Vassos 2022). The Ontario government voted down legislation for 10 permanent paid sick days (Dobson 2021).[1] Insufficient regulatory protection fuels home–workplace tensions and reflects structural fault lines evident in funding gaps and labor markets that devalue care work done largely by racialized women.

Intimate Community Unionism as a Way Forward

If the current crisis is syndemic, reflecting troubling synergies between the care crisis, health crisis, poverty, and discrimination (Rico and Pautassi, chapter 7, this volume), we need multilevel changes in the organization of home care. Several studies argue that alliances between home care workers and aging or disabled people receiving home care are key to achieving quality care and work (Delp and Quan 2002; Duffy 2010; Folbre 2006; Little 2015). To address the uniqueness of home care, I argue that we need an intimate community unionism made up of democratic alliances between labor organizations and groups of receivers to address tensions in the labor process, and structural fault lines at the labor market and state levels (Cranford 2020). COVID-19 exposed the danger of narrow, insufficient funding, and labor market precarity, yet understanding of how these fault lines exacerbate tensions between workers like Joyce and her receiver-employer remain hidden in the home. As such, input from collectivities of workers, receivers, and allies into a new home care system is more important than ever.

Widespread, long-standing relegation of social home care to inadequately funded subsystems (or private pay), which was exacerbated during COVID-19, underscores the need for voices of workers and receivers in reforming funding models. Feminists have long argued for universal government funding (Duffy, Armenia, and Stacey 2015b; Grant et al. 2004). More specifically, we need to include the viewpoints of aging and disabled people and workers in program design and facilitate their ongoing ability to influence how support is provided, in line with what Tronto (2013; chapter 1, this volume) calls "democratic caring." What would funding look like if it were designed by immigrant women workers and aging women receivers? Studies that have interviewed them show that it would value how housework and emotional support are intertwined with support for aging bodies, thus going well beyond the medical model (Aronson 2004; Cranford 2020).

COVID-19 exposed the depth of racialized and gendered labor market precarity of home care workers, and democratic coalitions between workers and receivers could push for labor market intermediaries suited to the various employment relations in home care. COVID-19 exacerbated turnover, and better funding would go a long way toward addressing this by increasing wages to parity with personal support workers in hospitals and long term care residential care (LTRC). COVID-19 also made more evident that earnings sufficient to make a living require adequate and stable work hours. However, while the multiple jobs of LTRC workers are mostly a product of inadequate funding and employers' unwillingness to hire full-time, permanent workers, in home care these realities are coupled with the receiver's intermittent needs. So we need labor market intermediaries to meet the needs of diverse groups of receivers and help a multiracial workforce find multiple jobs. We need nonprofit intermediaries, given the track record of for-profit agencies producing precariousness, which increased during COVID-19 (Mojtehedzadeh 2021). State-funded, democratically run intermediaries would facilitate worker and receiver input and protect public services from profit.

Finally, COVID-19 exacerbated tensions in the labor process, ranging from health and safety risks to racialized frictions over the line between help with daily activities and servitude. Such tensions must be recognized and negotiated if coalitions organizing for broader funding and nonprofit intermediaries are to endure. Top-down union strategies that flatten home care worker and receiver leadership threaten hard-won alliances because they do not recognize particular home care conflicts (Cranford, Hick, and Birdsell Bauer 2018; Rivas 2007). Community-based labor organizing provides inspiration for engaging deeply and continuously with workers and receivers to address tensions in the labor process because it focuses on grassroots leadership development (Chun et al., forthcoming; Moore 2018). Many home care workers work through agencies, and here too there are examples where both workers and receivers have collective representation allowing them to negotiate labor process tensions over what is done and how, but this requires ongoing coalition work that is fostered by broad, social funding and nonprofit delivery (Cranford 2020). Democratic alliances between home care receivers, workers, and allies are key to creating the awareness and political will necessary to make multilevel, systemic changes for quality care and work during COVID-19 and beyond.

NOTE

1. In May 2020, the prime minister said that "discussion with the provinces" would continue so as to ensure that "every worker in Canada who needs it has access to 10 days of paid sick leave a year" (Wilson 2020). Yet, in December 2021, Bill C-3 was passed, providing only federally regulated sectors up to 10 days of sick pay, which does not include home care workers (Canada 2021).

17

End-of-Life Considerations during COVID-19

CINDY L. CAIN

Public concerns about COVID-19 place death front and center, especially as we use mortality rates as one measure of the spread and effects of the disease. However, current discussions do not fully reflect end-of-life considerations, such as how we balance quality and quantity of life, what forms of expertise are offered by end-of-life care workers, or how all care workers are affected by the experiences of COVID-19 death.

This chapter shows how explicitly considering end-of-life carework changes our perspectives on how to respond to this pandemic. I use existing literature, publicly available data, news reports, and interviews with end-of-life care workers to argue that we need new frameworks, policy changes, and ethical reorientation to mitigate the problems we currently see in COVID-19 care.

End-of-Life Care Principles and Challenges of COVID-19

In the United States, about half of all people who die over the age of 65 are supported by hospice or palliative care, both of which emphasize quality of life over quantity of life (NHPCO 2020). People dying in their own homes are typically supported by hospice services, which include home visits from an interdisciplinary health care team, staffed with nurses, nursing aides, social workers, chaplains, and therapists. Seeing care recipients in their own home especially helps people who are seriously ill or frail and has the added benefit of contextualizing care recipients within their family unit (Cain 2015). For people dying in an inpatient setting, palliative care is a growing medical specialty that prioritizes relief of pain and other types of suffering. Palliative care is currently growing as a complement to curative care, with some pushing for its integration even beyond the end-of-life context (Meghani 2004). In both hospice and palliative care, these principles of tending to suffering, using a diverse set of professionals, contextualizing the patient within the family, and balancing quality of life with quantity of life deepen our understanding of how to support people with COVID-19.

The highly contagious nature of COVID-19 makes traditional ways of providing hospice and palliative care more challenging. In an effort to reduce contact with too many providers, the Centers for Medicare & Medicaid Services (CMS)—the major payer of end-of-life care in the United States—has relaxed requirements for face-to-face visits and referrals to some providers (CMS 2020c). While limiting visits and the number of people directly involved in care is protective of patients and care workers, this policy has an unintended side effect of shutting out psychosocial support workers (such as social workers, therapists, and chaplains), who are sometimes viewed as unnecessary for the basic minimum of care (Cain 2019).

This constricting of end-of-life care services is exactly what should *not* happen during a life-threatening pandemic. Instead, several palliative care experts argue that we should prioritize all aspects of palliative care to help triage care, align life-saving decisions with patients' preferences, and communicate with family members (Curtis, Kross, and Stapleton 2020; Mercadante 2020). In my research, a palliative care provider explained how she was positioned to help a family deal with the unexpected death of a young man: "A really difficult patient situation was of a 31-year-old who ended up dying. And his parents were there and his fiancé was there. And because of COVID, of course, the visiting was extremely limited, and they were very angry at the communication from the hospital. And they asked for the [palliative care] consult. Probably, partly because of that, they told me that no one had communicated enough information until I came along and explained everything that had happened during the hospital stay."

In fact, it is precisely at this moment, when we are experiencing what some experts call a "tsunami of suffering" that we most need end-of-life experts who have an expansive definition of pain and who understand the role of medicine in prolonging or mitigating suffering (Radbruch et al. 2020, 1467). This includes suffering of family members and care workers, in addition to the care recipient. Hospice and palliative care workers are also experts in navigating organizational issues during difficult times, such as creating policies and protocols, training staff, reallocating resources as needs change, and supporting other care workers (Etkind et al. 2020). In this situation, the palliative care provider could not save the patient's life, but she could help to bridge the realities of an overstretched hospital system and the family's sense of loss.

When one is serving people at the end of life, emotional connections are a central feature of improving patients' and family members' experiences and creating a sense of worthwhile work (Cain 2015; Fox 2006). However, necessary safety precautions, such as personal protective equipment (PPE, especially face masks) may make it more difficult for workers to read or communicate emotions. A palliative care provider explained that her connections to patients have been harder to establish since COVID-19:

[COVID-19] changed our regular work because initially we stopped seeing anybody in isolation to help preserve PPE. We didn't go into any isolation rooms at all, irrespective of the need to talk to the patient or anything. And then we were going in some [rooms] but not going in COVID rooms, and we stopped doing the physical exam. You know, because there was a waiver for that in terms of billing. . . . So, you're getting less in touch with the patient. I sit farther away from patients in the room. There is a bit of a disconnect with people. Yeah, the masks in general just create a disconnecting thing. And, facial expressions as well. Patients don't have masks on but everybody else in the hospital does.

A primary goal of palliative and hospice care is to help care recipients to think through how to balance quality of life and quantity of life. In routine end-of-life care, this balance is challenged when something that could potentially lengthen life comes at a cost to quality of life; or, conversely when something that could improve quality of life comes at a cost to quantity of life. COVID-19 presents new challenges in considering this balance of quality and quantity of life. One of the most visible examples of this has been the stories of people dying in hospitals with only phone or video contact with family members. While it may be reasonable to isolate COVID-19 patients to protect family members, other patients, and care workers, it is undeniable that this has created extremely difficult situations for those left behind (Wallace et al. 2020). Perhaps with more PPE available and insights from palliative care experts, other solutions may become apparent. We now know that transmission is drastically reduced by maintaining physical distance, being outside, and wearing facial coverings. These options likely are not feasible for someone at the end of life with COVID-19, but they may be possible for people at earlier stages, such as before they need a ventilator. During the height of the pandemic, many news stories reported people dropping their loved ones off at the hospital, knowing that they may never see them again.

Policies that limit visitation in an effort to prevent infection are especially heart-breaking when we consider people living in congregate care settings who do not have COVID-19 but are living under policies that prohibit visitors of any kind. Some palliative care experts are now saying that we need to think more creatively about how to solve the issue of visitors, especially as we know the threat of COVID-19 is not soon ending (Abbasi 2020; Verbeek et al. 2020). In September 2020, some of these restrictions were lifted at the national level, with CMS (2020a) writing, "Although visitation restrictions have partially protected the physical health of residents, the practice also has resulted in unintended harm. Residents experience loneliness, anxiety, and depression due to prolonged separation from families and loved ones. These measures also compromise the ability of families and guardians to validate resident well-being and safety, and caused significant distress for families" (32).

However, organizations have been slower to change their own rules, especially as space and supplies constraints still exist. One long-term care worker explained that even though the ban on visitors was relaxed, there were still challenges from safety precautions.

> There's only one person that's allowed to come to visit. And they're sup-posed to be quarantined for two weeks before and two weeks after. So hon-estly, there's not a ton of visitors. They did try mandating that visitors get a test within 72 hours, but it was impossible. So, they removed that, but they did try and it was really bad. If you have a visitor come, that same visitor can keep coming. And you can't have two visitors at the same time. So, if the visitor is coming, [they can come] every day they want, but if you want a new visitor, then that person has to stop coming. And the new visitor is the person that's coming, so it's one visitor per person.

In trying to create an option where visitors are allowed but infections are con-trolled, some organizations have created policies and procedures that may be overly burdensome and have an unintended effect of further curbing social con-tact. This worker credits the policies with reducing the overall number of visits. Simultaneously, residents were kept separate from one another as much as possi-ble, reducing social interaction even further. Here too, hospice and palliative care providers may play a role in helping to weigh considerations of quality of life and quantity of life and offer creative solutions for maximizing protection while still allowing residents to connect with important others.

As this pandemic continues, we are finding that policies about fully closing or fully opening places where people congregate are probably not sustainable. Principles coming from high-quality end-of-life care are instructive for thinking about alternative approaches. These principles are centered on understanding individuals as part of family units where care and quality of life are enhanced by integrating the whole unit, creating individualized and tailored options for con-tinued contact, and understanding that trade-offs between quantity of life and quality of life are part of the decision-making process of people with serious ill-nesses. Simultaneously, however, we must be attuned to the increased workloads and exposure potential for end-of-life care workers as they take on new responsi-bilities in the pandemic (Powell and Silveira 2020).

Supporting End-of-Life Care Workers

The previous section discussed how principles from hospice and palliative care could inform care for people with COVID-19, even given the challenges created by the highly contagious pandemic. If these principles were more effectively integrated into care systems, the quality of life for vulnerable adults would be improved, even in the case that death is the outcome. Importantly, however, these same principles could also be used to improve the quality of work for end-of-life care workers. Front-line care workers, often held up as "heroes" in the battle against COVID-19, still receive relatively poor pay and benefits (Dill and Hodges 2019). While carework is devalued economically (Romero and Pérez 2016; Peng, chapter 3, this volume), COVID-19 substantially increases the risks to care workers.

Care workers who most often serve people at the end of life include those working in patients' homes, geriatric settings, long-term care settings, hospice and palliative care, or emergency services. These workers are accustomed to the difficult physical and emotional work of caring for very sick people and their family members (James 1992). However, COVID-19 is exacerbating the physical and emotional toll. Physically, care workers have not had enough access to essential PPE, such as face masks, face shields, gloves, or gowns (Nguyen et al. 2020; Ranney, Griffeth, and Jha 2020). Because the work of caring for others involves close contact, shortages in PPE are devastating for care workers. For example, care workers in institutional settings for older adults, such as nursing homes or other forms of congregate care, are disproportionately exposed to and likely to be infected with COVID-19. Both residents and staff have high rates of infection, and residents are especially at high risk of fatality (Barnett and Grabowski 2020). In response to this devastation, CMS requires all nursing homes to report COVID-19 cases, related deaths, and key safety measures. These data reveal that before vaccines were widely available, about one-third of all COVID-19–related deaths occurred in long-term care facilities, with these estimates not even taking into account deaths of staff members and visitors (Kaiser Family Foundation 2020). Scholars now believe that nurses and nursing assistants working in nursing homes are among the most vulnerable essential workers worldwide (McGilton et al. 2020).

The harmful effects to workers are not just those directly related to being infected with COVID-19. Because of shortages of supplies and the helplessness of not knowing how to help care recipients, many frontline care workers are likely experiencing emotionally challenging situations. One kind of emotional challenge is moral distress, which comes from having a sense of what one should do to help another, but feeling constrained by what is possible (McCarthy and Deady 2008). Often those constraints are related to organizational resources, rules, or procedures. Moral distress may especially be present when workers perceive that the care systems are not individualized enough to meet the specific needs of patients. For example, one primary care doctor explained her frustration with much of health care: "There is nothing more discouraging than recognizing that people can't see the big picture. They can't think outside of this box. They need to fit into my rules and fit into my standard of work instead of saying my standard of work needs to meet these people where they're at."

This quote characterizes the widely held experience of wanting to do what is perceived would be helpful, but the larger context of care does not allow it. In the case of COVID-19, the lack of cure or even widely effective and available therapeutics sets up a care interaction that is likely to cause moral distress resulting from not being able to help.

Another source of potential moral distress comes from being the person assigned to make decisions about how to ration scarce resources. For example, there have been serious concerns about resources for testing and treating COVID-19. Many health system and statewide approaches to handling COVID-19 are premised on a utilitarian principle of reducing the total impact of the disease (Pattison 2020). Accordingly, many have tried to model who would benefit most from existing resources and plan to ration in line with these models. The case of ventilators made national news when it was revealed that some states had explicit policies that advised not to use ventilators on people with disabilities, those over a set age, or those who had poorer health on key measures (Mauldin, chapter 5, this volume). A medical ethicist at the University of Pennsylvania wrote a *New York Times* piece titled, "The Way We Ration Ventilators Is Biased—Not Every Patient Has a Fair Chance" (Schmidt 2020), which, along with other media coverage, put pressure on health systems to reconsider their rationing policies. However, standards that have biases embedded within them are common issues in end-of-life care. How we value different lives becomes embedded in decision-making processes in health care.

End-of-life care workers have found themselves in positions to shape these policies, but this can create some additional ethical concerns. One new palliative care provider explained that his job responsibilities shifted to include writing a protocol for allocating resources as their hospital filled with COVID-19 patients. As he had only been on the job for a few months, he reported not feeling prepared for this level of responsibility: "I was involved in some of the protocol development, like from an ethical standpoint, and just kind of thinking about if we were to get overrun. [From a] ventilator standpoint, or managing end of life issues, just symptom management, I've developed some protocols and things like that. And also I helped with the COVID committee to come up with sort of an allocation protocol, if we were going to need it. We haven't needed it. Thank goodness, which was my hope."

Medical ethicists have argued that these protocols should include ways to distribute feelings of responsibility and alleviate concerns about equity (Binkley and Kemp 2020). While end-of-life care workers do often have more experience thinking about these ethical issues, participating in decisions like this can place additional moral distress on individual care workers. Supportive work policies would acknowledge, appreciate, and mitigate the anguish and exhaustion that results.

The context of work affects how supported care workers feel as well. For example, early evidence from Canada demonstrates that residents in for-profit care facilities are about twice as likely to be infected with COVID-19 and die than residents in nonprofit facilities (Oved et al. 2020). Another study reports that unionized nursing homes had lower mortality rates, likely because unions were able to advocate for better working conditions and more safety precautions (Dean, Venkataramani, and Kimmel 2020). Even given evidence that congregate care settings are ground zero for COVID-19 (Barnett and Grabowski 2020), we do not currently have consistent data about care workers and their exposures and deaths from COVID-19 (Kaiser Family Foundation 2020). Deeper analyses of organizational conditions that allow workers to flexibly meet care recipient needs and reduce the physical and emotional toll on care workers are needed.

As stories of what is happening in nursing homes have come out, news coverage has sometimes held up particular care workers as the "heroes" of the pandemic. These news stories discussed workers "going above and beyond the call of duty," and we have seen many examples of singing, cheering, and showing symbolic support for frontline care workers. This symbolic valuing is problematic in two ways. First, holding up these workers who go "above and beyond the call of duty" as heroes sets an impossibly high standard, especially for workers who also have caregiving responsibilities in their own families. It is not just when they are being exceptional that we should value their work. Second, the symbolic support cannot be a replacement for improvements in work conditions, safety precautions, compensation, and other benefits. We need to change the focus to protecting workers with the best science possible and instituting more general protections for the physical and mental health of care workers (Peng, chapter 3, this volume).

Moving toward Interconnected Thinking

COVID-19 has turned deaths into a number that ticks by on the evening news, but most reports lack understanding of the deep issues that affect how COVID-19–related deaths are experienced, or how principles and expertise coming from end-of-life care can be helpful. In fact, much of the action to deal with the pandemic has been isolated, examining each problem that has arisen only within its own context. This isolated thinking misses an opportunity to think creatively about how to solve problems of quality of life, quality of work, and supporting care workers.

Our current approach is largely driven by a panicked response, which perpetuates unequal access to resources and lacks appreciation for the systemic ways that deaths, care, and work all intersect. In an effort to save as many lives as possible, our current approach also falls back on existing processes and structures that have embedded biases. Our approach has been to create blanket rules and procedures regarding some end-of-life contexts, without acknowledging how these may perpetuate existing inequalities. It is time to reconsider policies and practices with an eye toward ethical principles of equity, interconnectedness, mutuality, and true democracy (Tronto, chapter 1, this volume).

A future orientation may include coordinated action, like cooperation between those committed to improving the quality of end-of-life care and those working to reduce inequality in who is infected and who cares for vulnerable others. These missions are aligned if our definition of quality care includes the principles of equity and justice, and we are willing to examine our starting assumptions about how to reward care workers.

A future orientation would see these issues as interconnected systems. Built into a future orientation would also be a rigorous process of analyzing biases in existing systems and processes. These systems include not only how we treat those in need of care but also how we support care workers. For example, measures meant to protect care recipients are connected to the quality of care worker settings.

Workers who are well supported and protected will likely feel less distressed and more able to align care with recipients' visions of quality of life. On the other hand, unsafe conditions further harm recipients, family members, and care workers. Understanding biases as artifacts of imperfect systems, we can begin to build new approaches, which are then subject to continual review for bias. It is not likely that we will create perfect processes from the beginning, and all processes have unintended consequences. The goal should be to create approaches that are reviewed and reworked as needed.

Ethically, this future orientation would start with principles of equity and justice and infuse our current end-of-life care systems with feminist ethics of care, including mutuality, interconnectedness, and appreciation of the value of caring.

18

COVID-19 and the Rise of the Care Robots

HELEN DICKINSON AND CATHERINE SMITH

A range of nations around the world report either currently experiencing or antic-ipating a care crisis. The use of robots has been seen as one way to respond to this, as these technologies are able to undertake several of the roles that human carers currently fulfill. However, there are concerns that the implementation of these technologies runs ahead of evidence-informed research into the experiences and needs of carers and those cared for, including considerations of their ethical implications (Smith et al. 2020). The advent of the COVID-19 pandemic led to calls for the use of robot technologies to intensify, and existing applications are being more widely implemented. It seems highly likely that one of the longer-term impacts of the COVID-19 pandemic will be greater investment in robot technologies and perhaps greater willingness to use these in care settings than we would otherwise have seen in the shorter term.

The increasing use of robot technologies in care services raises a number of questions within a context that care has largely been undervalued and distributed in an unjust way (Tronto, chapter 1, this volume). For example, will the expansion of robotic technologies in the context of the COVID-19 pandemic lead to a more just redistribution of care as some aspects of these processes are able to be auto-mated? We have seen the ways in which frontline care workers (typically ignored) have been acknowledged for their crucial work in the pandemic (e.g., England's "clap for our carers"). We have also seen the phenomenon of "caremongering" (Moscrop 2020) emerge in some jurisdictions. As a play on the antithesis of scare-mongering, caremongering refers to people coming together on local social media groups to meet the needs of people who are not able to get out or access essen-tials. Perhaps these are just some indications of a desire to redistribute care respon-sibilities. But if so, what role is there for robot technologies in fulfilling this?

This chapter details some of the uses of robots in care in different parts of the world during the pandemic and what this means for care services. Our argument is structured as follows. First, we explore the pre-pandemic crisis in care and ethical concerns in robot usage in care. We then examine the different ways in which robots were employed in the rapid response to lockdown and the social isolation that were part of the COVID-19 response in many places. In exploring these issues and linking to ethics of care scholarship, it is evident that there are important care network and practice considerations in employing new technologies. We ultimately conclude that, so far, we see little to suggest that these technologies will significantly disrupt care patterns to the extent that they will redistribute unequal care responsibilities. Moreover, in ensuring that such technologies do not exacerbate inequities, we need to account for moral and relational aspects in discussions of the design and application of these technologies.

Care Services in Crisis

In numerous care systems around the world, it has become almost commonplace to define this sector as in crisis (Himmelstein et al. 2017; Hodgkin et al. 2017; Ward, Ray, and Tanner 2020). We argue that the care crisis is a culmination of at least three points, which we outline in the paragraphs that follow.

The case has been made for a *demographic* crisis. It is well established that many countries face a shift in patterns of aging. Japan is the country that exemplifies this trend most, with Arai and colleagues (2015) describing it as a "super-aged" country, where the percentage of those over 65 reached 25 percent in 2013 and is expected to exceed 30 percent in 2025 and nearly 40 percent by 2060. This shift brings concerns that there will be insufficient individuals to care for the older population, and the government response has been to fill this gap through increased female workforce participation and robots. Although Japan is somewhat of an anomaly in developed countries, with its restrictive immigration policies (Peng 2017b), other countries face similar problems over a slightly longer time scale (Sharkey and Sharkey 2012). It is not simply the sheer number of people requiring care that poses a challenge for governments. Increased numbers of older people within a population, alongside improved life expectancies for people with disability (Guzman-Castillo et al. 2017), mean that we are seeing greater demand for care services within a population that is older, sicker, and has higher numbers of chronic and complex conditions. This demand crisis compounds a difficult situation in many countries, which have care services already struggling within a fiscally constrained environment (Pearson and Ridley 2017).

The sector is also described as experiencing a *workforce* crisis, with this issue manifest through both the number of individuals available within a particular area and the presence of appropriately skilled and disposed individuals (Hodgkin et al. 2017; Kamal et al. 2017). This latter is of particular importance given that a number of countries have experienced scandals of abuse in residential aged care and disability services. Australia, for example, has recently undergone two Royal Commissions (formal public inquiries). The first looked into aged care quality and safety following widespread reports concerning the abuse of older people in residential care, and another investigated the neglect and abuse of people with disability. Sadly, these abuses are not restricted to either these care settings or Australia (Byrne 2018), and while abuse has long existed in care relationships, there is some suggestion that these issues have become more frequent in a context of privatization as providers give priority to commercial agendas (Greener 2015).

Contemporary care is also suffering from a *value* crisis. Care in both paid and unpaid forms of work is central to a working economy and can be understood as a core social infrastructure (Glinsner et al. 2018; Rayner and Espinoza 2016; Tronto 2015). Over recent decades care has become commodified through neoliberal market rhetoric and activity (Fraser 2014) and in the process has been viewed more as a responsibility of governments. This situation is problematic because when care is seen as only an allocation of resources, there is no measure of whether care has been successful in meeting the needs of the people cared for. If the measure of success is merely that a service has been provided, the voice of those cared for becomes irrelevant (Tronto 2013). Discursive relational work is understood as key to competence in this domain, yet this work is often underaccounted for in official mandates and is both driven and informed by intrapersonal affective mandates, such as love and compassion, which are taken for granted and undercompensated in precarious, contracted work. In devaluing care and care workers, carework has become lowly regarded and low paid, often taken up by those already living at the margins of society (Robinson 2011).

Robots might plausibly play a role in responding to some of these crises of care, although, as we argue later in the chapter, not entirely or without generating care dilemmas of their own.

The Use of Robots in Care Services

In everyday language, lots of different things are called robots, capturing the broad array of applications of these technologies. Consequently, van Wynsberghe (2015) argues that "robots may be one of the most difficult technological innovations to define" (39). To capture the breadth of debate concerning robots in care settings we draw on a definition from Richards and Smart (2016) who define these technologies broadly as a "constructed system that displays both physical and mental agency, but is not alive in the biological sense" (6).

Robots are a relatively nascent technology in the context of care services. In larger institutions we have seen the use of robots to undertake tasks such as meal delivery, collection of dirty linen, delivery of clean linen, distribution of medical and housekeeping supplies (Stoyles 2017), and distribution of pharmaceuticals (Berdot et al. 2016). Such technologies are typically embedded within larger institutions as their costs are currently prohibitive for smaller settings or individual homes. Social or socially assistive robots (SARs) can be further categorized as companion robots that are designed to meet social needs, and service-type robots that function to both physically assist and also provide social interaction (Vandemeulebroucke,

Dierckx de Casterlé, and Gastmans 2018). SARs might undertake physically demanding chores in a servant-like capacity, as part of a safety mechanism to alert other humans to incidents such as falls, or to changes in physical measures, such as temperature, heart rate, or blood pressure. They may also provide cognitive assistance in remembering to do things like move around, eat, or take medications, or provide entertainment and companionship, alleviating boredom and loneliness.

Robots may have some positive impacts in the context of care services, such as delivering efficiencies and enhancing effectiveness, quality, and safety (Australian Centre for Robotic Vision 2018). Yet robotic technologies variously bring a corresponding number of practical and ethical concerns (Sharkey and Sharkey 2012), and they pose challenges not just for users of care services but also for care professionals, families, provider organizations, and governments. As the Australian Human Rights Commission (2018) notes, "Like any tool, technology can be used for good or ill . . . modern technology carries unprecedented potential on an individual and global scale" (7). New technologies are therefore disjunctive: offering significant advantages alongside the potential for misuse, including unintended consequences that need careful consideration to ensure such developments do not negatively affect particular groups. History shows that disruptive technologies require careful policy as well as legal and administrative scrutiny during their implementation.

Robot technologies are integrated into practices of care in both physical and social roles with varying degrees of government foresight and legislation. Evidence-informed research into ethical implications and the experiences and needs of carers and those cared for often lags the use of technologies. Concerns have been raised regarding a whole range of issues from data security and privacy, the ability of hackers to access these technologies, and users becoming too reliant on these technologies (Gunkel 2012; Sharkey and Sharkey 2012; Smith et al. 2020; Sparrow and Howard 2017). The use of robots also raises questions such as the boundaries between humans and machines, what good care looks like, and who owns responsibility for those outcomes (van Wynsberghe 2016). Decisions about practices of care with and by robots ultimately require reflection on what care is and how it is best achieved for human beings to flourish (Shatzer 2013). The literature on technology implementation demonstrates that it should not be assumed that robots can simply be slotted into services; work must be undertaken to ensure that they fit with the prevailing model of care (Aarons, Hurlburt, and McCue Horwitz 2010; Cook et al. 2012). Without this alignment, they have less chance of successful implementation (Greenhalgh 2018).

COVID-19 and Care Robots

The COVID-19 pandemic has accelerated development and implementation of the technologies and applications outlined in the previous section. U.S. and European governments have announced significant funding for manufacturers developing devices that can help combat COVID-19 (Lomas 2020; Newmarker 2020). The pandemic has essentially helped to make the case for the expansion of these technologies, despite their expense and potential risks, on the basis that we have significant workforce shortages or that there are risks in humans being in close proximity to one another. Robots cannot contract COVID-19 or become sick; this is clearly an advantage over humans who may not be able to work because they are ill or worry that they have the virus and may infect others. This is even more important where care is required among individuals who may be immunocompromised and at greater risk of becoming seriously ill if they contract COVID-19.

Some of the technologies used throughout the pandemic have in effect replaced human effort. For example, one obvious application for robotics relates to disinfecting spaces, on the basis that robots do not get tired or risk being infected (Wired.com 2020), with drones being repurposed from other duties into such a role in a variety of places (Franco 2020). Robots have also been used to deliver food and equipment in quarantine hotels and to keep shop shelves stocked so people are able to access supplies (Annunziata 2020; Cuthbertson 2020). Robots can even be used to take temperatures of individuals or to detect people with high fevers in social spaces (Marr 2020), and they have also been developed to perform tests and take swabs from people who are suspected of being infected (Pollard 2020). Robots are also being used to help police and regulate individuals in other ways. In China drones are being used to track individuals who are supposed to be in quarantine (Doffman 2020), and in Singapore robots were used in parks to remind people to socially distance (Stankiewicz 2020).

Many of the applications suggested so far are in essence relatively transactional in the sense that they fulfill one particular activity or another. But these have also had applications in social contexts. Social isolation has moved from being a fringe issue affecting a few more marginalized groups, to something many of us have had to deal with. This has been even more pronounced in aged care settings, where we have seen many of these closed to visitors for fear of spreading infection among a vulnerable population. Social robots are programmed to do things like remind people to take medications, engage people in doing exercises, and entertain through dances and other movements (Hulspas 2020). Some robots are also used to connect individuals to their families, having a camera, microphone, and screen and enabling them to see their loved ones through this process. There has also been a reported substantial increase in the purchase of sex (companion) robots during lockdown (Cookney 2020).

Some commentators have argued that the COVID-19 moment might be just what the robotics industry needs to take hold in a more significant way. Hanson Robotics, for example, had plans to mass produce their artificial intelligence–powered humanoid robot Sophia during 2021, despite criticism from other roboticists that the technology is not ready to do what will be expected of a human-sized, human-appearing personal care robot (Fearon 2021). Many of these robotic technologies have not been created purely for the pandemic, but their potential application has been made clearer due to the limitations imposed by restrictions associated with COVID-19. While many organizations are thinking carefully about where to cut money in budgets, only 15 percent of companies are planning to cut investments for automation, artificial intelligence, and industrial Internet of Things (Trevedei 2020). Howard and Borenstein (2020) suggest that having been forced to adopt robots in the COVID-19 emergency, employers and consumers may get used to these, and they may become a new normal if and when life returns to some normalcy. Prior to the pandemic there were a number of concerns expressed about automation of particular functions because these might lead to loss of jobs, but this emergency may have overcome what would have otherwise been a more significant debate about the introduction of these technologies.

Where Next for Care Robots?

In concluding this chapter, we consider where care robots might go next and what this tells us about care and its distribution. It is important to note that the use of robots is not pervasive across all care services and within different jurisdictions. For the time being, the cost of many of these technologies is significant, although the investments being made over the pandemic period could serve to bring this down over time. In many care settings, financial margins are slim, and it may not be feasible to invest significant amounts of money in these technologies just yet. Such analysis suggests that this decision is purely one of economic value, which we believe could prove problematic. At the point that these technologies become cost effective it raises questions as to what the impact will be on workers. Although robots have typically been sold as tools to augment workers' skills, the COVID-19 pandemic has reframed this, making the case that humans are the problem. But we question the degree to which it is easy to separate human from technical acts of care and what this tells us about how we value care and caregivers.

One of the selling points of these technologies to care providers is the idea that robots can undertake the more "mundane" aspects of care roles that employees do not always enjoy doing. Activities such as reminding people to take medications, carrying equipment and supplies, and lifting individuals are all potential actions that could be undertaken effectively by robots. While in one sense it may seem simple or straightforward to strip out these activities and have these provided by robots, with the remaining facets of care provided by humans, it is unlikely to be quite this easy in practice. There are several other functions that carers fulfill while, for example, taking blood pressure or reminding people to take medication. There are important facets of information gathering going on; for example, How does Mrs. Sanchez look today? Does she seem alert? Are there any visible signs that something might be different? If a robot is not programmed to undertake this function, then this sort of information might be lost and along with it an important opportunity to intervene with preventive activities. Moreover, these opportunities are, for some more socially isolated individuals, one of the few chances in a day that they might have to interact with another person and therefore fulfill an important social function and one that we have seen through the pandemic is a key influence on human well-being. If we value only the transactional activities of care processes, then we miss aspects that are highly valued by those receiving the care. Yet all too often care recipients are not involved in the design of these technologies so we do not pick up these broader functions.

The impacts of mass social isolation provide an unfortunate but informative insight into the need for human connection during the pandemic, and the deterioration of mental health in such conditions even where people are digitally connected has been evident. We can now demonstrate how keeping care ethics central (Held 2006) and "seeing and responding to need, taking care of the world by sustaining the web of connection so that no one is left alone" (Gilligan 1993, 62) as key principals to guide the use of robots in carework.

In considering whether in the future robots can deliver care services solely or in collaboration with humans it raises an important question about what it is that we mean by care in the first place. Some commentators are clear that robots cannot care. Turkle (2017) argues that care is a two-way process, a relational activity. Care is imbued with emotional labor, not just from the caregiver to the care receiver, but in both directions. In her analysis this means that robots cannot care, they can merely perform a facsimile of care. The implication in this analysis is that robots cannot care about us, and more widespread use of robots in care processes could leave individuals feeling as though they are connected, even though they are in fact alone.

Should humans become less involved in care processes it could have a significant impact on women, low-income earners, and recently arrived migrants given their preponderance in care roles. In essence this raises a question as to who takes care of carers. Continuing to consider what it means to give, take, and receive care is a question of moral and relational thinking (Sevenhuijsen 2003) and involves making decisions about how to care as a community. While some robotic technologies might deal with aspects of the "care crisis," we ultimately concur with Harding (2017) who argues that "empirical and conceptual work on care and feminist perspective on re-valuing care" makes "the case for a fundamental re-appraisal of how we resource and regulate" (1) the care sector. Arguably, with the broader application of these technologies, we have the opportunity to do this, but in doing so, ethical and relational considerations need to be central to this debate. So far, we would argue that these have been absent as technology developers and governments and care providers too often view value solely in terms of the bottom line.

19

Challenging Gender Regimes through Employee Voice in Carework

KATHERINE RAVENSWOOD

This chapter addresses employee voice in two sectors: residential aged care (nursing homes) and community support. It illustrates the way in which continuing gender discrimination results in a lack of voice for health care assistants in these sectors. This could have potentially large impacts on the safety of health care assistants and their clients during the current pandemic. Health care assistants provide care and support in activities of daily living and regular health care; for example, showering and dressing, assisting with a feeding tube or catheters, wound care, and medication. In community support this is conducted in the client's home with no supervision, and the client could be an older person, a person with a disability, or a person needing palliative care. In residential aged care, health care assistants work under the supervision of registered nurses and within their teams to provide care to older people. This chapter argues that health care assistants' voice will not be heeded until the organization of this carework is transformed, gender regimes are dismantled, and health care assistants and the carework they do is respected and valued fairly.

COVID-19 has not had the same catastrophic impact in Aotearoa[1]/New Zealand (henceforth Aotearoa), thus far, on health and health systems as seen in some countries globally. Aotearoa has no land borders and a relatively small population of approximately 5 million people (Statistics New Zealand n.d.). Aotearoa's government structure relies on a single legislature (i.e., not federal and state levels) (New Zealand Government 2020). The country has also taken a stricter approach than some with four separate lockdowns to date in February 2022. Its cumulative case rate per million people on January 31, 2022, was 3,242. This compares to 80,266 for Canada, 100,060 for Australia, 225,136 for the United States, and 254,488 for the United Kingdom (Our World in Data n.d.). The majority of cases have been those that are "imported" through people entering the country and being tested in managed isolation (Ministry of Health 2020). Furthermore, despite closed borders and strict lockdowns, the economic impact has been less severe than predicted (The Treasury 2020).

However, among the community transmission cases of COVID-19 in Aotearoa's first wave of infections, 11 percent of total cases were health care workers, with more than 57 percent of these infected at work. More health care assistants than workers in other health occupations in Aotearoa were infected, and the biggest clusters were in residential aged care (Ministry of Health 2020). The data show a clear risk for health care assistants. While health care assistant cases were concentrated in residential aged care, community and disability support workers were also infected. As indicated by Ito Peng (chapter 3, this volume) and Cynthia J. Cranford (chapter 16, this volume), this is a highly diverse workforce that relies on migrant labor. Aotearoa's infection statistics exemplify this, with "ethnic minority" health care assistants overrepresented in infections among health care workers (Ministry of Health 2020).

While this chapter focuses on Aotearoa, the gender regimes that devalue carework are similar and occur globally, evidenced throughout this volume (e.g., Cranford, chapter 16; Armstrong and Klosterman, chapter 6). Despite specific differences between countries and their funding environment for residential aged care and community support there are many similarities in the regulatory environment, especially across countries such as New Zealand and Australia (Kaine and Ravenswood 2013; Ravenswood and Kaine 2015), Canada, and the United Kingdom (Cranford, chapter 16, this volume).

Residential Aged Care and Community Care in Aotearoa

Carework in Aotearoa is subject to the same cost focus as elsewhere: in the market it is something done by women, at the lowest cost possible. The women who work in these sectors subsidize the wealth of the State and their employers.

Similarly to Cranford's description of community care in Ontario, a marketized approach to aged care is entrenched in Aotearoa. Residential aged care and community care services are generally state funded and contracted out through government agencies to privately owned companies. This approach is one that maintains carework as low value, low status, and low skill, thus justifying the low wages and often poor working conditions of both residential aged care and community care in New Zealand (Ravenswood and Harris 2016; Tronto, chapter 1, this volume).

Although both these sectors perpetuate gender norms of carework, within the organization of community care, health care assistants arguably experience poorer working conditions than those in residential aged care. They experience less access to guaranteed weekly hours, training, higher levels of pay, and so on (Ravenswood, Douglas, and Ewertowska 2021). As Mauldin (chapter 5, this volume) explains of community-based disability services, the nature of community care in Aotearoa means that health care assistants often work alone, in isolation from colleagues and managers, and invisible to policymakers and the public (Ayalon 2012). This invisibility perpetuates the ingrained perception that community care is mostly glorified housework, not personal care, including administering some medications and medical procedures.

In the last decade, health care assistants in Aotearoa took collective action to challenge their working conditions and the gender discrimination that influenced those conditions. In community care, health care assistants and their unions took action to challenge the lack of payment for both their time and their fuel costs of traveling between clients. Their action resulted in the Home and Community Support (Payment for Travel Between Clients) Settlement Act 2016 and the Guaranteed Hours Funding Framework (Ministry of Health 2017). The former provides for payment at the adult minimum wage for travel between clients, and compensation for some of the fuel costs (though not vehicle insurance or maintenance) of travel between clients. The latter is a policy that has informed ongoing work to ensure that health care assistants have guaranteed minimum hours per week.

Residential aged care health care assistants, joined by community care, took action under the Equal Pay Act of 1972, asserting that the low wages in these sectors were caused by historical, ongoing gender discrimination in Aotearoa. This led to the Care and Support Workers (Pay Equity Settlement) Act of 2017, which prescribes the hourly pay rates for health care assistants depending on their qualifications. It also requires employers to provide an opportunity for health care assistants to increase their care worker qualifications, and thus move up the pay scale.

Despite these considerable successes, health care assistants and their union representatives are still excluded from input on decisions such as those for the contracts for service and the associated funding models that drive the wages and work conditions in practice. Furthermore, managerial attitudes toward the work and health care assistants do not appear to have shifted significantly, and often health care assistants are still treated as low status and unskilled (Douglas and Ravenswood 2019). Consequently, health care assistants lack not only a voice in strategic decisions in the sector (Ravenswood and Markey 2018), they are often denied the opportunity to influence when they work and for how many hours (Ravenswood and Harris 2016), closed off from input on care decisions for their clients, and excluded from decisions including the level of care and staffing requirements with aged care funders (Ravenswood and Kaine 2015).

The Impact of COVID-19 on Residential Aged Care and Community Care

Three elements highlight the impact of COVID-19 on these two care sectors in Aotearoa: first, how the pandemic affected the social status of health care assistants; second, the impact on health care assistant safety; and third, how it has changed the way that health care assistants and their unions build solidarity.

In Aotearoa, the first lockdown saw health care assistants become essential workers, which perhaps led to greater media interest in their experiences of work.

For residential aged care, however, increased visibility led to media stories that while highlighting health care assistants' heroism, worked to reinforce the idea that carework is a calling (Palmer and Eveline 2012), and in the case of pandemics, a saintly sacrifice. The media highlighted gendered ideals of devoted carers, working together and creating a family with the residents that they cared for (Dodson and Zincavage 2007). One example was the decision by health care assistants and other staff to reside at the rest home they served for the duration of the lockdown in order to provide consistent care for their residents. Most of the workers reportedly made this choice for safe care provision for their clients, which had consequences for their families. For example, one worker shared that her child was extremely vulnerable to COVID-19 infection. Left unsaid was that to maintain her job and income, she had to sacrifice family time for her work (Checkpoint 2020). In some instances, greater social recognition meant increased stigma: some health care assistants who worked in infected rest homes faced exclusion and stigma within the broader society (Jackways et al. 2020).

Media attention was useful for community care health care assistants who were struggling with inadequate supplies of personal protective equipment (PPE). Low status and a lack of visibility for community support workers stymied their opportunity to be heard when they voiced concerns about a lack of PPE. Some employers said that health care assistants did not require PPE unless they were told it was necessary (Broughton 2020). Ministry of Health policy advised that PPE was not necessary for community support health care assistants unless the client was infected or self-isolating. Guidelines in March 2020 placed priority on workers using "hand hygiene" for *noncontact care*. In a job where most of the care is personal contact care, health care assistants could not ask for and receive PPE during a pandemic (Sharpe 2020). Media stories provided an opportunity for health care assistants in community support to gain greater exposure of their plight and to highlight their concerns for their own and their clients' safety.

However, overall health care assistants have not been recognized for their work during the pandemic, despite initial media attention to their work. In addition to their knowledge and safety being ignored, their lack of visibility was reinforced through instances of their essential worker status being challenged. During the first lockdown in March and April 2020, travel was only allowed for essential trips to a local supermarket, a medical appointment, or to work in essential jobs, which included hospital and supermarket staff. Essential workers were able to travel within their city for work (unlike others in the first lockdown) and could take advantage of "priority" queues at supermarkets. However, community and disability support health care assistants had their essential status challenged by security staff at supermarkets, and some were stopped and had their travel questioned by police (Bennie 2020). As Bennie (2020) stated, this treatment reflects the lack of understanding of the work, and the invisibility and low status of the clients and those who provide their care.

Despite the potential for greater recognition of their work during the COVID-19 pandemic, as Peng argues (chapter 3, this volume), health care assistants were not heard when voicing safety concerns. For example, the impact of infections on health care assistants was greater than that on other health workers in Aotearoa. Health care assistants who were infected in community-based care, rather than institutional settings, were overlooked in the media and other reporting—becoming just a number.

In contrast with community care, specific health and safety guidelines for infection control were communicated to rest homes in Aotearoa earlier in the pandemic. However, these guidelines did not reflect the reality of the work, despite health care assistants having raised issues regarding workload and staffing for years prior to COVID-19. Early guidelines included enhanced cleaning in rest homes with COVID-19 infections, as well as assigning health care assistants to work only with infected or uninfected residents in care "bubbles." While eminently sensible, the guidelines did not account for the current practice of high workloads, nor the funding and accreditation rules that had minimal staffing requirements that would not support these additional infection control requirements (Ravenswood 2020), let alone staff being unable to work because they had contracted COVID-19 (Jackways et al. 2020).

Government-sponsored independent reviews were conducted in Aotearoa subsequent to the first lockdown and outbreak of COVID-19 in 2020. These included two reviews into residential aged care, including how fast COVID-19 spread through some, but not other, rest homes. Other authorities, including the auditor general, reviewed the supply and provision of PPE. While the residential aged care reviews included interviews with "staff," it was unclear how many were health care assistants, and it appears that any engagement with health care assistants was via employers and managers, as opposed to engaging with unions and their members (Jackways et al. 2020). Recommendations from the reviews focused on pandemic-specific decisions and did not include recommendations to increase capacity or funding as part of providing safe and quality care that is sustainable during and after pandemics.

The auditor general's review into PPE focused solely on supply and distribution to hospitals, general practices, and, to some extent, rest homes in Aotearoa. It did not encompass guidelines for usage in community care and did not examine the supply and distribution to community care providers. Just as the health care assistant voice had been excluded from key decisions around funding and work models in both residential aged care and community care *prior* to COVID-19, health care assistants' voice continues to be excluded. COVID-19 has exacerbated the inequalities in community care, and, as Rico and Pautassi (chapter 7, this volume) argue, has shifted even greater care burdens onto women.

This is a somewhat bleak picture of the impact of COVID-19 on health care assistants in residential aged care and community care. However, this crisis created opportunities for health care assistants to unite in a way unforeseen by policymakers, spurred by the circumstances of increased internet use in a physically distanced society. Health care assistants in Aotearoa connected with other health care assistant unionists in Australia, the United States, Spain, Switzerland, and Ireland (McCully and Ravenswood 2020). These relationships created a greater sense of unity, which has been enduring and galvanized by global union campaigns, such as the UNI Global Union campaign Caring for Those Who Care (McCully and Ravenswood 2020). At the workplace level in Aotearoa, health care assistants worked together in ways they had not done previously: conducting their own client screening checks and coordinating with other local health care assistants to ensure that they were all safe on the job (McCully and Ravenswood 2020).

The Concept of Employee Voice

Industrial relations, with its focus on how macrolevel policy and regulation affects workplaces and individuals, tends to investigate employee voice as a spectrum of how much employees are included in decision making, and the types of decisions they can influence, from task level through to strategic decisions in the workplace (Wilkinson et al. 2014). Employee voice is often categorized into either individual or collective voice—when individuals or groups of employees have input into decisions made (Wilkinson et al. 2014).

In practice, individual employee voice is often used as a managerial tool to increase employee engagement and performance (Barry and Wilkinson 2016). This is achieved through focusing on low-level activity, such as sharing information with employees and limiting autonomy in how they conduct their work. Consequently, individual employee voice often aims to improve organizational outcomes, rather than improve the workplace experiences and working conditions of employees (Donaghey et al. 2011; Josserand and Kaine 2016).

In contrast to individual voice, collective voice is more likely to result in improved employee outcomes (Ravenswood and Markey 2018). Unions are a common example of collective voice that include bargaining for employment contracts and campaigning for improved work conditions. Ideally, employee voice could allow employees input on their working conditions *and* the strategic direction of the organization they work for, including sector or industry policy, such as service contracts or funding.

As a framework for studying power relationships, employee voice should be examined within the full institutional, regulatory, and organizational context in which carework takes place (Kaine and Ravenswood 2019). In relation to carework, and specifically in residential aged care, Ravenswood and Markey (2018) argue that gender regimes are core to the institutional, regulatory, and organizational context that frequently mutes care workers' voices. Gender regimes are the same practices and norms that have long rendered carework as low-status and low-value work (England, Budig, and Folbre 2002; Folbre and Nelson 2000; Palmer and Eveline 2012).

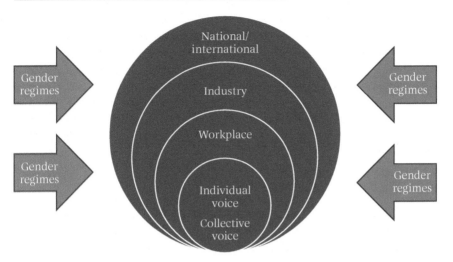

FIGURE 19.1 Employee voice.

As Marchington (2015) argues, employee voice entails complex relationships between workplace, sector, and state regulation. Figure 19.1 illustrates how individual and collective voice is affected by gender regimes within workplace, sector, national, and international contexts (Ravenswood and Markey 2018). In residential aged care and community care, health care assistants are often denied their individual voice because of gendered inequalities and devaluation of their work that is seen as low skilled (Ravenswood and Harris 2016). Following this gendered view, at the sector level health care assistants are excluded from decisions on service agreements, which dictate staffing levels and workload. At a national level they are excluded from decisions on sector funding models. Health care assistants face significant challenges in breaking down the gender regimes that underlie the use of voice mechanisms in their sectors.

Centering Health Care Assistant Voice

Health care assistant collective voice has become stronger and more active in Aotearoa. Health care assistants and their unions achieved groundbreaking changes to funding and policy, increasing their wages significantly. They challenged ongoing gender discrimination in their wages and won. Prior to the pandemic, unions campaigned together to publicize the need for safer staffing levels (E tū and New Zealand Nurses Organization 2019). During COVID-19 their actions around the lack of PPE, health care assistant and client safety concerns garnered media attention when employers and government did not recognize these issues as problems. It could be argued that the heightened risk and lack of support during the pandemic created a situation in which health care assistants strengthened their own support networks and capacity to be heard.

Despite their skill, knowledge, and active voice, gender regimes thwart their calls from being heeded. Health care assistants, as frontline employees, have the most consistent contact with their clients, and therefore the most practical knowledge of care provision. Indeed, research suggests that treating health care assistants with respect, as skilled and knowledgeable providers, and involving them in client care, health, and safety planning ensures the well-being of both clients and workers (Palesy 2018; Palesy and Billett 2017). Yet their knowledge and skill are consistently ignored because of the gendered organizational inequalities. The funding models that outsource these sectors to private employers are themselves based on the same discriminatory perceptions of carework, and neoliberal ideology (or as Tronto neologizes wealth-care) that aims to keep costs to a minimum to increase profit and reduce government expenditure. At all levels, health care assistants are often excluded from decisions because they are devalued as women doing low-wage carework.

Ravenswood and Kaine (2015) argue that the state has the power, but perhaps not the willingness, to lead the way in valuing and respecting health care assistants. Through changes to existing regulation, the government could reduce its reliance on the power of employer voice (Ravenswood and Markey 2018). They could include health care assistant voice in policy, funding, and strategic decisions for these sectors. Rather than privileging employers' voice in audits and reviews of the sector they could approach health care assistants directly and through their union representatives. These changes would begin to dismantle the gendered organizational regimes that label these workers as inferior and the work as low value.

With the emergence of new COVID-19 variants and greater community transmission in Aotearoa, the use and provision of PPE and safe staffing levels for infection control will be crucial to avoiding widespread infection among residential aged care and community care clients, staff, and their families. All of these insights draw on the knowledge and skill of health care assistants and have significant ramifications for residential aged care and community care. It is time that we value these workers, their skills, and their knowledge, and make sure that they are heard. Not doing so will mean that the government and employers fail to learn from COVID-19 lessons and remain derelict in their duty to protect health care assistants and care recipients both now and into the future.

NOTE

1.   The Māori name for New Zealand. Aotearoa and New Zealand are commonly used interchangeably.

20

Building a Care Infrastructure in the United States

JULIE KASHEN

Alicia Cleveland had to leave her work as a nanny to care for her own three children when schools closed during the COVID-19 pandemic. Given the preexisting medical conditions of her children, she had no choice. Yet the loss of income was a significant challenge. Alicia, a member of the National Domestic Workers Alliance, is one of the millions of caregivers—both paid and unpaid—whose lives have been upended by the COVID-19 pandemic (Gibson 2020).

Janelle Jones (2020) wrote, "You don't have to think too hard to imagine a world bereft of care; the COVID-19 pandemic has created a natural experiment in this devastating reality." COVID-19 has shone the spotlight on the reality that caregiving undergirds the functioning of our society and economy. The underpaid and undervalued care jobs done by a predominantly female and disproportionately Black, Indigenous, Latinx, Asian, and immigrant workforce, sustain our communities and economic engines. So much of our underinvestment in care, and the people who provide it, is tied to the racist and sexist past and present of the United States. The lack of a public system for providing high-quality, affordable, well-compensated care across generations, which I will refer to as a care infrastructure,[1] has made the impact of COVID-19 disastrous for millions of families, especially families of color. In the United States, the existing policy framework was profoundly inadequate and precarious prior to the pandemic. The crisis has devastated it.

This chapter focuses on why the United States—and countries throughout the world—must name the historical intersecting oppressions holding policy and culture change back, cut through the deficiencies and silos they helped create, and work through policy and culture change to weave the threads together into a publicly funded care infrastructure that creates both good care jobs and reliable care options for families.

I begin by describing how intersecting oppressions have led to (1) an "every family and caregiver for themselves" approach; (2) an undervaluing of care work, and (3) silos between care consumers and the care workers as well as across care solutions at different life stages, noting how these have all been exacerbated by the COVID-19 pandemic. I then describe how cutting across silos is a win for all: good for families, equity, and economic growth. Finally, I conclude with a plan for how to successfully build the care infrastructure long overdue in the United States.

The Intersecting Oppressions Keeping Care Fragmented and Undervalued

Sexism, racism, xenophobia, ableism, ageism, classism, and other intersecting oppressions have led to an every-family-and-caregiver-for-themselves approach that has been exacerbated by the COVID-19 pandemic. As Ai-jen Poo, the executive director of the National Domestic Workers Alliance said, "In the experience of [the domestic/care] workforce, you can really see the ways that our society and our culture are still very much structured by a hierarchy of human value, whether it's race or gender" (Tippet 2020). These hierarchies have been embedded into U.S. public policy to systemically limit power and resources for women, people of color, immigrants, people with disabilities, older people, LGBTQIA people, and others, and especially for those at the intersections of those identities. The result is that those who hold the power (especially formal positions of influence) and resources (especially wealth) make the rules, and those rules favor the powerful and resourced people's ability to continue to hold onto their power and resources.[2]

Fragmentation and the Scarcity Myth

Maintaining that status quo is often easier than disrupting it, and those with power and resources have many tools at their disposal to maintain it, including defining the cultural narrative and the political power to influence public policy. Both culture and policy have been used to support an "every family and caregiver for themselves" approach, stoke divisions between those who provide the care and those who receive it, and create silos across care solutions at different life stages.

For example, the messages that care (1) is an individual responsibility, not a collective one, (2) is women's work, and (3) does not deserve economic value, have been repeated by supposed experts, policy leaders, pop culture stories, magazines, and more for decades (Kashen and Mabud 2020). In many ways, the COVID-19 pandemic, combined with the lack of a care infrastructure in place prior to the pandemic, reinforced these cultural norms. The nature of the COVID-19 pandemic, and how easily the virus spreads, forced individuals, families, and communities—already being told they are "on their own"—into greater isolation. Those in nursing homes were limited from having visitors due to the risk of the viral spread. Too many died living in those types of congregate care settings, including both patients and staff members (Mauldin, chapter 5, this volume). Parents could no longer rely on schools or childcare, which shut down or reduced their hours or enrollment numbers for safety. Nor could they rely on grandparents without putting them at risk, since older people are at greater risk of getting seriously ill or dying from COVID-19. Those providing paid care have been forced to put themselves and their families at risk.

For many, the pandemic has reinforced the "every family for themselves" myth. This makes it harder to build widespread support for public policy change. Individuals socialized to believe that they are supposed to be fully on their own first need to see that these are public problems with public solutions and then engage in the collective call for change. And those who do the work and receive low or no pay for it, or manage the extensive responsibilities of both caring and participating in the paid workforce, have limited time and financial resources to engage in changing public policies.

These factors are made worse by division, another very effective (and despicable) tool for sustaining the status quo. When the caring majority is siloed into those providing the care and those receiving it, those paid to care and those not, and those caring for children and those caring for aging adults or supporting the independent living of people with disabilities, it is harder to make the case that we are all in this together and need collective solutions. It creates a scarcity myth and a fight for resources (Dayen 2020).

These siloes pit care consumers against those providing care. For example, separating services and care means that when the U.S. government funds its largest public health insurance program for people with low incomes (Medicaid) to provide home care services it does not make sure that there is enough money to cover the cost of livable wages, benefits, and paid time off. It does not cover the cost of providing paid sick days to home care workers while ensuring that the consumer can still receive care. Similarly, it means that when the government invests in helping families to afford childcare it doesn't cover the costs of making childcare jobs good, family-supporting jobs.

Those creating these false divisions also aim to have childcare, long-term care, and paid leave advocates fighting against each other for limited resources instead of working together to build political power and will for a full care agenda. The scarcity myth makes trade-offs feel inevitable when they are, in fact, policy choices.

Undervaluing Care

History shows how the vicious cycle of institutionalized sexism and racism has led to the lack of a care infrastructure and the undervaluing of those who provide care. Caregiving has long been undervalued labor. As Akosionu and colleagues also discuss (chapter 4, this volume), starting with the institution of chattel slavery that forced Black women to nurse and take care of the children of white landowners—to the detriment of their own children—racism and sexism have long played a role in the care of children (Vogtman 2017). Once chattel slavery was outlawed, work in the home, known as domestic work, was still one of the limited occupations U.S. laws and customs made available to Black women. That changed in the 1960s as a result of the positive impact of the civil rights movement, the organizing of Black women, and the opportunities created by their efforts. Yet this history also left a long legacy, and to this day, Black and immigrant women remain a disproportionately significant part of the domestic workforce (Nadasen and Williams 2014).

Alongside this undervaluing of care, labor laws codified in the New Deal of the 1930s exempted caregivers. In an explicitly racist move, some members of Congress would not support these labor rights and protections if they included farmworkers and domestic workers, thus they were passed with unfair exclusions. Domestic workers and farmworkers have since been fighting for, and in many cases winning, inclusion in these laws (on the local, state, and federal level) (Dayen 2020). Yet the legacy of this combination of undervaluing care jobs and excluding care workers from crucial labor laws remains today. The result is that the government continues to treat care as an individual responsibility to be met by the unpaid labor of women of all races and the underpaid labor of women of color.

Pre-pandemic, the typical domestic workers—the nannies, home care workers, and house cleaners who care for our loved ones and keep our homes clean and orderly—were paid $12.01 per hour (Wolfe et al. 2020). This is on average just 74 cents for every dollar that their peers are paid, when compared to demographically similar workers (Wolfe et al. 2020). For the childcare and early-learning workforce who work across settings (in homes and centers), the median hourly wage is $12.12 (Gould and Blair 2020). Few care workers have health insurance coverage or retirement savings (Wolfe et al. 2020). This means they are often struggling to make ends meet. The devastating effects of the pandemic have been especially destructive for their health and financial stability. For example, while home care workers were showing up to work and risking their and their families' health at the height of the pandemic, the childcare sector lost more than 350,000 jobs in a single month at the beginning of the pandemic, and many of those jobs have not yet returned (Malik 2021).

As long as caregiving is not treated as a public good, and caregivers are paid far less than what their work is worth, those with power and resources will continue to hold power and resources. After all, when unpaid caregiving falls on women, it is harder for them to get higher paying jobs and promotions and to focus on providing for their own families. When childcare workers, home care workers, and personal care assistants remain underpaid, they struggle to pay their bills and make ends meet. These challenges have ripple effects on their ability to participate in civic engagement, run for office, donate to candidates, and take on leadership and decision-making roles in every sphere.

How to Turn the Corner Together: Breaking Down the Silos

Building a robust care infrastructure that cuts across silos and lifts up the people who care as valuable and central to care services will help disrupt the cycle of institutionalized racism and sexism. It will also support equitable economic growth, creating jobs quickly, spurring growth in other sectors and ensuring financial stability for individuals, families, and communities (Kalipeni and Kashen 2020).

The COVID-19 Spotlight and Opportunity

While many people experienced isolation as the pandemic reached its peak, others started to see themselves as part of a greater crisis. They saw their caregiving challenges reflected across colleagues, friends, and neighbors. The media began to write about the ways in which these challenges affected millions of families. By seeing that they were not alone, individuals began to question the cultural assumption that care is an individual challenge to be solved alone, which opened the door to public engagement.

In addition, people relying on care experienced a renewed appreciation for the people who are paid to provide care. Parents at home facilitating remote learning or caring for their children appreciated the work of teachers and early educators more than ever. The home care workers showing up every day despite the potential contagion risks reminded the families they care for just how important their work is. It never made sense to separate care services from the people who provide the care, and this crisis moment further reminds us of that.

Furthermore, advocates came together in new ways to break down silos, including by forming the Care Can't Wait Coalition to organize, advocate, and build power together across care issues. This helped to change the public conversation from one of scarcity to one of abundance and possibility. The possibilities that come from these strengthened connections are significant. They include benefits for families and communities, and equitable economic growth.

Benefits for Families and Communities

The millions of workers with family care responsibilities need support—either to participate in paid work, knowing that their family members are safe and nurtured or to participate in caregiving, knowing that their economic security will remain intact. Ensuring that families can both work and care will also help create economic stability and asset building, which can help disrupt the intergenerational poverty that disproportionately affects Black, Indigenous, and Latinx families.

Higher compensation for carework is important unto itself. Paying better wages to the people who provide care and improving the quality of those jobs are key parts of combating the racist and sexist structures that have defined care as low value. In turn, improving working conditions will allow the women of color in these jobs to increase their own well-being, build assets, and ultimately gain more power and resources, which will further help upend the hierarchies. At the same time, improving jobs in these ways has major benefits for the consumers.

Factors such as how well care workers are paid, how they are treated and valued, what kind of training and preparation they receive, what kind of care they can afford for their own families, and what kind of voice they have at work all greatly affect how care is delivered (Kashen, Potter, and Stettner 2016). When children receive high-quality care, it helps establish strong social, emotional, and cognitive foundations. It allows parents to work with the peace of mind that their children are in safe, nurturing care. Similarly for people in home health care or relying on personal attendants to support the daily activities of life—the greater the investment in the person providing the services, the more likely the services will be safer, more attentive, and of higher quality. The more consumers and care workers see themselves as part of the same interdependent team—as people who all need a significant public investment in care—the stronger the efforts to achieve a collective approach will be (Dayen 2020).

Equitable Economic Growth

In addition, investing in care infrastructure will yield millions of jobs in the care sector and support the employment of caregivers, including parents. These elements are crucial for an equitable economic recovery. Treating care as the valuable public good that it is will create the scaffolding needed to ensure greater stability and opportunities. It will ensure that women of color can fully participate in the rebuilding of the U.S. economy. It will disrupt current systems that lead Black women in particular to age into poverty and homelessness (Christ and Gronniger 2018). Centering the women who care in policy solutions will make a dent in the hierarchy and begin the path to topple it.

Building a Care Infrastructure Is a Win for All

Here is the plan for how to successfully build the care infrastructure long overdue in the United States.

As we build back from the current crisis, we must start with a foundation of a robust care infrastructure. That includes childcare for all, paid leave for all, and a holistic plan for long-term services and supports that prioritizes home and community-based services and integrates quality care and quality jobs seamlessly. In other words, we need significant public investments in a care system that recognizes "services" to mean "the people who provide care" and treats them accordingly, and a care system that values paid caregivers and attendants and family caregivers across generations.

First, it is long past due to build a childcare and early education system. Without action, the United States is at risk of losing billions of dollars in economic activity from the combination of reduced parental labor force participation, the impact of child care disruptions on employers and state tax revenue, and the shrinkage of the child care and early learning sector (Kashen et al. 2022). As of this writing, the House of Representatives has passed historic, transformative child care and preschool legislation (Guarino 2021), and it remains to be seen whether the Senate will pass something similar or maintain the unacceptable status quo.

The United States has addressed this before. During World War II, policymakers established affordable childcare options to meet the needs of the women working in factories while the men were abroad at war (Cohen 2015). It was a successful program that demonstrated how effective it is when the government treats childcare as a collective responsibility. When the program was dismantled after the war, Eleanor Roosevelt noted, "Many thought [the child care centers] were purely a war emergency measure. A few of us had an inkling that perhaps they were a need which was constantly with us, but one that we had neglected to face in the past" (Suskind 2020). That need has once again been long neglected.

As in the 1940s, this is a moment to take responsibility to build a childcare system to ensure that all families have safe, affordable, high-quality, convenient childcare options in their own homes, family care homes, or childcare centers. Such a system must meet families' diverse needs and values and provide the resources, including better compensation, needed for the early educators and staff who do this essential work. It should be sustainable and last well beyond the immediate crisis.

In addition to having good options for care for children, our workplace must support family caregivers when they want or need to take time to care, whether it is for a newborn or a newly adopted child or for their own illness or that of a loved one. The COVID-19 pandemic made clear just how important these policies are. Congress put emergency paid leave policies into place during the pandemic, and one study showed that states that gained access to paid sick leave through the emergency congressional measures saw 400 fewer confirmed COVID-19 cases per day. For every 1,300 workers who gained 2 weeks of paid sick days, one COVID-19 case was prevented per day (Pichler, Wen, and Ziebarth 2020).

Everyone should be able to meet their care obligations without risking financial insecurity. Families also need the guarantee of permanent paid sick leave and comprehensive paid family and medical leave—and they need it regardless of the size or type of employer they work for, or the type of work they do (Kashen 2019b).

Most aging people and people with disabilities do not have good affordable home and community-based care options, or even affordable congregate care options. The services are unaffordable, families are forced to spend down their entire savings to receive support to cover the costs, and caregivers are paid too little. A new, holistic system of long-term care that builds and expands on existing laws to provide sustainable long-term services and supports—especially for home and community-based services—is the only way to support dignity and independence for people of all ages and abilities. Public funds must also help cover the costs of making home care jobs good jobs, raising standards and ensuring dignity for domestic workers (Kashen 2019a).

Most caregivers, the people who take care of our aging parents and our young children, are unpaid or underpaid. It is time to increase compensation and provide health care, retirement security, and other benefits, including paid time off, and to ensure a voice and path to collective power building for all care workers. Additional policies are needed to support family caregivers, such as providing them with respite care, and to ensure that family caregivers can receive Social Security credit for serving as caregivers of dependent relatives.

Most people want the best care possible for their children or older loved ones and believe that the value of that care, or support for daily living, is priceless. Yet most families also cannot afford to compensate early educators, home care workers, or personal care assistants in a way that makes care jobs good jobs. This is why we need an approach that includes families, employers, and the government. The government must contribute with significant public investment that includes the cost of good compensation, including livable wages, benefits, labor protections, a voice at work, and paid time off. Building back from the pandemic presents us with the responsibility to demand what we all need—whether we are people who need care, provide care to our loved ones, or are paid to care for others.

Acknowledgment

The author wishes to thank Haeyoung Yoon, senior policy director for the National Domestic Workers Alliance, for her input.

NOTES

1. A care infrastructure is a system with significant public investment that recognizes care as both an individual and social responsibility, values care workers, and supports family members to both care and provide financially for each other. It includes childcare, paid family and medical leave, and long-term services and supports.

2. These issues are discussed further in the report I coauthored with Rakeen Mabud for the Time's Up Impact Lab: "Nevertheless It Persists: Disrupting the Vicious Cycle of Institutionalized Sexism," https://timesupfoundation.org/work/times-up-impact-lab/neverthe less-it-persists-disrupting-the-vicious-cycle-of-institutionalized-sexism/?utm_source =structural-sexism-launch-pr&utm_medium=email&utm_campaign=structural-sexism -launch.

Epilogue

Care in Crisis: Convergences and Divergences

MIGNON DUFFY, AMY ARMENIA, AND KIM PRICE-GLYNN

As the authors in this volume have shown, the care crisis did not emerge from the COVID-19 pandemic; rather, a long history of global neglect of care preceded the arrival of this virus. This underinvestment, based in the wealth care ideology that prioritizes market forces over human flourishing, has been facilitated by long-standing inequalities that stigmatize dependence, disability, and the need for care and place the work of care on unpaid and paid carers with little power or leverage. The combination of these systemic weaknesses turned a pandemic into a syndemic and a crisis into a catastrophe.

At this writing, while the pandemic has shifted, it is an ongoing crisis in much of the world. A vaccine was developed in record time, a testament to the potential of science when there is adequate public investment. However, the vaccine's distribution remains hampered by the very same global, racial, and economic inequalities that have been described in this volume. More than two years into this pandemic, parts of the world struggle with lack of access to vaccination that could stem the virus's transmission. And even the way we talk about a postvaccine world is shaped by ableist visions that if deaths have become limited to older adults and those with preexisting conditions then we can lift all restrictions on movement and behavior (Mauldin, chapter 5, this volume). We live in a time of great uncertainty—about how the virus itself will continue to develop, about the long-term economic impacts of the global shocks, and about the consequences of this historic moment for care around the world.

Amid these uncertainties, we offer this volume as a glimpse into some of the potentials and possibilities of this unprecedented time for care. While the collection of chapters does not offer a comprehensive international comparative framework, there are important lessons to be learned from the convergences and divergences that emerge from the stories told in these pages.

The convergences are perhaps easiest to see. Across the globe, the authors in this book have described the systematic devaluation of care that preceded and will outlast the pandemic emergency—whether we call it wealth-care or examine the silencing of care voices in the creation of pandemic policy or notice the lack of attention to personal protective equipment and other basic safety measures. We have also seen a clear and perhaps hardening of the gendered division of carework, supported by global and racialized structures as well. Across an incredible variety of contexts, women shouldered the shifts and increases in carework during the pandemic—whether it was in South African families or countries in Latin America or Europe where child care was suddenly shut down.

More hopefully, another convergence that emerges from these stories is the rising public awareness of care as a social problem. In some cases, such as the United States, this was explicitly named as the public discourse began to include phrases like "care infrastructure." In many places around the world, care workers were deemed essential workers. In other places, like some countries in Latin America, gender as a priority disappeared in the policy language of the moment. This shows that rising discourse about care may or may not always have good outcomes—but we are talking about it.

There are important lessons in the divergences as well. Although the larger narrative is about the inadequacy of care structures across the globe, there are important variations across these stories. Workers in unions were more protected from the fallout of the pandemic than workers who were not in unions. Workers in nonprofit and government agencies were more protected than workers in for-profit institutions. Home-based workers and unpaid workers experienced more precarity than those in institutions.

One of the most important lessons to emerge is the importance of policies that prioritized care and were gender aware and care aware in contrast to policies that were care blind or gender blind. Gender-blind and care-blind policies, such as those followed in Israel or Latin America, had a negative impact on women and carers. While migrant workers found themselves in precarious circumstances during the pandemic, some countries added flexibility to their immigration policies, motivated by a need for care workers. In some contexts, such as in Canada, the government redeployed national resources in novel ways to meet care needs, like sending the military into nursing homes.

In these convergences and divergences, we see ongoing frustrations but also hope. We see the potential of Ito Peng's fourth R: revaluing and public investment (chapter 3, this volume). We see that resources matter and can be effective, when matched with supportive culture and care-aware policy. We see the potential for valuing care in public discourse as a step toward valuing care in more material ways. Revaluation is a long-term goal and will involve both mobilization in times of crisis and maintaining advocacy and voice in more "normal" times.

It remains to be seen what the long-term impacts of the COVID-19 crisis will be on care policy around the world. And for many countries mired in poverty or facing austerity governments, large-scale public investment in care is not an immediate option. But the ability to build broad coalitions across long-standing advocacy organizations and the incorporation of a public goods/infrastructure frame may be key to leveraging the increased visibility of paid care into real transformative change.

ACKNOWLEDGMENTS

This volume was conceived, born, and raised during the very crisis that it covers. We are thankful for, and in awe of, the authors of the chapters, who contributed their expertise and thought during a global pandemic, at times without childcare or open schools, in lockdowns or during remote work, through their own and their families' bouts with COVID. The book itself is a testament to the innovation and commitment that we need to improve our systems of care during and beyond this crisis.

After completing the first drafts of the chapters, we gathered most of the volume's contributors to take part in a series of web meetings. Participating authors discussed their chapters individually and together with other authors to promote conversation across chapters. We are so thankful for their generous time and reflections. These conversations were illuminating and provocative, engaging the central ideas of the book and fostering interconnections within the book.

We thank Peter Mickulas, senior editor at Rutgers University Press, for his excitement at the ideas we bring to him, including this book series and this volume, and the care and expertise of his staff in bringing this book to press.

As we worked on this book during a time of global loss, we suffered an irreplaceable loss ourselves. Debi Osnowitz was an extraordinary scholar, editor, and human, and we knew when we conceived of the idea of a global volume that it was her guiding hand we needed to help us make it whole. Debi worked closely with a number of our authors to make their chapters clearer and to smooth the language throughout, and the volume is certainly better for her work and insight. Sadly, partway through our process, she passed away unexpectedly. Those of us who were fortunate enough to know her feel her absence daily.

As members of the Carework Network, we are fortunate to surround ourselves with a larger group of scholars who are critically involved in care research and advocacy. The Carework Network provides us with a community for learning and engagement that nurtures our work.

We are grateful for the support of colleagues at Rollins College, the University of Connecticut, and the University of Massachusetts Lowell. Financial support for this work came from Rollins College Office of the Dean of Faculty and the University of Connecticut Scholarship Facilitation Fund.

Our families have made this work possible during unprecedented times. We are fortunate to have family members who step up and get things done so that we have time to work and think. Our gratitude goes out to our partners, Kerry Donohoe, Scott Englehart, and Eric Price-Glynn, and our kids Ben and Becca, Elena, and Lucas and Lillian for providing support and encouragement throughout this process.

REFERENCES

Aarons, Gregory A., Michael Hurlburt, and Sarah McCue Horwitz. 2010. "Advancing a Conceptual Model of Evidence-Based Practice Implementation in Public Service Sectors." *Administration and Policy in Mental Health and Mental Health Services* 38 (1): 4–23.

Abbasi, Jennifer. 2020. "Social Isolation—the Other Covid-19 Threat in Nursing Homes." *JAMA* 324 (7): 619–620.

Abramowitz, Sharon A., Kristen E. McLean, Sarah L. McKune, Kevin L. Bardosh, Mosoka Fallah, Josephine Monger, Kodjo Tehoungue, and Patricia A. Omidian. 2015. "Community-Centered Responses to Ebola in Urban Liberia: The View from Below." *PLoS Neglected Tropical Diseases* 9 (4). https://doi.org/10.1371/journal.pntd.0003706.

Abrego, Leisy, and Ralph LaRossa. 2009. "Economic Well-Being in Salvadoran Transnational Families: How Gender Affects Remittance Practices." *Journal of Marriage and Family* 71 (4): 1070–1085.

Ackerly, Brooke A. 2018. *Just Responsibility: A Human Rights Theory of Global Justice.* New York: Oxford University Press.

Adams, Adrienne E., Angela K. Littwin, and McKenzie Javorka. 2020. "The Frequency, Nature, and Effects of Coerced Debt among a National Sample of Women Seeking Help for Intimate Partner Violence." *Violence against Women* 26 (11): 1324–1342.

Adams-Prassl, Abi, Teodora Boneva, Marta Golin, and Christopher Rauh. 2020. "Inequality in the Impact of the Coronavirus Shock: Evidence from Real Time Surveys." *Journal of Public Economics* 189: 104245. https://doi.org/10.1016/j.jpubeco.2020.104245.

Addati, Laura, Umberto Cattaneo, Valeria Esquivel, and Isabel Valarino. 2018. *Care Work and Care Jobs for the Future of Decent Work.* Geneva: International Labour Organization.

Alhmidi, Maan. 2020. "Admitted to Canada under Pilot Program, Refugee Nurses Ready for Work as PSWs." *Toronto Star*, September 19. https://www.thestar.com/news/canada/2020/09/19/admitted-to-canada-under-pilot-program-refugee-nurses-ready-for-work-as-psws.html.

Allegretto, Sylvia, and Lawrence Mishel. 2018. *The Teacher Pay Penalty Has Hit a New High: Trends in the Teacher Wage and Compensation Gaps through 2017.* Economic Policy Institute Report, September. https://irle.berkeley.edu/files/2018/09/Teacher-pay-penalty-has-hit-a-new-high.pdf.

Allen, Kate. 2020. "This Black PSW with COVID-19 Was Sent Home from Hospital: Two Days Later He Died." *Toronto Star*, May 23. https://www.thestar.com/news/gta/2020/05/23/this-black-psw-with-covid-19-was-sent-home-from-hospital-two-days-later-he-died.html.

Alon, Titan, Matthias Doepke, Jane Olmstead-Rumsey, and Michèle Tertilt. 2020. "The Impact of COVID-19 on Gender Equality." National Bureau of Economic Research Working Paper 26947, April. https://www.nber.org/papers/w26947.

Altintas, Evrim and Oriel Sullivan. 2017. "Trends in Fathers' Contributions to Housework and Childcare under Different Welfare Policy Regimes." *Social Politics* 24 (1): 81–108.

Altman, Barbara M. 2016. "Conceptual Issues in Disability: Saad Nagi's Contribution to the Disability Knowledge Base." In *Sociology Looking at Disability: What Did We Know and When Did We Know It, Research in Social Science and Disability*, vol. 9, edited by Sara Green and Sharon Barnartt, 57–95. Bingley, UK: Emerald Group Publishing Limited.

Amin, Iftekhar, and Stan Ingman. 2014. "Elder Care in the Transnational Setting: Insights from Bangladeshi Transnational Families in the United States." *Journal of Cross-Cultural Gerontology* 29 (3): 315–328.

Amnesty International. 2020. "Global: Amnesty Analysis Reveals over 7,000 Health Workers Have Died from COVID-19." Amnesty International, September. https://www.amnesty.org/en/latest/news/2020/09/amnesty-analysis-7000-health-workers-have-died-from-covid19/.

Andersen, Torben M., Philipp J. Schröder, and Michael Svarer. 2020. "Designing Reopening Strategies in the Aftermath of COVID-19 Lockdowns: Some Principles with an Application to Denmark." IZA Policy Paper 158, May, 1–17. https://www.iza.org/publications/pp/158/designing-reopening-strategies-in-the-aftermath-of-covid-19-lockdowns-some-principles-with-an-application-to-denmark.

Anderson, Bridget, and Isabel Shutes, eds. 2014. *Migration and Care Labor: Theory, Policy and Politics*. New York: Palgrave Macmillan.

Anderson, Roy M., Hans Heesterbeek, Don Klinkenberg, and T. Déirdre Hollingsworth. 2020. "How Will Country-Based Mitigation Measures Influence the Course of the COVID-19 Epidemic?" *Lancet* 395 (10228): 931–934. https://doi.org/10.1016/S0140-6736(20)30567-5.

Andrew, Alison, Sarah Cattan, Monica Costa Dias, Christine Farquharson, Lucy Kraftman, Sonya Krutikova, Angus Phimister, and Almudena Sevilla. 2020. "The Gendered Division of Paid and Domestic Work under Lockdown." IZA Discussion Paper 13500, July, 1–32. https://docs.iza.org/dp13500.pdf.

Annunziata, Marco. 2020. "The Robots That Help Get Food on the Shelves in the Covid-19 Crisis." *Forbes*, April 21. https://www.forbes.com/sites/marcoannunziata/2020/04/21/the-robots-that-help-get-food-on-the-shelves-in-the-covid-19-crisis/#15ce5d5b583f.

Arai, Hidenori, Yasuyoshi Ouchi, Kenji Toba, Tamao Endo, Kentaro Shimokado, Kazuo Tsubota, Seiichi Matsuo, Hidezo Mori, Wako Yumara, Masayuki Yokode, Hiromi Rakugi, and Shinichi Ohshima. 2015. "Japan as the Front-Runner of Super-Aged Societies: Perspectives from Medicine and Medical Care in Japan." *Geriatrics & Gerontology International* 15 (6): 673–687.

Armstrong, Pat, Carol Amaratunga, Jocelyne Bernier, Karen Grant, Ann Pederson, and Kay Willson, eds. 2002. *Exposing Privatization: Women and Health Care Reform*. Aurora, ON: Garamond Press.

Armstrong, Pat, and Hugh Armstrong. 2005. "Public and Private: Implications for Care Work." *Sociological Review* 53 (2): 169–187.

———. 2016. *About Canada: Health Care*. 2nd ed. Halifax: Fernwood Publishing.

———, eds. 2020. *The Privatization of Care: The Case of Nursing Homes*. New York: Routledge.

Armstrong, Pat, Hugh Armstrong, Jacqueline Choiniere, Ruth Lowndes, and James Struthers. 2020. *Re-imagining Long-Term Residential Care in the COVID-19 Crisis*. Canadian Centre for Policy Alternatives, April. https://policyalternatives.ca/publications/reports/re-imagining-long-term-residential-care-covid-19-crisis.

Armstrong, Pat, Hugh Armstrong, and M. Patricia Connelly. 1997. "The Many Forms of Privatization." *Studies in Political Economy* 53 (1): 3–9.

Armstrong, Pat, and Ruth Lowndes, eds. 2018. *Creative Teamwork: Developing Rapid, Site-Switching Ethnography*. New York: Oxford University Press.

Aronson, Jane. 2004. "'Just Fed and Watered': Women's Experiences of the Gutting of Home-Care." In *Caring For/Caring About: Women, Home-Care and Unpaid Caregiving*, edited by

Karen R. Grant, Carol Amaratunga, Pat Armstrong, Madeline Boscoe, Ann Pederson, and Kay Wilson, 167–184. Aurora, ON: Garamond Press.

Aronson, Jane, and Sheila M. Neysmith. 1996. "'You're Not Just in There to Do the Work': Depersonalizing Policies and the Exploitation of Home-Care Workers' Labor." *Gender and Society* 10 (1): 59–77.

Arza, Camila, and Juliana Martínez Franzoni. 2018. "A Long Decade of Gendering Social Policy in Latin America: Transformative Steps and Inequality Traps." In *Handbook on Gender and Social Policy*, edited by Sheila Shaver, 408–429. London: Edward Elgar Publishing.

Aspinwall, Nick. 2020. "Taiwan's COVID-19 Success Story Continues as Neighbors Fend Off New Outbreaks." *The Diplomat*, September. https://thediplomat.com/2020/09/taiwans-covid-19-success-story-continues-as-neighbors-fend-off-new-outbreaks/.

Atkinson Jamie, Margaret O'Brien, and Alison Koslowski. 2020. "United Kingdom Country Note." In *International Review of Leave Policies and Research 2020*, edited by A. Koslowski, S. Blum, I. Dobrotić, G. Kaufman, and P. Moss, 583–600. http://www.leavenetwork.org/lp_and_r_reports/.

Attiah, Karen. 2021. "Wealthy Nations Are Gobbling up Vaccines: This Moral Failure Will Come Back to Haunt Us." *Washington Post*, February 1. https://www.washingtonpost.com/opinions/2021/02/01/covid-vaccines-access-poor-rich-countries/.

Austen, Siobhan, Therese Jefferson, Rachel Ong, Rhonda Sharp, Gill Lewin, and Valerie Adams. 2016. "Recognition: Applications in Aged Care Work." *Cambridge Journal of Economics*, 40, 1037–1054. https://doi.org/10.1093/cje/bev057.

Australian Centre for Robotic Vision. 2018. *A Robotics Roadmap for Australia 2018*. Brisbane: Australian Centre for Robotic Vision. https://apo.org.au/sites/default/files/resource-files/2018-06/apo-nid176691_1.pdf.

Australian Human Rights Commission. 2018. *Human Rights and Technology Issues Paper*. Sydney: Australian Human Rights Commission. https://humanrights.gov.au/our-work/rights-and-freedoms/publications/human-rights-and-technology-issues-paper-2018.

Ayalon, Liat. 2012. "Suicidal and Depressive Symptoms in Filipino Home Care Workers in Israel." *Journal of Cross-Cultural Gerontology* 27 (1): 51–63. https://doi.org/10.1007/s10823-011-9156-8.

Baldassar, Loretta. 2007. "Transnational Families and Aged Care: The Mobility of Care and the Migrancy of Ageing." *Journal of Ethnic and Migration Studies* 33 (2): 275–297.

———. 2014. "Too Sick to Move: Distant 'Crisis' Care in Transnational Families." *International Review of Sociology* 24 (3): 391–405.

———. 2016. "De-demonizing Distance in Mobile Family Lives: Co-presence, Care Circulation and Polymedia as Vibrant Matter." *Global Networks* 16 (2): 145–163.

Baldassar, Loretta, Mihaela Nedelcu, Laura Merla, and Raelene Wilding. 2016. "ICT-Based Co-Presence in Transnational Families and Communities: Challenging the Premise of Face-to-Face Proximity in Sustaining Relationships." *Global Networks* 16 (2): 133–144.

Banerjee, Rupa, Philip Kelly, Ethel Tungohan, GABRIELA-Ontario, Migrante-Canada and Community Alliance for Social Justice. 2017. *Assessing the Changes to Canada's Live-in-Caregiver Program: Improving Security or Deepening Precariousness?* Pathways to Prosperity Project, December. http://p2pcanada.ca/files/2017/12/Assessing-the-Changes-to-Canadas-Live-In-Caregiver-Program.pdf.

Bango, Julio. 2020. Cuidados en América Latina y el Caribe en Tiempos de COVID-19. Hacia Sistemas Integrales para fortalecer la respuesta y la recuperación. BRIEF v 1.1. 19.08.2020, ONU Mujeres, ECLAC.

Bárcena, Alicia. 2020. *Latin America Is the World's Most Unequal Region: Here's How to Fix It.* Santiago: ECLAC.

Barnett, Michael L., and David C. Grabowski. 2020. "Nursing Homes Are Ground Zero for COVID-19 Pandemic." *JAMA Health Forum* 1 (3). https://doi.org/10.1001/jamahealthforum .2020.0369.

Barnett, Steven, and Kwanghee Jung. 2020. *Understanding and Responding to the Pandemic's Impacts on Preschool Education: What Can We Learn from Last Spring?* New Brunswick, NJ: National Institute for Early Education Research.

Barnett, Steven, Kwanghee Jung, and Milagros Nores. 2020. *Young Children's Home Learning and Preschool Participation Experiences during the Pandemic.* New Brunswick, NJ: National Institute for Early Education Research.

Barry, Michael, and Adrian Wilkinson. 2016. "Pro-social or Pro-management? A Critique of the Conception of Employee Voice as a Pro-social Behaviour within Organizational Behaviour." *British Journal of Industrial Relations* 54 (2): 261–284. https://doi.org/10.1111/bjir .12114.

Bartlett, Lora. 2004. "Expanding Teacher Work Roles: A Resource for Retention or a Recipe for Overwork?" *Journal of Education Policy* 19 (5): 565–582.

Bassok, Daphna, Molly Michie, Deiby Mayaris Cubides-Mateus, Justin B. Doromal, and Sarah Kiscaden. 2020. *The Divergent Experiences of Early Educators in Schools and Child Care Centers during COVID-19: Findings from Virginia.* Virginia: EdPolicyWorks.

Bassok, Daphna, Amy E. Smith, Anna J. Markowitz, and Justin B. Doromal. 2021. *Child Care Staffing Challenges during the Pandemic: Lessons from Child Care Leaders in Louisiana.* Virginia: EdPolicyWorks.

Bastidas Aliaga, María. 2021 "Gender Inequality during the Pandemic: Perspectives of Women Workers in Latin America and the Caribbean." *International Journal of Labour Research* 10 (1–2): 92–106.

Baughman, Reagan A., Bryce Stanley, and Kristin E. Smith. 2020. "Second Job Holding among Direct Care Workers and Nurses: Implications for COVID-19 Transmission in Long-Term Care." *Medical Care Research and Review* 79 (1): 151–160.

Baxter, Mary. 2020. "Why Don't We Know How Many Home-Care Workers have COVID-19?" TVO, July 15. https://www.tvo.org/article/why-dont-we-know-how-many-home-care -workers-have-covid-19.

Belanger, Daniele, and Rachel Silvey, eds. 2020. "An Im/mobility Turn: Power Geometries of Care and Migration." Special issue, *Journal of Ethnic and Migration Studies* 46 (16): 3423–3440. https://doi.org/10.1080/1369183X.2019.1592396.

Bengali, Shashank, and Ralph Jennings. 2020. "These Governments Tamed COVID-19: They're Keeping Social Distancing in Place." *Los Angeles Times*, November 17. https://www.latimes .com/world-nation/story/2020-06-17/social-distancing-remains-as-asia-eases-covid-19 -lockdowns.

Benjamin, Orly. 2016. *Gendering Israel's Outsourcing: The Erasure of Employees' Caring Skills.* New York: Palgrave-McMillan.

Bennie, Garth. 2020. *NZDSN Submission Notes for Epidemic Response Committee.* Wellington, New Zealand: New Zealand Disability Support Network.

Berckmoes, Lidewyde H., and Valentina Mazzucato. 2018. "Resilience among Nigerian Transnational Parents in the Netherland: A Strength-Based Approach to Migration and Transnational Parenting." *Global Networks* 18 (4): 589–607.

Berdot, Sarah, Virginie Savoldelli, Vincent Zaugg, Emmanuel Jaccoulet, Patrice Prognon, Laeticia Minh, Maï Lê, and Brigitte Sabatier. 2016. "Return on Investment after Implementation of a Centralized Automated Storage System in a Hosptial Pharmacy." *Journal of Pharmacy and Pharmacology*, 4, 526–532.

Bernstein, Hamutal, Michael Karpman, Dulce Gonzalez, and Stephen Zuckerman. 2020. *Immigrant Families Hit Hard by the Pandemic May Be Afraid to Receive the Help They Need.* Urban

Institute. https://www.urban.org/urban-wire/immigrant-families-hit-hard-pandemic-may
-be-afraid-receive-help-they-need.

Bettio, Francesca, and Janneke Plantenga. 2004. "Comparative Care Regimes in Europe." *Feminist Economics* 10 (1): 85–113.

Bhaskar, Ranjit. 2020. "Looking Ahead: What Immigrant Health Workers on the Frontlines Mean for Canada." New Canadian Media, September 4. https://newcanadianmedia.ca/looking-ahead-what-immigrant-health-workers-on-the-front-lines-mean-for-canada/.

Binkley, Charles E., and David S. Kemp. 2020. "Ethical Rationing of Personal Protective Equipment to Minimize Moral Residue during the Covid-19 Pandemic." *Journal of the American College of Surgeons* 230 (6): 1111–1113.

Blofield, Merike, Fernando Filgueira, Cecilia Giambruno, and Juliana Martínez Franzoni. 2021. "Beyond States and Markets: Families and Family Regimes in Latin America." In *Latin American Social Policy Developments in the Twentieth-First Century*, edited by Natálya Sátiro, Eloísa del Pino, and Carmen Midaglia, 255–285. London: Palgrave.

Blofield, Merike, Cecilia Giambruno, and Fernando Filgueira. 2020. *Policy Expansion in Compressed Time: Assessing the Speed, Breadth and Sufficiency of Post-COVID-19 Social Protection Measures in 10 Latin American Countries.* Santiago de Chile: ECLAC.

Blofield, Merike, and Michael Touchton. 2019. "Moving Away from Maternalism? The Politics of Parental Leave Reforms in Latin America." *Comparative Politics* 53 (1): 1–24.

Blum, Sonja, and Ivana Dobrotić. 2021. "Childcare-Policy Responses in the COVID-19 Pandemic: Unpacking Cross-Country Variation." *European Societies* 23 (1): 545–563.

Boniol, Mathieu; Michelle McIsaac, Lihui Xu, Tana Wuliji, Khassoum Diallo, and Jim Campbell. 2019. "Gender Equity in the Health Workforce: Analysis of 104 Countries." Health Workforce Working paper 1. World Health Organization. https://apps.who.int/iris/handle/10665/311314.

Bourgeault, Ivy. 2015. "Double Isolation: Immigrants and Older Adult Care Work in Canada." In *Caring on the Clock: The Complexities and Contradictions of Paid Care Work*, edited by Mignon Duffy, Amy Armenia, and Clare L. Stacey, 117–126. New Brunswick, NJ: Rutgers University Press.

Bowden, Olivia. 2020. "More Canadian Women Have COVID-19 and Are Dying as a Result: Here's Some Possible Reasons Why." *Global News.* https://globalnews.ca/news/6920505/more-women-have-coronavirus/.

Branch, Enobong. 2011. *Opportunity Denied: Limiting Black Women to Devalued Work.* New Brunswick, NJ: Rutgers University Press.

Braunstein, Elissa, Stephanie Seguino, and Levi Altringer. 2019. "Estimating the Role of Social Reproduction in Economic Growth." CWE-GAM Working Paper Series 19-02, April. https://doi.org/10.17606/rv6p-6f66.

Brewster, Amanda L., Traci L. Wilson, Suzanne R. Kunkel, Sandy Markwood, and Tanya B. Shah. 2020. "To Support Older Adults amidst the COVID-19 Pandemic, Look to Area Agencies on Aging." *Health Affairs* (blog), April 8. https://www.healthaffairs.org/do/10.1377/hblog20200408.928642/full/.

Broughton, Cate. 2020. "Coronavirus: Home Care Workers Stockpiling Masks, Gloves and Hand Sanitiser." Stuff. https://www.stuff.co.nz/national/health/coronavirus/120412322/coronavirus-home-care-workers-stockpiling-masks-gloves-and-hand-sanitiser.

Brown, Catherine, Ulrich Boser, and Perpetual Baffour. 2016. *Workin' 9 to 5: How School Schedules Make Life Harder for Working Parents.* Center for American Progress Report, October 11. https://www.americanprogress.org/issues/education-k-12/reports/2016/10/11/145084/workin-9-to-5-2/

Brown, Wendy. 2015. *Undoing the Demos: Neoliberalism's Stealth Revolution.* Brooklyn: Zone Books.
———. 2019. *In the Ruins of Neoliberalism.* New York: Columbia University Press.

Bryceson, Deborah, and Ulla Vuorela. 2002. "Transnational Families in the Twentieth-First Century." In *The Transnational Families: New European Frontiers and Global Networks*, edited by Deborah Bryceson and Ulla Vuorela, 3–30. New York: Berg.

Budig, Michelle J., Melissa J. Hodges, and Paula England. 2019. "Wages of Nurturant and Reproductive Care Workers: Individual and Job Characteristics, Occupational Closure, and Wage-Equalizing Institutions." *Social Problems* 66 (2): 294–319. https://doi.org/10.1093/socpro/spy007.

Bujard, Martin, Inga Laß, Sabine Diabaté, Harun Sulak, and Norbert F. Schneider. 2020. *Eltern während der Corona-Krise: Zur Improvisation gezwungen.* Wiesbaden: Bundesinstitut für Bevölkerungsforschung.

Bureau of Labor Statistics (BLS). 2021. *Labor Force Statistics from the Current Population Survey.* https://www.bls.gov/cps/cpsaat11.htm.

Burwick, Andrew, Elizabeth Davis, Lynn Karoly, Theresa Schulte, and Kathryn Tout. 2020. "Promoting Sustainability of Child Care Programs during the COVID-19 Pandemic: Considerations for States in Allocating Financial Resources." Special Topics Paper. Mathematica. https://www.acf.hhs.gov/opre/report/promoting-sustainability-child-care-programs-during-covid-19-pandemic.

Button, Kirsty. 2017. "The Impact of Intergenerational Negotiations and Power Dynamics on the Burden of Care Experienced by Low-Income Grandmothers." CSSR Working Paper 400, Centre for Social Science Research, University of Cape Town.

Byrne, Gary. 2018. "Prevalence and Psychological Sequelae of Sexual Abuse among Individuals with an Intellectual Disability: A Review of the Recent Literature." *Journal of Intellectual Disabilities* 22 (3): 294–310.

Cain, Cindy L. 2015. "Orienting End-of-Life Care: The Hidden Value of Hospice Home Visits." In *Caring on the Clock: The Complexities and Contradictions of Paid Care Work*, edited by Mignon Duffy, Amy Armenia, and Clare L. Stacey, 67–78. New Brunswick, NJ: Rutgers University Press.

———. 2019. "Agency and Change in Healthcare Organizations: Workers' Attempts to Navigate Multiple Logics in Hospice Care." *Journal of Health and Social Behavior* 60 (1): 3–17.

Calarco, Jessica M., Emily Meanwell, Elizabeth Anderson, and Amelia Knopf. 2020. "Let's Not Pretend It's Fun": How Disruptions to Families' School and Childcare Arrangements Impact Mothers' Well-Being." *SocArXiv* Preprint. https://doi.org/10.31235/osf.io/jyvk4.

Campbell, Fernanda Q., Pratima A. Patil, and Kristin McSwain. 2020. "Boston's Child-Care Supply Crisis: What a Pandemic Reveals." Boston: The Boston Foundation.

Canada. 2020. *A Stronger and More Resilient Canada: The Speech from the Throne.* September 23. https://www.canada.ca/en/privy-council/campaigns/speech-throne/2020/speech-from-the-throne.html.

———. 2021. *Legislation to Provide Ten Days of Paid Sick Leave and Enhance Protections for Health Care Workers Receives Royal Assent.* https://www.canada.ca/en/employment-social-development/news/2021/12/legislation-to-provide-ten-days-of-paid-sick-leave-and-enhance-protections-for-health-care-workers-receives-royal-assent.html.

———. n.d. *Pathways for Caregivers.* Accessed May 24, 2022. https://www.canada.ca/en/immigration-refugees-citizenship/corporate/publications-manuals/operational-bulletins-manuals/permanent-residence/economic-classes/pathways-for-caregivers.html#pr-1.

Canada-National Defence. 2020. "Update on Canadian Armed Forces' Response to COVID-19 Pandemic." May 7. https://www.canada.ca/en/department-national-defence/news/2020/05/update-on-canadian-armed-forces-response-to-covid-19-pandemic.html.

Canadian Broadcasting Corporation (CBC). 2014. "Changes Needed for Canada's Live-In Caregiver Program." *CBC News*, August 14. https://www.cbc.ca/news/canada/manitoba/changes-needed-for-canada-s-live-in-caregiver-program-1.2736840.

Canadian Institute for Health Information (CIHI). 2020. "Pandemic Experience in the Long-Term Care Sector: How Does Canada Compare with Other Countries?" CIHI, June. https://www.cihi.ca/sites/default/files/document/covid-19-rapid-response-long-term-care-snapshot-en.pdf.

Canadian Press and News Staff. 2021. "Ontario to Allow Fully-Vaccinated Long-Term Care Staff to Work in More Than One Facility." City News Everywhere, April 24. https://toronto.citynews.ca/2021/04/24/ontario-to-allow-fully-vaccinated-long-term-care-staff-to-work-in-more-than-one-facility/.

Carbone, June, and Naomi Cahn. 2014. *Marriage Markets: How Inequality Is Remaking the American Family*. New York: Oxford University Press.

The Care Collective, Andreas Chatzidakis, Jamie Hakim, Jo Littler, Catherine Rottenberg, and Lynne Segal. 2020. *The Care Manifesto: The Politics of Interdependence*. London: Verso.

Caregivers' Action Centre, Vancouver Committee for Domestic Workers and Caregivers' Rights, Caregiver Connections, Education and Support Organization, Migrant Workers Alliance for Change. 2020. *Behind Closed Doors: Exposing Migrant Care Worker Exploitation during COVID-19*. October. https://migrantrights.ca/wp-content/uploads/2020/10/Behind-Closed-Doors_Exposing-Migrant-Care-Worker-Exploitation-During-COVID19.pdf.

care-macht-mehr.com. 2020. "Clean Up Time! Redesigning Care after Corona." https://care-macht-mehr.com/clean-up-time-redesigning-care-after-corona/.

Carli, Linda L. 2020. "Women, Gender Equality and COVID-19." *Gender in Management* 35 (7/8): 647–655.

Carlson, Daniel L, Richard Petts, and Joanna Pepin. 2020. "Changes in Parents' Domestic Labor during the COVID-19 Pandemic." *SocArXiv*, May 6. doi:10.1111/soin.12459.

Casey, V. 2021. "Home Care Facing Crisis following Worker Exodus: Ontario Has Seen over 3,000 Skilled Staff Leave for Other Health-Care Jobs." *Toronto Star Toronto*, November 1, 2021, A.3.

Center for Public Representation. 2020. "Money Follows the Person Receives Short-Term Funding as Part of COVID-19 Relief Package." https://medicaid.publicrep.org/feature/money-follows-the-person/.

Center on Reinventing Public Education (CRPE). 2020. *Fall 2020: The State of School Reopening*. Center on Reinventing Public Education. https://www.crpe.org/current-research/covid-19-school-closures.

Centers for Disease Control and Prevention (CDC). 2019. "CDC: 1 in 4 US Adults Live with a Disability | CDC Online Newsroom | CDC." https://www.cdc.gov/media/releases/2018/p0816-disability.html.

———. 2020a. "COVID-19 Racial and Ethnic Health Disparities." https://www.cdc.gov/coronavirus/2019-ncov/community/health-equity/racial-ethnic-disparities/disparities-deaths.html.

———. 2020b. "Interim Operational Considerations for Public Health Management of Healthcare Workers Exposed to or with Suspected or Confirmed COVID-19: Non-U.S. Healthcare Settings." https://www.cdc.gov/coronavirus/2019-ncov/hcp/non-us-settings/public-health-management-hcw-exposed.html.

Centers for Medicare & Medicaid Services (CMS). 2020a. "Coronavirus Commission on Safety and Quality in Nursing Homes." Baltimore, MD: U.S. Centers for Medicare and Medicaid Services. Accessed October 12, 2022. https://www.cms.gov/files/document/covid-final-nh-commission-report.pdf.

———. 2020b. *COVID-19 Nursing Home Data*. Baltimore, MD: Department of Health and Human Services.

———. 2020c. "Hospice: CMS Flexibilities to Fight Covid-19." Baltimore, MD: U.S. Centers for Medicare and Medicaid Services.

Cha, Ariana Eunjung. 2020. "Quadriplegic Man's Death from Covid-19 Spotlights Race, Disability and Family." *Washington Post*, July 7. https://www.washingtonpost.com/health/2020/07/05/coronavirus-disability-death/.

Chami, Ralph, Ekkehard Ernst, Connel Fullenkamp, and Anne Oaking. 2018. "Is There a Remittance Trap?" *Finance & Development*, September, 44–47. https://www.imf.org/external/pubs/ft/fandd/2018/09/is-there-a-remittance-trap-chami.htm.

Charlesworth, Sara, and Jenny Malone. 2017. "Re-Imagining Decent Work for Home-care Workers in Australia." *Labor and Industry* 27 (4): 284–301.

Chaudry, Ajay, Taryn Morissey, Christina Weiland, and Hirokazu Yoshikawa. 2017. *Cradle to Kindergarten: A New Plan to Combat Inequality.* 2nd ed. New York, NY: Russell Sage Foundation.

Chazan, May. 2015. *The Grandmothers' Movement: Solidarity and Survival in the Time of AIDS.* Montreal, QC: McGill-Queen's University Press.

Checkpoint. 2020. "Covid-19 Lockdown: Rest Home Staff Move in with Residents." Radio New Zealand. https://www.rnz.co.nz/national/programmes/checkpoint/audio/2018741276/covid-19-lockdown-rest-home-staff-move-in-with-residents.

Christ, Amber, and Tracey Gronniger. 2018. "Older Women & Poverty." Justice in Aging, December. https://www.justiceinaging.org/wp-content/uploads/2018/12/Older-Women-and-Poverty.pdf.

Chun, Jennifer Jihye, Cynthia Cranford, Yang-sook Kim, and Jennifer Nazareno. Forthcoming. "Confronting Servitude within the Welfare State: Homecare Labor Markets and Asian Immigrant Women Workers." *Signs: Journal of Women in Culture and Society.*

Ciobanu, Ruxandra Oana, Tineke Fokkema, and Mihaela Nedelcu. 2017. "Ageing as a Migrant: Vulnerabilities, Agency and Policy Implications." *Journal of Ethnic and Migration Studies* 43 (2): 164–181.

Clair, Robin, P. 1998. *Organizing Silence: A World of Possibilities.* New York: SUNY Press.

Coffey, Clare, Patricia Espinoza Revollo, Rowan Harvey, Max Lawson, Anam Parvez Butt, Kim Piaget, Diana Sarosi, and Julie Thekkudan. 2020. *Time to Care: Unpaid and Underpaid Care Work and the Global Inequality Crisis.* London: Oxfam.

Cohen, Barney, and Jane Menken. 2006. "Executive Summary." In *Aging in Sub-Saharan Africa: Recommendations for Furthering Research*, edited by Barney Cohen and Jane Menken, 1–8. Washington, DC: The National Academies Press.

Cohen, Jeffrey H. 2011. "Migration, Remittances, and Household Strategies." *Annual Review of Anthropology* 40 (1): 103–114.

Cohen, Rhaina. 2015. "Who Took Care of Rosie the Riveter's Kids?" *The Atlantic*, November 18. https://www.theatlantic.com/business/archive/2015/11/daycare-world-war-rosie-riveter/415650/.

Collins, Caitlyn, Liana Christin Landivar, Leah Ruppanner, and William J. Scarborough. 2021a. "COVID-19 and the Gender Gap in Work Hours." *Gender, Work & Organization* 28 (S1): 101–112.

Collins, Caitlyn, Leah Ruppanner, Liana Christin Landivar, and William J Scarborough. 2021b. "The Gendered Consequences of a Weak Infrastructure of Care: School Reopening Plans and Parents' Employment During the COVID-19 Pandemic." *Gender & Society* 35 (2): 180–193.

Comas-Herrera, Adelina, Joseba Zalakaín, Elizabeth Lemmon, David Henderson, Charles Litwin, Amy T. Hsu, Andrea E. Schmidt, Greg Arling, and Jose-Luis Fernández. 2020. *Mortality Associated with COVID-19 in Care Homes: International.* International Long-Term Care Network. Last updated October 14, 2020. https://ltccovid.org/wp-content/uploads/2020/10/Mortality-associated-with-COVID-among-people-living-in-care-homes-14-October-2020-3.pdf.

Commission on a Gender Equal Economy. 2020. *Creating a Caring Economy: A Call to Action.* London: Women's Budget Group. https://wbg.org.uk/wp-content/uploads/2020/10/WBG -Report-v10.pdf.

Comunidad Mujer. 2020. Estadísticas de Género. https://www.comunidadmujer.cl/estudios /estadisticas-de-genero/.

Congressional Budget Office. 2015. *Rising Demand for Long-Term Services and Supports for Elderly People.* Washington, DC: Congressional Budget Office. https://www.cbo.gov/publication /44363.

Contenta, Sandro. 2020. "A Young Boy's Home-care Needs Highlight the Dangers of Spreading COVID-19." *Toronto Star,* April 11. https://www.thestar.com/news/canada/2020/04/11/a -young-boys-home-care-needs-highlight-the-dangers-of-spreading-covid-19.html.

Conway, Claire. 2015. "Poor Health: When Poverty Becomes Disease." UC San Francisco, January. https://www.ucsf.edu/news/2016/01/401251/poor-health-when-poverty-becomes-disease.

Cook, Joan M., Casey O'Donnell, Stephanie Dinnen, James C Coyne, Josef I Ruzek, and Paula P. Schnurr. 2012. "Measurement of a Model of Implementation for Health Care: Toward a Testable Theory." *Implementation Science,* 7, 59.

Cookney, Franki. 2020. "Sex Dolls Sales Surge in Quarantine, but It's Not Just About Loneliness." *Forbes,* May 21. https://www.forbes.com/sites/frankicookney/2020/05/21/sex-doll -sales-surge-in-quarantine-but-its-not-just-about-loneliness/#27cadff217of.

Craig, Lyn. 2020. "Coronavirus, Domestic Labour and Care: Gendered Roles Locked Down." *Journal of Sociology* 56 (4): 684–692.

Craig, Lyn, and Brendan Churchill. 2021. "Dual-Earner Parent Couples' Work and Care during COVID-19." *Gender, Work & Organization,* 28, 66–79.

Cranford, Cynthia J. 2020. *Home Care Fault Lines: Understanding Tensions and Creating Alliances.* Ithaca, NY: ILR Press.

Cranford, Cynthia, and Jennifer Jihye Chun. Forthcoming. "Multi-level Analysis of Home-Care Labor." In *Research Handbook on Intersectionality,* edited by Mary Romero and Reshawna Chapple.

Cranford, Cynthia, Angela Hick, and Louise Birdsell Bauer. 2018. "Lived Experiences of Social Unionism: Toronto Homecare Workers in the late 2000s." *Labor Studies Journal* 43 (1): 74–96.

Cranford, Cynthia, and Diana Miller. 2013. "Emotion Management from the Client's Perspective: The Case of Personal Home-care." *Work, Employment and Society* 27 (5): 785–801.

Crawford, April, Kelly A. Vaughn, Cathy L. Guttentag, Cheryl Varghese, Yoonkyung Oh, and Tricia A. Zucker. 2021. "'Doing What I Can, but I Got No Magic Wand': A Snapshot of Early Childhood Educator Experiences and Efforts to Ensure Quality during the COVID-19 Pandemic." *Early Childhood Education Journal* 49 (5): 829–840. https://doi.org/10.1007/s10643 -021-01215-z.

Crawly, Mike. 2021. "Ontario's COVID-19 Paid Sick Days to Extend into 2022." *CBC News,* December 7. https://www.cbc.ca/news/canada/toronto/covid-19-ontario-paid-sick-days-extension-1 .6276367.

Crețan, Remus, and Duncan Light. 2020. "COVID-19 in Romania: Transnational Labour, Geopolitics, and the Roma 'Outsiders.'" *Eurasian Geography and Economics* 61 (4–5): 559–572. https://doi.org/ 10.1080/15387216.2020.1780929.

CTV News. 2021. "'They Are Not Machines': Deaths of Health-Care Workers Underline the Strain of COVID-19." January 7. https://www.ctvnews.ca/health/coronavirus/they-re-not -machines-deaths-of-health-care-workers-underline-the-strain-of-covid-19-1.5258509.

Curtis, J. Randall, Erin K. Kross, and Renee D. Stapleton. 2020. "The Importance of Addressing Advance Care Planning and Decisions about Do-Not-Resuscitate Orders during Novel Coronavirus 2019 (Covid-19)." *JAMA* 323 (18): 1771–1772.

Cuthbertson, Anthony. 2020. "Coronavirus: 'Little Peanut' Robot Delivers Food to People in Quarantine." *Independent*, January 29. https://www.independent.co.uk/life-style/gadgets -and-tech/news/coronavirus-quarantine-robot-china-little-peanut-food-delivery -a9308166.html.

Czymara, Christian S., Alexander Langenkamp, and Tomás Cano. 2020. "Cause for Concerns: Gender Inequality in Experiencing the COVID-19 Lockdown in Germany." *European Societies* 23 (S1): S68-S81. https://doi.org/10.1080/14616696.2020.1808692.

Da, Wei Wei. 2003. "Transnational| Grandparenting: Childcare Arrangements among Migrants from the People's Republic of China to Australia." *Journal of International Migration & Integration* 4 (1): 79–103.

Daily, Sarah, and Asiya Kazi. 2020. *Supporting Families and Child Care Providers during the Pandemic with a Focus on Equity*. Washington, DC: Child Trends.

Daly, Tamara. 2015. "Dancing the Two-step in Ontario's Long-Term Care Sector: More Deterrence-Oriented Regulation=Ownership and Management Consolidation." *Studies in Political Economy* 95 (1): 29–58.

Daly, Tamara, Pat Armstrong, and Ruth Lowndes. 2015. "Liminality in Ontario Long-Term Care Facilities: Private Companions Work in the Space 'Betwixt and Between.'" *Competition and Change* 9 (3): 246–263.

Daly, Tamara, and Marta Szebehely. 2012. "Unheard Voices, Unmapped Terrain: Care Work in Long-Term Residential Care for Older People in Canada and Sweden." *International Journal of Social Welfare* 21 (2): 139–148.

Dang, Hai-Anh H., and Cuong Viet Nguyen. 2020. "Gender Inequality during the COVID-19 Pandemic: Income, Expenditure, Savings, and Job Loss." *World Development* 140 (April): 105296.

D'Arcy, Laura P., Yasuko Sasai, and Sally C. Stearns. 2012. "Do Assistive Devices, Training, and Workload Affect Injury Incidence? Prevention Efforts by Nursing Homes and Back Injuries among Nursing Assistants." *Journal of Advanced Nursing* 68 (4): 836–845. https://doi .org/10.1111/j.1365-2648.2011.05785.x.

Datta, A. Rupa, and Joshua Borton. 2020. *How Much of Children's Early Care and Education Participation in 2012 Was Publicly Funded?* OPRE Report #2020-69. National Survey of Early Care and Education at the University of Chicago.

Dayen, David. 2020. "An Interview with Ai-jen Poo." The American Prospect, October 21. https://prospect.org/familycare/an-interview-with-ai-jen-poo/.

De Henau, Jerome, and Susan Himmelweit. 2020 "The Gendered Employment Gains of Investing in Social vs. Physical Infrastructure: Evidence from Simulations across Seven OECD Countries." IKD Working Paper 84, April. http://www.open.ac.uk/ikd/sites/www.open.ac .uk.ikd/files/files/working-papers/DeHenauApril2020v3.pdf.

Dean, Adam, Atheendar Venkataramani, and Simeon Kimmel. 2020. "Mortality Rates from Covid-19 Are Lower in Unionized Nursing Homes: Study Examines Mortality Rates in New York Nursing Homes." *Health Affairs* 39 (11). https://doi.org/10.1377/hlthaff.2020.01011.

Deetz, Stanley A. 1992. *Democracy in an Age of Corporate Colonization: Developments in Communication and the Politics of Everyday Life*. New York: SUNY Press.

Delp, Linda, and Katie Quan. 2002. "Homecare Worker Organizing in California: An Analysis of a Successful Strategy." *Labor Studies Journal* 27 (1): 1–23.

Diliberti, Melissa Kay, and Julia H. Kaufman. 2020. *Will This School Year Be Another Casualty of the Pandemic? Key Findings from the American Educator Panels Fall 2020 COVID-19 Surveys*. RRA168-4. Santa Monica, CA: RAND Corporation. https://www.rand.org/pubs/research _reports/RRA168-4.html.

Dill, Janette, Odichinma Akosionu, J'Mag Karbeah, and Carrie Henning-Smith. 2020. "Addressing Systemic Racial Inequity in the Health Care Workforce." *Health Affairs* (blog), September 10. https://www.healthaffairs.org/do/10.1377/hblog20200908.133196/full/.

Dill, Janette, and Melissa J. Hodges. 2019. "Is Healthcare the New Manufacturing? Industry, Gender, and 'Good Jobs' for Low- and Middle-Skill Workers." *Social Science Research* 84 (November): 102350. https://doi.org/10.1016/j.ssresearch.2019.102350.

Dobson, Sarah. 2021. "Ontario Conservatives Vote Down Paid Sick Days." HRReporter, April 26. https://www.hrreporter.com/focus-areas/compensation-and-benefits/ontario-conservatives-vote-down-paid-sick-days/355346.

Dodson, Lisa, and Rebekah M. Zincavage. 2007. "'It's Like a Family': Caring Labor, Exploitation, and Race in Nursing Homes." *Gender & Society* 21 (6): 905–928. https://doi.org/10.1177/0891243207309899.

Doffman, Zak. 2020. "This New Coronavirus Spy Drone Will Make Sure You Stay at Home." *Forbes*, March 5. https://www.forbes.com/sites/zakdoffman/2020/03/05/meet-the-coronavirus-spy-drones-that-make-sure-you-stay-home/#26e437061669.

Donaghey, Jimmy, Niall Cullinane, Tony Dundon, and Adrian Wilkinson. 2011. "Reconceptualising Employee Silence: Problems and Prognosis." *Work, Employment and Society* 25 (1): 51–67. https://doi.org/10.1177/0950017010389239.

Doolittle, Robyn. 2020. "Ontario Long-Term Care Homes Warn They Are Not Equipped to Handle Second COVID-19 Wave." *Globe and Mail*, September 21. https://www.theglobeandmail.com/canada/article-ontario-long-term-care-homes-warn-they-are-not-equipped-to-handle/.

Doucet, Andrea, and Pat Armstrong. 2021. "A Conversation with Pat Armstrong about Creative Team Work: Developing Rapid Site-Switching Ethnography." *Families, Relationships and Societies* 10 (1): 179–188.

Douglas, Julie, and Katherine Ravenswood. 2019. *The Value of Care: Understanding the Impact of the 2017 Pay Equity Settlement on the Residential Aged Care, Home and Community Care and Disability Support Sectors.* Auckland, New Zealand: New Zealand Work Research Institute.

Dreby, Joanna. 2010. *Divided by Borders: Mexican Migrants and Their Children.* Berkeley: University of California Press.

Duffy, Mignon. 2005. "Reproducing Labor Inequalities: Challenges for Feminists Conceptualizing Care at the Intersections of Gender, Race and Class." *Gender & Society*, 19 (1): 66–82.

———. 2007. "Doing the Dirty Work: Gender, Race, and Reproductive Labor in Historical Perspective." *Gender & Society* 21 (3): 313–336.

———. 2010. "'We Are the Union': Care Work, Unions, and Social Movements." *Humanity and Society* 34 (2): 125–140.

———. 2011. *Making Care Count: A Century of Gender, Race, and Paid Care Work.* New Brunswick, NJ: Rutgers University Press.

Duffy, Mignon, Randy Albelda, and Clare Hammonds. 2013. "Counting Care Work: The Empirical and Policy Applications of Care Theory." *Social Problems* 60 (2): 145–167.

Duffy, Mignon, Amy Armenia, and Clare L. Stacey. eds. 2015a. *Caring on the Clock: The Complexities and Contradictions of Paid Care Work.* New Brunswick, NJ.: Rutgers University Press.

Duffy, Mignon, Amy Armenia, and Clare Stacey. 2015b. "Making Paid Care Work." In *Caring on the Clock: The Complexities and Contradictions of Paid Care Work*, edited by Mignon Duffy, Amy Armenia, and Clare L. Stacey, 287–291. New Jersey: Rutgers University Press.

Dugarova, Esuna. 2020. *Unpaid Care Work in Times of the COVID-19 Crisis: Gendered Impacts, Emerging Evidence and Promising Policy Responses.* Report prepared for the UN Expert Group meeting Families in Development: Assessing Progress, Challenges and Emerging Issues. Focus on Modalities for IYF+30. https://www.un.org/development/desa/family/wp-content/uploads/sites/23/2020/09/Duragova.Paper_.pdf.

Durán, María-Ángeles. 2008. "Diez buenas razones para medir el trabajo no remunerado en el cuidado de la salud. In *La economía invisible y las desigualdades de género. La importancia de medir y valorar el trabajo no remunerado*, 147–148. Washington, DC: Editora.

Dworkin, Anthony Gary. 2008. "School Reform and Teacher Burnout." In *Schools and Society: A Sociological Approach to Education*, edited by Jeanne H. Ballantine and Joan Z. Spade, 119–126. Los Angeles, CA: Pine Forge Press.

Dwyer, Rachel E. 2013. "The Care Economy? Gender, Economic Restructuring, and Job Polarization in the U.S. Labor Market." *American Sociological Review* 78 (3): 390–416.

E tū, and New Zealand Nurses Organisation. 2019. *In Safe Hands?—a 2019 Report into Aged Care Staffing.* https://www.flexmediagroup.co.nz/in-safe-hands/index.html.

Eaton, Joe. 2020. "COVID Crisis in Long-Term Care: Who Is to Blame?" AARP. http://www.aarp.org/caregiving/health/info-2020/covid-19-nursing-homes-who-is-to-blame.html.

Eaton, Liberty, Alan J. Flisher, and Leif E. Aarø. 2003. "Unsafe Sexual Behaviour in South African Youth." *Social Science and Medicine* 56 (1):149–165.

Economic Commission for Latin America and the Caribbean (ECLAC). 2013. *Social Panorama of Latin America 2012.* (LC/G.2557-P). Santiago, Chile.

———. 2014. *Social Panorama of Latin America, 2013.* (LC/G.2557-P). Santiago, Chile.

———. 2016. *Equality and Women's Autonomy in the Sustainable Development Agenda.* (LC/G.2686/Rev.1). Santiago, Chile.

———. 2017. *Social Panorama of Latin America 2016.* (LC/PUB.2017/12-P). Santiago, Chile.

———. 2019. *Latin American Economic Outlook 2019: Development in Transition.* (LC/PUB.2019/14). Santiago, Chile.

———. 2020a. *Care in Latin America and the Caribbean during the COVID-19: Towards Comprehensive Systems to Strengthen Response and Recovery.* Santiago, Chile.

———. 2020b. *Economic Survey of Latin America and the Caribbean: Main Conditioning Factors of Fiscal and Monetary Policies in the Post-COVID-19 Era.* (LC/PUB.2020/12-PS). Santiago, Chile.

———. 2020c. *Observatorio COVID-19 en América Latina y el Caribe.* https://www.cepal.org/es/temas/covid-19.

———. 2021. *The Recovery Paradox in Latin America and the Caribbean Growth amid Persisting Structural Problems: Inequality, Poverty and Low Investment and Productivity.* Special Report N11. Santiago, Chile.

Economic Commission for Latin America and the Caribbean and Pan American Health Organization (ECLAC and PAHO). 2021. *The Prolongation of the Health Crisis and Its Impact on Health, the Economy and Social Development.* COVID-19 Report. Santiago, Chile.

Educators for Excellence. 2020. "Voices from the Virtual Classroom: A Survey of America's Teachers on COVID-19 Related Education Issues." Educators for Excellence. e4e.org/virtualvoices.

EdWeek. 2020. *Survey Tracker: Monitoring How K–12 Educators Are Responding to Coronavirus.* EdWeek Research Center, April. https://www.edweek.org/teaching-learning/survey-tracker-monitoring-how-k-12-educators-are-responding-to-coronavirus/2020/04.

Ehrenreich, Barbara, and Deidre English. 1979. *For Her Own Good: 150 Years of Experts' Advice to Women.* Garden City, NY: Anchor Books.

Ehrenreich, Barbara, and Arlie R. Hochschild, eds. 2003. *Global Women: Nannies, Maids and Sex Workers in the New Economy.* New York: Metropolitan Books.

Eisler, Riane. 2007. La verdadera riqueza de las naciones: Creando una economía de las naciones. La Paz: Fundación Solón.

Ellsberg, Mary, and Myra Betron. 2010. "Preventing Gender-Based Violence and HIV: Lessons from the Field: AIDSTAR-One: Spotlight on Gender." https://aidsfree.usaid.gov/sites/default/files/preventing_gbv_hiv.pdf.

Elson, Diane. 2017. "Recognize, Reduce, and Redistribute Unpaid Care Work: How to Close the Gender Gap." *New Labor Forum* 26 (2): 52–61.

Eng, Susan. 2020. "We Can Do Better Caring for Our Frail and Elderly." *Toronto Star*, contributors opinion, June 24. https://www.thestar.com/opinion/contributors/2020/06/24/we-can-do-better-caring-for-our-frail-and-elderly.html.

England, Paula. 2005. "Emerging Theories of Care Work." *Annual Review of Sociology* 31 (1): 381–399.

England, Paula, Michelle Budig, and Nancy Folbre. 2002. "Wages of Virtue: The Relative Pay of Care Work." *Social Problems* 49 (4): 455–473.

Esquivel, Valeria, and Andrea Kaufmann. 2017. *Innovation in Care: New Concepts, New Actors, New Policies.* Berlin: Friedrich Ebert Stiftung.

Estabrooks, Carole A., Sharon E. Straus, Colleen M. Flood, Janice Keefe, Pat Armstrong, Gail J. Donner, Véronique Boscart, Francine Ducharme, James L. Silvius, and Michael C. Wolfson. 2020. "Restoring Trust: COVID-19 and the Future of Long-Term Care in Canada. *FACETS* 5 (1): 651–691. doi:10.1139/facets-2020-0056.

Etkind, Simon N., Anna E. Bone, Natasha Lovell, Rachel L. Cripps, Richard Harding, Irene J. Higginson, and Katherine E. Sleeman. 2020. "The Role and Response of Palliative Care and Hospice Services in Epidemics and Pandemics: A Rapid Review to Inform Practice during the Covid-19 Pandemic." *Journal of Pain and Symptom Management* 60 (1): e31–e40.

Eurostat. 2020a. "Data on Percent of Part-Time Employed Parents of Children under Six." https://ec .europa.eu/eurostat/databrowser/view/lfst_hhptechi$DV_616/default/table?lang=de.

———. 2020b. "Data on Share of Children under Six in Daycare Facilities." https://ec.europa.eu /urostat/databrowser/view/ilc_caindformal$DV_404/default/table?lang=de.

Ewing-Nelson, Claire. 2020. One in Five Child Care Jobs Have Been Lost Since February, and Women Are Paying the Price. Washington, DC: National Women's Law Center.

Fasani, Francesco, and Jacopo Mazza. 2020. "Immigrant Key Workers: Their Contribution to Europe's COVID-19 Response." IZA Policy Paper 155. https://www.iza.org/publications/pp /155/immigrant-key-workers-their-contribution-to-europes-covid-19-response.

Fearon, Robin. 2021. "Robot Army: Caring Technology Enters Mass Production to Fight Pandemic." Discovery.com. https://www.discovery.com/science/robot-army—caring -technology-enters-mass-production-to-fight-pa.

Feng, Zhiyu, and Krishna Savani. 2020. "Covid-19 Created a Gender Gap in Perceived Work Productivity and Job Satisfaction: Implications for Dual-Career Parents Working from Home." *Gender in Management* 35 (7/8): 719–736.

Ferguson, Rob. 2021. "Ontario For-Profit Nursing Homes Have 78% More COVID Deaths." *Toronto Star*, January 20. https://www.thestar.com/politics/provincial/2021/01/20/ontarios -for-profit-nursing-homes-have-78-more-covid-19-deaths-than-non-profits-report-finds .html.

Filgueira, Fernando, and Juliana Martínez Franzoni. 2017. "The Divergence in Women's Economic Empowerment: Class and Gender under the Pink Tide." *Social Politics* 24 (4): 370–398.

———. 2019. "Growth to Limits of Female Labor Participation in Latin America's Unequal Care Regime." *Social Politics* 26 (2): 245–275.

Flood, Sarah, Miriam King, Renae Rodgers, Steven Ruggles, J. Robert Warren, and Michael Westberry. 2022. Integrated Public Use Microdata Series, Current Population Survey: Version 10.0 (dataset). Minneapolis, MN: IPUMS. https://doi.org/10.18128/D030.V10.0.

Folbre, Nancy. 1994. *Who Pays for the Kids? Gender and the Structure of Constraints.* New York: Routledge.

———. 2006. "Demanding Quality: Worker/Consumer Coalitions and 'High Road' Strategies in the Care Sector." *Politics and Society* 34 (1): 11–31.

Folbre, Nancy, Leila Gautham, and Kristin Smith. 2021. "Essential Workers and the Care Penalty in the U.S." *Feminist Economics* 27 (1–2): 173–187.

Folbre, Nancy, and Julie A. Nelson. 2000. "For Love or Money—or Both?" *Journal of Economic Perspectives* 14 (4): 123–140. https://doi.org/10.1257/jep.14.4.123.

Fox, John. 2006. "'Notice How You Feel': An Alternative to Detached Concern among Hospice Volunteers." *Qualitative Health Research* 16 (7): 944–961.

Franco, Elise. 2020. "Crisis Innovators: 5 Companies Fighting Back against Covid-19." Bizjour-
    nals, August 25. https://www.bizjournals.com/charlotte/inno/stories/inno-insights/2020
    /08/25/meet-five-crisis-innovators-fighting-covid.html.

Frankfurt, Harry G. 1988. *The Importance of What We Care About: Philosophical Essays.* Cam-
    bridge: Cambridge University Press.

Franklin, Paula. 2020. "Our Failure to Prevent Known Risks: Occupational Safety and Health
    in the Healthcare Sector during the COVID-19 Pandemic." ETUI Policy Brief N°11/2020.
    Brussels: European Trade Union Institute (ETUI).

Fraser, Nancy. 1994. "After The Family Wage Gender Equity and the Welfare State." *Political
    Theory* 22 (4): 591–618.

———. 2014. *Transnationalizing the Public Sphere.* Cambridge: Polity Press.

———. 2016. "Progressive Neoliberalism Versus Reactionary Populism: A Choice That Femi-
    nists Should Refuse." *NORA—Nordic Journal of Feminist and Gender Research* 24 (4): 281–284.
    https://doi.org/10.1080/08038740.2016.1278263.

Frederick, Angela, and Dara Shifrer. 2018. "Race and Disability: From Analogy to Inter-
    sectionality." *Sociology of Race and Ethnicity* 5 (2): 200–214. https://doi.org/10.1177/2332
    649218783480.

Freytas-Tamura, Kimiko de. 2020. "'They Call Me a Criminal': Nursing Home Workers Who
    May Spread the Virus." *New York Times*, September 10. https://www.nytimes.com/2020/09
    /10/us/virus-florida-nursing-homes-contract-workers.html.

Friedman, Brittany. 2020. "Carceral Immobility and Financial Capture: A Framework for the
    Consequences of Racial Capitalism." *UCLA Criminal Justice Law Review* 4 (1): 177–185.

Friedman, Carli, and Laura VanPuymbrouck. 2019. "The Relationship between Disability Prej-
    udice and Medicaid Home and Community-Based Services Spending." *Disability and
    Health Journal* 12 (3): 359–365. https://doi.org/10.1016/j.dhjo.2019.01.012.

Garland-Thomson, Rosemarie. 2002. "Integrating Disability, Transforming Feminist Theory."
    NWSA Journal 14 (3): 1–32.

Gebeloff, Robert, Danielle Ivory, Matt Richtel, Mitch Smith, Karen Yourish, Scott Dance, Jackie
    Fortiér, Elly Yu, and Molly Parker. 2020. "The Striking Racial Divide in How Covid-19 Has
    Hit Nursing Homes." *New York Times*, May 21. https://www.nytimes.com/2020/05/21/us
    /coronavirus-nursing-homes-racial-disparity.html.

Gentilini, Ugo, Mohamed Almenfi, Ian Orton, and Pamela Dale. 2020. Social Protection and
    Jobs Responses to COVID-19: A Real-Time Review of Country Measures. Washington, DC:
    World Bank.

Gherardi, Natalia. 2020. "No hay cuarentena que valga: la persistencia de violencias por
    razones de género." In *Covid-19 y derechos humanos. La pandemia de la desigualdad*, edited
    by Juan Pablo Bohoslavsky, 497–517. Buenos Aires: Editorial Biblos.

Gibson, Kate, 2020. "Pandemic Leaves Domestic Workers Facing Tough Choices, Often With-
    out a Safety Net." *CBS News*, September 18. https://www.cbsnews.com/news/pandemic
    -domestic-workers-face-difficult-choices-covid-19-unemployment/.

Gilligan, Carol. 1993. *In a Different Voice: Psychological Theory and Women's Development.* Cam-
    bridge, MA: Harvard University Press.

Giroux, Henry A. 2005. "The Terror of Neoliberalism: Rethinking the Significance of Cultural
    Politics." *College Literature* 32 (1): 1–19.

Gitlow, Lynn, and Kathleen Flecky. 2005. "Integrating Disability Studies Concepts into Occu-
    pational Therapy Education Using Service Learning." *American Journal of Occupational
    Therapy* 59 (5): 546–553.

Glenn, Evelyn Nakano. 1992. "From Servitude to Service Work: Historical Continuities in the
    Racial Division of Paid Reproductive Labor." *Signs: Journal of Women in Culture and Soci-
    ety* 18 (1): 1–43.

———. 2010. *Forced to Care: Coercion and Caregiving in America.* Boston: Harvard University Press.

Glinsner, Barbara, Birgit Sauer, Myriam Gaitsch, Penzm Otto, and Johanna Hofbauer. 2018. "Doing Gender in Public Services: Affective Labour of Emplyment Agents." *Gender, Work & Organization* 26 (7): 983–999. https://doi.org/https://doi.org/10.1111/gwao.12263.

Goering, Sara. 2008. "'You Say You're Happy, But . . .': Contested Quality of Life Judgments in Bioethics and Disability Studies." *Journal of Bioethical Inquiry* 5 (2–3): 125–135. https://doi.org/10.1007/s11673-007-9076-z.

Gomaa, Ahmed E., Loren C. Tapp, Sara E. Luckhaupt, Kelly Vanoli, Raymond Francis Sarmiento, William M. Raudabaugh, Susan Nowlin, and Susan M. Sprigg. 2015. "Occupational Traumatic Injuries among Workers in Health Care Facilities—United States, 2012–2014." *MMWR. Morbidity and Mortality Weekly Report* 64 (15): 405.

Goodin, Robert E. 1985. *Protecting the Vulnerable: A Reanalysis of Our Social Responsibilities.* Chicago: University of Chicago Press.

Goodley, Dan, and Rebecca Lawthom. 2019. "Critical Disability Studies, Brexit and Trump: A Time of Neoliberal–Ableism." *Rethinking History* 23 (2): 233–251. https://doi.org/10.1080/13642529.2019.1607476.

Goodman, Peter S. 2020. "They Crossed Oceans to Lift Their Families Out of Poverty: Now, They Need Help." *New York Times*, July 27. https://www.nytimes.com/2020/07/27/business/global-remittances-coronavirus.html.

Gottfried, Heidi, and Jennifer Jiyhe Chun. 2018. "Carework in Transition: Transational Circuits of Gender, Migration and Care." *Critical Sociology* 44 (7–8): 997–1012. https://doi.org/10.1177/0896920518765931.

Gould, Elise, and Hunter Blair. 2020. "Who's Paying Now? The Explicit and Implicit Costs of the Current Early Care and Education System." Economic Policy Institute (EPI) and the Center for the Study of Child Care Employment at U.C. Berkeley, January 15 https://cscce.berkeley.edu/whos-paying-now-the-explicit-and-implicit-costs-of-the-current-early-care-and-education-system/.

Grabowski, David C., and Vincent Mor. 2020. "Nursing Home Care in Crisis in the Wake of COVID-19." *JAMA* 324 (1): 23–24. https://doi.org/10.1001/jama.2020.8524.

Grant, Karen R., Carol Amaratunga, Pat Armstrong, Madeline Boscoe, Ann Pederson, and Kay Willson, eds. 2004. *Caring For/Caring About: Women, Home-Care and Unpaid Caregiving.* Aurora, ON: Garamond Press.

Grant, Kelly, and Erin Anderssen. 2020. "'These People Are Dying, Gasping for Air': Care Home Workers Are at the Frontlines of Canada's COVID-19 Outbreaks." *Globe and Mail*, April 7. https://www.theglobeandmail.com/canada/article-these-people-are-dying-gasping-for-air-care-home-workers-are-at/.

Greener, Joe. 2015. "Embedded Neglect, Entrenched Abuse: Market Failure and Mistreatment in Elderly Residential Care " In *Social Policy Review 27: Analysis and Debate in Social Policy*, edited by Z. Irving, M. Fenger, and J. Hudson, 131–149. Bristol: Policy Press.

Greenhalgh, Trisha. 2018. "How to Improve Success of Technology Projects in Health and Social Care." *Public Health Research Practice* 28 (3): e2831815.

Greve, Bent, Paula Blomquist, Bjørn Hvinden, and Minna van Gerven. 2021. "Nordic Welfare States—Still Standing or Changed by the COVID-19 Crisis?" *Social Policy and Administration* 55 (2): 295–311. https://doi.org/10.1111/spol.12675.

Grimes, Laura, Katie Savin, Joseph A. Stramondo, Joel Michael Reynolds, Marina Tsaplina, Teresa Blankmeyer Burke, Angela Ballantyne, Eva Feder Kittay, Devan Stahl, Jackie Leach Scully, Rosemarie Garland-Thomson, Anita Tarzian, Doron Dorfman, and Joseph J. Fins. 2020. "Disability Rights as a Necessary Framework for Crisis Standards of Care and the Future of Health Care." *Hastings Center Report* 50 (3): 28–32. https://doi.org/10.1002/hast.1128.

Guarino, Amanda, 2021. "Child Care and Pre-K in the Build Back Better Act: A Look at the Leg-islative Text." First Five Years Fund, December 14. https://www.ffyf.org/child-care-and -pre-k-in-the-build-back-better-act-a-look-at-the-legislative-text/.

Guevarra, Anna Romina. 2014. "Supermaids: The Racial Branding of Global Filipino Care Labor." In *Migration and Care Labor: Theory, Policy and Politics*, edited by Bridget Ander-son and Isabel Shutes, 130–150. London: Palgrave.

Gunkel, David J. 2012. *The Machine Question: Critical Perspectives on AI, Robots, and Ethics.* Lon-don: MIT Press.

Guo, Man, Jinyu Liu, Ling Xu, Weiyu Mao, and Iris Chi. 2016. "Intergenerational Relationships and Psychological Well-Being of Chinese Older Adults with Migrant Children: Does Internal or International Migration Make a Difference?" *Journal of Family Issues* 36 (10): 1351–1376.

Gurdasani, Deepti, Nisreen A. Alwan, Trisha Greenhalgh, Zoë Hyde, Luke Johnson, Martin McKee, Susan Michie, Kimberly A. Prather, Sarah D. Rasmussen, Stephen Reicher, Paul Roderick, and Hisham Ziauddeen. 2021. "School Reopening without Robust COVID-19 Mitigation Risks Accelerating the Pandemic." *The Lancet* 397 (10280): 1177–1178. https:// doi.org/10.1016/S0140-6736(21)00622-X.

Guthrie, Brandon L., Diana M. Tordoff, Julianne Meisner, Lorenzo Tolentino, Wenwen Jiang, Sherrilynne Fuller, Dylan Green, Diana Louden, and Jennifer M. Ross. 2020. "Summary of School Re-opening Models and Implementation Approaches during the COVID-19 Pan-demic." https://globalhealth.washington.edu/file/6393/download.

Guzman-Castillo, Maria, Sara Ahmadi-Abhari, Piotr Bandosz, Simon Capewell, Andrew Step-toe, Archana Singh-Manoux, Mika Kivimaki, Martin J. Shipley, Eric J. Brunner, and Mar-tin O'Flaherty. 2017. "Forecasted Trends in Disability and Life Expectancy in England and Wales up to 2025: A Modelling Study." *The Lancet Public Health* 2 (7): e307–e313.

Hall, Katherine, and Dorrit Posel. 2019. "Fragmenting the Family? The Complexity of House-hold Migration Strategies in Post-Apartheid South Africa." *IZA Journal of Development and Migration* 10 (4): 1–20.

Hamilton, Laura S., David Grant, Julia H. Kaufman, Melissa Diliberti, Heather L. Schwartz, Ger-ald P. Hunter, Claude Messan Setodji, and Christopher J. Young. 2020. *COVID-19 and the State of K–12 Schools: Results and Technical Documentation from the Spring 2020 American Educator Panels COVID-19 Surveys.* RAND Corporation. https://doi.org/10.7249/RRA168-1.

Hank, Karsten, and Anja Steinbach. 2021. "The Virus Changed Everything, Didn't It? Couples' Division of Housework and Childcare before and during the Corona Crisis." *Journal of Family Research* 33 (1): 99–114. https://doi.org/10.20377/jfr-488.

Harding, Rosie. 2017. "A Relational Re(view) of the UK's Social Care Crisis." *Palgrave Communi-cations* 3 (17096): 1–5.

Harknett, Kristen, Daniel Schneider, and Sigrid Luhr. 2022. "Who Cares If Parents Have Unpre-dictable Work Schedules? Just-in-Time Work Schedules and Child Care Arrangements." *Social Problems* 69 (1): 164–183.

Harrington, Brooke. 2016. *Capital without Borders: Wealth Managers and the One Percent.* Cam-bridge: Harvard University Press.

Harvey, David 2005. *A Brief History of Neoliberalism.* New York: Oxford.

Haug, Nina, Lukas Geyrhofer, Alessandro Londei, Elma Dervic, Amelie Desvars-Larrive, Vit-torio Loreto, Beate Pinior, Stefan Thurner, and Peter Klimek. 2020. "Ranking the Effec-tiveness of Worldwide COVID-19 Government Interventions." *Nature Human Behaviour,* 4, 1303–1312. https://doi.org/10.1038/s41562-020-01009-0.

Hays, Sharon. 2003. *Flat Broke with Children: Women in the Age of Welfare Reform.* Oxford: Oxford University Press.

Held, Virginia. 2006. *The Ethics of Care: Personal, Political and Global.* Oxford: Oxford Univer-sity Press.

Hellgren Zenia. 2015. "Markets, Regimes, and the Role of Stakeholders: Explaining Precariousness of Migrant Domestic/Care Workers in Different Institutional Frameworks." *Social Politics: International Studies in Gender, State & Society* 22 (2): 220–241.

Hertz, Rosanna, Jane Mattes, and Alexandria Shook. 2020. When Paid Work Invades the Family: Single Mothers in the COVID-19 Pandemic. *Journal of Family Issues* 42 (9): 2019–2045.

Hess, Cynthia, and Ariane Hegewisch. 2019. *The Future of Care Work: Improving the Quality of America's Fastest-Growing Jobs*. Washington, DC: Institute for Women's Policy Research.

Himmelstein, David U., Steffie Woolhandler, Mark Almberg, and Clare Fauke. 2017. "The U.S. Health Care Crisis Continues: A Data Snapshot." *International Journal of Health Services* 48 (1): 28–41.

Himmelstein, Kathryn E. W., and Atheendar S. Venkataramani. 2019. "Economic Vulnerability among US Female Health Care Workers: Potential Impact of a $15-per-Hour Minimum Wage." *American Journal of Public Health* 109 (2): 198–205.

Hine, Darlene Clark. 1989. Black Women in White: Racial Conflict and Cooperation in the Nursing Profession, 1890–1950. Bloomington: Indiana University Press.

Hipp, Lena, and Mareike Bünning. 2021. "Parenthood as a Driver of Increased Gender Inequality during COVID-19? Exploratory Evidence from Germany." *European Societies* 23 (S1): S658–S673. https://doi.org/10.1080/14616696.2020.1833229.

Hoang, Lan Anh, and Brenda Yeoh, eds. 2015. *Transnational Labour Migration, Remittances and the Changing Family in Asia*. Basingstoke: Palgrave Macmillan.

Hodgkin, Suzanne, Jeni Warburton, Pauline Savy, and Melissa Moore. 2017. "Workforce Crisis in Residential Aged Care: Insights from Rural, Older Workers." *Australian Journal of Public Administration* 76 (1): 93–105.

Holden, Emily, and Daniel Strauss. 2020. "The Mystery of Which US Businesses Are Profiting from the Coronavirus Bailout." *The Guardian*, June 9. https://www.theguardian.com/us-news/2020/jun/09/us-congress-billions-coronavirus-aid-relief-package.

Hong, Nicole. 2020. "3 Hospital Workers Gave Out Masks: Weeks Later, They All Were Dead." *New York Times*, May 4. https://www.nytimes.com/2020/05/04/nyregion/coronavirus-ny-hospital-workers.html.

Horn, Vincent, and Cornelia Schweppe, eds. 2015. *Transnational Aging: Current Insights and Future Challenges*. London: Routledge.

Horst, Cindy, Marta Bivand Erdal, Jorgen Carling, and Karin Afeef. 2014. "Private Money, Public Scrutiny? Contrasting Perspectives on Remittances." *Global Networks* 14 (4): 514–532.

Horton, Richard. 2020. "Offline: COVID-19 Is Not a Pandemic." *The Lancet* 396 (September 26): 874.

Howard, Ayanna, and Jason Borenstein. 2020. "AI, Robots and Ethics in the Age of Covid-19." MIT Sloan Management Review, May 12. https://sloanreview.mit.edu/article/ai-robots-and-ethics-in-the-age-of-covid-19/.

Hsu, Amy, Whitney Berta, Peter C. Coyte, and Audrey Laporte. 2016. "Staffing in Ontario's Long-Term Care Homes: Differences by Profit Status and Chain Ownership." *Canadian Journal on Aging* 315 (2): 175–189.

Hulspas, Marcel 2020. "Will That Robot Be Taking Care of Us Later?" WIN, February 4 https://www.win-nieuws.nl/2020/02/04/will-that-robot-be-taking-care-of-us-later/.

Hussein, Shereen, and Karen Christensen. 2017. "Migration, Gender and Low-paid Work: On Migrant Men's Entry Dynamics into the Feminized Social Care Work in the UK." *Journal of Ethic and Migration Studies* 43 (5): 749–765.

Ilkkaracan, Ipek. 2016. "The Purple Economy Complementing the Green: Towards Sustainable and Caring Economies." Presented at Gender and Macroeconomics: Current State of Research and Future Directions, March 9, New York, NY.

Immigration, Refugees and Citizenship Canada. 2021. "Minister Mendicino Launches Plan to Accelerate Caregiver Application Processing." April 15. https://www.newswire.ca/news

-releases/minister-mendicino-launches-plan-to-accelerate-caregiver-application-process
ing-891765884.html.

Ingersoll, Richard, Henry May, and Greg Collins. 2017. *Minority Teacher Recruitment, Employ-ment, and Retention: 1987 to 2013*. Palo Alto, CA: Learning Policy Institute.

Institute of Medicine, Committee on the Future Health Care Workforce for Older Americans. 2008. *Retooling for an Aging America: Building the Health Care Workforce*. Washington DC: The National Academies Press.

International Centre on Nurse Migration (ICNM). 2022. *Sustain and Retain in 2022 and Beyond: The Global Nursing Workforce and the COVID-19 Pandemic*. January. https://www.emergency
-live.com/it/wp-content/uploads/2022/01/Nurse-Sustain-and-Retain-in-2022-and
-Beyond-The-global-nursing-workforce-and-the-COVID-19-pandemic.pdf.

International Labour Organization (ILO). 2011. *Domestic Workers across the World: Global and Regional Statistics and the Extent of Legal Protection*. Geneva: ILO.

———. 2013. *Domestic Workers across the Globe: Global and Regional Statistics and the Extent of Legal Protection*. Geneva: ILO.

———. 2015. *ILO Global Estimates on Migrant Workers*. Geneva: ILO.

———. 2017. *World Social Protection Report: Universal Social Protection to Achieve the Sustainable Development Goals*. Geneva: ILO.

———. 2018. *Care Work and Care Jobs for the Future of Decent Work*. Geneva: ILO.

———. 2019. *Panorama Laboral 2019*. Lima, Peru: Oficina Regional para América Latina y el Caribe de la Organización Internacional del Trabajo.

———. 2020a. *COVID and the Education Sector*. Geneva: ILO.

———. 2020b. *COVID-19 and Care Workers Providing Home or Institution-Based Care*. Geneva: ILO.

———. 2020c. *The COVID-19 Response: Getting Gender Equality Right for a Better Future for Women at Work*. Geneva: ILO.

———. 2020d. *Domestic Workers in Latin America and the Caribbean during the Covid-19 Crisis*. Geneva: ILO.

———. 2020e. *A Gender-Responsive Employment Recovery: Building Back Fairer*. Geneva: ILO.

———. 2020f. *ILO Monitor: COVID-19 and the World of Work*. 3rd ed., updated estimates and analysis. Geneva: ILO.

———. 2020g. *Impact of the COVID-19 Crisis on Loss of Jobs and Hours among Domestic Workers*. Geneva: ILO.

———. 2020h. *Impactos en el mercado de trabajo y los ingresos en América Latina y el Caribe1*. Geneva: ILO.

———. 2020i. *Social Protection Responses to the COVID-19 Crisis: Country Responses and Policy Con-siderations*. Geneva: ILO.

———. 2021a. *ILO Monitor: COVID-19 and the World of Work*. 5th ed., updated estimates and analysis. Geneva: ILO.

———. 2021b. *ILO Monitor: COVID-19 and the World of Work*. 7th ed., updated estimates and analysis. Geneva: ILO.

———. 2021c. *An Uneven and Gender-Unequal COVID-19 Recovery: Update on Gender and Employ-ment Trends 2021*. Geneva: ILO.

———. 2022. *World Employment and Social Outlook: Trends 2022*. Geneva: ILO.

International Labour Organization and United Nations Development Programme (ILO/UNDP). 2009. *Decent Work in Latin America and the Caribbean: Work and Family, Towards New Forms of Reconciliation*. Santiago, Chile: ILO/UNDP.

International Monetary Fund (IMF). 2021. *World Economic Outlook: Managing Divergent Recov-eries*. Washington, DC: IMF. https://www.imf.org/en/Publications/WEO/Issues/2021/03/23
/world-economic-outlook-april-2021.

Iversen, Torben, and Frances Rosenbluth. 2013. "The Political Economy of Gender in Service Sector Economies." In *The Political Economy of the Service Transition*, edited by Anne Wren, 306–326. Oxford: Oxford University Press.

Jackways, Tanya, Riana Manuel, Phil Wood, Peter Moodie, John Holmes, and Frances Hughes. 2020. *Independent Review of COVID 19 Clusters in Aged Residential Care Facilities.* Wellington, New Zealand: Ministry of Health.

Jaga, Ameeta, and Ariane Ollier-Malaterre. 2022. "'You Can't Eat Soap': Reimagining COVID-19, Work, Family and Employment from the Global South." *Work, Employment and Society* 36 (4): 769–780. https://doi.org/10.1177/09500170211069806.

James, Nicky. 1992. "Care = Organisation + Physical Labour + Emotional Labour." *Sociology of Health & Illness* 14 (4): 488–509.

Jean-Jacques, Muriel, and Howard Bauchner. 2021. "Vaccine Distribution—Equity Left Behind?" *JAMA* 325 (9): 829–830. https://doi.org/10.1001/jama.2021.1205.

Jeffords, Shawn. 2020. "Ontario Home-Care Providers Push for Expanded Services to Fight Pandemic." *Toronto Star*, October 1. https://www.thestar.com/news/gta/2020/10/01/ontario-home-care-providers-push-for-expanded-services-to-fight-pandemic.html.

Jensen, Per H., Ralf Och, Birgit Pfau-Effinger, and Rasmus Møberg. 2017. "Explaining Differences in Women's Working Time in European Cities." *European Societies* 19 (2): 138–156.

Jenson, Janet. 1997. "Who Cares? Gender and Welfare Regimes." *Social Politics* 4 (2): 160–177.

Jokela, Merita. 2017. "The Role of Domestic Employment Policies in Shaping Precarious Work." *Social Policy & Administration* 51 (2): 286–307.

———. 2019. "Patterns of Precarious Employment in a Female-Dominated Sector in Five Welfare States—The Case of Paid Domestic Labor Sector." *Social Politics* 26 (1): 30–58.

Jones, Janelle. 2020. "The Failed Economics of Care Work." *American Prospect*, October 19. https://prospect.org/familycare/the-failed-economics-of-care-work/.

Josserand, Emmanuel, and Sarah Kaine. 2016. "Labour Standards in Global Value Chains: Disentangling Workers' Voice, Vicarious Voice, Power Relations, and Regulation." *Relations Industrielles / Industrial Relations* 71 (4): 741–767.

Kabeer, Naila. 2020. "Women's Empowerment and Economic Development: A Feminist Critique of Storytelling Practices in 'Randomista' Economics." *Feminist Economics* 26 (2): 1–26.

Kaine, Sarah, and Katherine Ravenswood. 2013. "Working in Residential Aged Care: A Trans-Tasman Comparison." *New Zealand Journal of Employment Relations* 38 (2): 33–46.

Kaine, Sarah, and Katherine Ravenswood. 2019. "Employee Voice in Practice: Aged Care in Australia and New Zealand." In *Employee Voice at Work, Work, Organization, and Employment*, edited by P. Holland, J. Teicher, and J. Donaghey, 183–200. Singapore: Springer.

Kaiser Family Foundation. 2020. "State Data and Policy Actions to Address Coronavirus." https://www.kff.org/report-section/state-covid-19-data-and-policy-actions-policy-actions/.

Kalipeni, Josephine, and Julie Kashen. 2020. "Building Our Care Infrastructure for Equity, Economic Recovery and Beyond." Caring Across Generations, September 1. https://caringacross.org/wp-content/uploads/2020/09/Building-Our-Care-infrastructure_FINAL.pdf.

Kalomo, Eveline N., and Fred H. Besthorn. 2018. "Caregiving in Sub-Saharan Africa and Older, Female Caregivers in the Era of HIV/AIDS: A Namibian Perspective." *GrandFamilies: The Contemporary Journal of Research, Practice and Policy* 5 (1): 33–48.

Kamal, Arif H., Janet H. Bull, Keith M. Swetz, Steven O. Wolk, Tait D. Shanafelt, and Evan R. Myers. 2017. "Future of the Palliative Care Workforce: Preview to an Impending Crisis." *American Journal of Medicine* 130 (2): 113–114.

Karl, Ute, and Sandra Torres. 2015. *Ageing in Contexts of Migration.* New York: Routledge.

Kashen, Julie. 2019a. "Domestic Workers Bill: A Model for Tomorrow's Workforce." The Century Foundation, December 17. https://tcf.org/content/report/domestic-workers-bill-a-model -for-tomorrows-workforce/.

———. 2019b. "10 Ways to Make Workplace Laws Work for Everyone." The Century Foundation, April 2. https://tcf.org/content/commentary/10-ways-make-workplace-laws-work -everyone/.

Kashen, Julie, Julie Cai, Hayley Brown, and Shawn Fremstad 2022. "How States Would Benefit If Congress Truly Invested in Child Care and Pre-K." The Century Foundation and the Center for Economic Policy Research, March 21. https://tcf.org/content/report/how-states -would-benefit-if-congress-truly-invested-in-child-care-and-pre-k/.

Kashen, Julie, and Rakeen Mabud. 2020, "Nevertheless It Persists: Disrupting the Vicious Cycle of Institutionalized Sexism." *Times Up Impact Lab*, July 14. https://timesupfoundation.org /work/times-up-impact-lab/nevertheless-it-persists-disrupting-the-vicious-cycle-of -institutionalized-sexism/#:~:text=In%20%E2%80%9CNevertheless%2C%20It%20 Persists%3A,in%20which%20institutionalized%20sexism%20has.

Kashen, Julie, Halley Potter, and Andrew Stettner. 2016. "Quality Jobs, Quality Care." The Century Foundation, June 13. https://tcf.org/content/report/quality-jobs-quality-child-care/.

Kelly, Christine. 2016. *Disability Politics and Care: The Challenge of Direct Funding*. Vancouver: UBC Press.

Kerr, Andrew, and Amy Thornton. 2020. "Essential Workers, Working From Home and Job Loss Vulnerability in South Africa." A Datafirst Technical Paper 41. Cape Town: DataFirst, University of Cape Town.

Ketchen, Sandra. 2021. "Ontario Is on the Verge of Home-Care Crisis: Strain Will Put Pressure on Long-Term-Care Homes, Rest of Health-Care System." *Toronto Star*, October 23.

Kidman, Rachel, and Jody J. Heymann. 2009. "The Extent of Community and Public Support Available to Families Caring for Orphans in Malawi." *AIDS Care* 21 (4): 439–447.

Kim, E. Tammy. 2020. "When You Are Paid 13 Hours for a 24-Hour Shift." *New York Times*, June 30. https://www.nytimes.com/2020/06/30/opinion/coronavirus-nursing-homes.html.

Kinder, Molly. 2020. "Essential but Undervalued: Millions of Health Care Workers Aren't Getting the Pay or Respect They Deserve in the COVID-19 Pandemic." Washington, DC: Brookings Institution. https://www.brookings.edu/research/essential-but-undervalued -millions-of-health-care-workers-arent-getting-the-pay-or-respect-they-deserve-in-the -covid-19-pandemic/.

Kinder, Molly, and Martha Ross. 2020. "Low-Wage Workers Have Suffered Badly From COVID-19 So Policymakers Should Focus on Equity." In *Reopening America and the World: Saving Lives and Livelihoods*, edited by John R. Allen and Darrel M. West, 30–35. Brookings Institution Press. https://www.brookings.edu/wp-content/uploads/2020/05/Brookings-Reopening -America-FINAL.pdf.

King, Russell, Eralba Cela, Tineke Fokkema, and Julie Vullnetari. 2014. "The Migration and Well-Being of the Zero Generation: Transgenerational Care, Grandparenting, and Loneliness amongst Albanian Older People." *Population, Space and Place* 20 (8): 728–738.

King, Russell, Aija Lulle, Dora Sampaio, and Julie Vullnetari. 2017. "Unpacking the Ageing– Migration Nexus and Challenging the Vulnerability Trope." *Journal of Ethnic and Migration Studies* 43 (2): 182–198.

King, Russell, and Julie Vullnetari. 2006. "Orphan Pensioner and Migrating Grandparents: The Impact of Mass Migration on Older People in Rural Albania." *Ageing and Society* 26 (5): 783–816.

Kirzinger, Ashley, Audrey Kearney, Liz Hamel, and Mollyann Brodie. 2021. *KFF/The Washington Post Frontline Health Care Workers Survey—Toll of the Pandemic*. Washington, DC: The Washington Post/Kaiser Family Foundation Survey Project.

Klarok, Florek. 2021. *Resilience of the Long-Term Care Sector—Early Key Lessons Learned from the Covid-19 Pandemic*. Brussels: European Public Service Union.

Klenk, Tanja, and Emmanuele Pavolini. 2015. "Editors' Introduction." In *Restructuring Welfare Governance: Marketization, Managerialism and Welfare State Professionalism*, edited by T. Klenk and E. Pavolini, 1–8. Northampton, MA: Edward Edgar Publishing.

Kleven, Henrik, Camille Landais, Sgaard, Jakob E. 2018. *Children and Gender Inequality: Evidence from Denmark*. NBER WP 24219. https://www.nber.org/system/files/working_papers/w24219/w24219.pdf.

Klostermann, Janna. 2020. "Care Has Limits: Women's Moral Lives and Revised Meanings of Care Work." Unpublished doctoral dissertation, Carleton University.

Knezevich, Alison. 2020. "Invisiblecare Aides: They Serve the Vulnerable, but Many Low-Wage Home Care Workers Are Overlooked in Pandemic, Baltimore Area Advocates Say." *Baltimore Sun*, June 8, 1.

Kraft, Matthew A., and Nicole S. Simon. 2020. *Teachers' Experiences Working from Home during the COVID-19 Pandemic*. Providence, RI: Teach Upbeat. https://education.brown.edu/sites/default/files/2020-06/Upbeat%20Memo%20-%20Kraft.pdf.

Kremer, Monique. 2007. *How Welfare States Care: Culture, Gender and Parenting in Europe*. Amsterdam: Amsterdam University Press.

Kröger, Teppo. 2009. "Care Research and Disability Studies: Nothing in Common?" *Critical Social Policy* 29 (3): 398–420. https://doi.org/10.1177/0261018309105177.

Kronfol, N. M., A. Rizk, and A. M. Sibai. 2015. "Ageing and Intergenerational Family Ties in Arab Countries." *Eastern Mediterranean Health Journal* 21 (11): 835–843.

Krumer-Nevo, Michal, Anastasia Gorodzeisky, and Yuval Saar-Heiman. 2017. "Debt, Poverty, and Financial Exclusion." *Journal of Social Work* 17 (5): 511–530.

Kuhlmann, Ellen, Michelle Falkenbach, Kasia Klasa, Emmanuele Pavolini, and Marius-Ionut Ungureanu. 2020. "Migrant Carers in Europe in Times of COVID-19: A Call to Action for European Health Workforce Governance and a Public Health Approach." *European Journal of Public Health* 30 (4): iv22–iv27.

Kulic, Nevena, Sani Dotti, Susanne Strauss, and Luna Bellani. 2021. "Economic Disturbances in the COVID-19 Crisis and Their Gendered Impact on Unpaid Activities in Germany and Italy." *European Societies* 23 (S1): S400–S416. https://doi.org/10.1080/14616696.2020.1828974.

Kulish, Nicholas, Sarah Kliff, and Jessica Silver-Greenberg. 2020. "The U.S. Tried to Build a New Fleet of Ventilators: The Mission Failed." *New York Times*, April 20. https://www.nytimes.com/2020/03/29/business/coronavirus-us-ventilator-shortage.html.

Kunzmann, Kevin. 2020, "PPE in the United States: What Went Wrong?" *Contagion Live: Infectious Diseases Today*. https://www.contagionlive.com/news/ppe-in-the-united-states-what-went-wrong.

Kuo, Caroline, Jane Fitzgerald, Don Operario, and Marisa Casale. 2012. "Social Support Disparities for Caregivers of AIDS-Orphaned Children in South Africa." *Journal of Community Psychology* 40 (6): 631–644.

Kurowski, Alicia, Jon Boyer, and Laura Punnett. 2015. "The Health Hazards of Health Care: Physical and Psychosocial Stressors in Paid Care Work." In *Caring on the Clock: The Complexities and Contradictions of Paid Care Work*, edited by M. Duffy, A. Armenia, and C. Stacey, 83–93. New Brunswick, NJ: Rutgers University Press.

Kurtz, Holly. 2020. "National Survey Tracks Impact of Coronavirus on Schools: 10 Key Findings." *Education Week*, April 10. https://www.edweek.org/teaching-learning/national-survey-tracks-impact-of-coronavirus-on-schools-10-key-findings/2020/04.

Lal, Arush, Ngozi A. Erondu, David L. Heymann, Githinji Gitahi, and Robert Yates. 2021. "Fragmented Health Systems in COVID-19: Rectifying the Misalignment between Global Health Security and Universal Health Coverage." *The Lancet* 397 (10268): P61–67.

Lamb, Sarah. 2009. *Aging and Indian Diaspora: Cosmopolitan Families in India and Abroad.* Bloomington: Indiana University Press.

Lan, Pei-chia. 2006. Global Cinderella: Migrant Domestics and Newly Rich Employers in Taiwan. Durham, NC: Duke University Press.

Landivar, Liana Christin, Leah Ruppanner, William J. Scarborough, and Caitlyn Collins. 2020. "Early Signs Indicate That COVID-19 Is Exacerbating Gender Inequality in the Labor Force." *Socius* 6: 1–3.

Lazar, M. 2005. *Feminist Critical Discourse Analysis: Gender, Power and Ideology in Discourse.* London: Palgrave Macmillan.

Lee, Emma, and Zachary Parolin. 2021. "The Care Burden during COVID-19: A National Database of Child Care Closures in the United States." Preprint. Open Science Framework. https://doi.org/10.31219/osf.io/t5d3q.

Leiblfinger, M., V. Prieler, K. Schwiter, J. Steiner, A. Benazha, and H. Lutz. 2020. "Impact of the COVID-19 Pandemic on Live-In Care Workers in Germany, Austria, and Switzerland." https://ltccovid.org/2020/05/14/impact-of-the-covid-19-pandemic-on-live-in-care-workers-in-germany-austria-and-switzerland/.

Leichsenring, Kai, Heidemarie Staflinger, and Annette Bauer. 2020. "The Situation of '24-Hour care' from the Perspective of Migrant Caregivers in Austria." April 8. https://ltccovid.org/2020/04/08/the-situation-of-24-hour-care-from-the-perspective-of-migrant-caregivers-in-austria/.

Leinaweaver, Jessaca. 2010. "Outsourcing Care: How Peruvian Migrants Meet Transnational Family Obligations." *Latin American Perspectives* 37 (5): 67–87.

Levanon, Asaf, Paula England, and Paul Allison. 2009. "Occupational Feminization and Pay: Assessing Causal Dynamics Using 1950–2000 US Census Data." *Social Forces* 88 (2): 865–891.

Levin, Bess. 2020. "Texas Lt. Governor: Old People Should Volunteer to Die to Save the Economy." *Vanity Fair*, March. https://www.vanityfair.com/news/2020/03/dan-patrick-coronavirus-grandparents.

Levitt, Peggy, and B. Nadya Jaworsky. 2007. "Transnational Migration Studies: Past Developments and Future Trends." *Annual Review of Sociology* 33 (April): 129–156.

Levitt, Peggy, Jocelyn Viterna, Armin Mueller, and Charlotte Lloyd. 2017. "Transnational Social Protection: Setting the Agenda." *Oxford Development Studies* 45 (1): 2–19.

Levy, Rhonda B., and George Vassos. 2022. "Ontario, Canada: Three Paid COVID Sick Days Extended until March 31, 2023." Littler Workplace Policy Institute, July 22. https://www.littler.com/publication-press/publication/ontario-canada-three-paid-covid-sick-days-extended-until-march-31-2023.

Lewis, Jane, and Anne West. 2017. "Early Childhood Education and Care in England under Austerity: Continuity or Change in Political Ideas, Policy Goals, Availability, Affordability and Quality in a Childcare Market?" *Journal of Social Policy* 46 (2): 331–348.

Lewis, Talila. 2019. "Longmore Lecture: Context, Clarity & Grounding." Talila A. Lewis. http://www.talilalewis.com/1/post/2019/03/longmore-lecture-context-clarity-grounding.html.

Li, Heidi Oi-Yee, and David Huynh. 2020. "Long-Term Social Distancing during COVID-19: A Social Isolation Crisis among Seniors?" *Canadian Medical Association Journal* 192 (21): E588.

Lightman, Naomi. 2017. "Discounted Labour? Disaggregating Care Work in Comparative Perspective." *International Labour Review* 156 (2): 243–267.

Little, Deborah. 2015. "Building a Movement of Caring Selves: Organizing Direct Care Workers." In *Caring on the Clock: The Complexities and Contradictions of Paid Care Work*, edited by Mignon Duffy, Amy Armenia, and Clare L. Stacey, 251–262. New Jersey: Rutgers University Press.

Lloyd, Liz, Albert, Banerjee, Charlene Harrington, Frode. F Jacobsen, and Marta Szebehely. 2014 "'It Is a Scandal!': Comparing the Causes and Consequences of Nursing Home Media Scandals in Five Countries." *International Journal of Sociology and Social Policy* 34 (1/2): 2–18.

Locke, Catherine. 2017. "Do Male Migrants 'Care'? How Migration Is Reshaping the Gender Ethics of Care." *Ethics and Social Welfare* 11 (3): 277–295.

Lomas, Natasha. 2020. "Startups Developing Tech to Combat Covid-19 Urged to Apply for Fast-Track EU Funding." *Techcrunch*, March 16. https://techcrunch.com/2020/03/16/startups -developing-tech-to-combat-covid-19-urged-to-apply-for-fast-track-eu-funding/.

Long, Michelle, and Matthew Rae. 2020. "Gaps in the Emergency Paid Sick Leave Law for Health Care Workers." KFF. https://www.kff.org/coronavirus-covid-19/issue-brief/gaps-in-emer gency-paid-sick-leave-law-for-health-care-workers/.

Longmore, Paul K. 1995. "Medical Decision Making and People with Disabilities: A Clash of Cultures." *Journal of Law, Medicine & Ethics: A Journal of the American Society of Law, Medicine & Ethics* 23 (1): 82–87.

Lorinc, John. 2020. "Do We Need to Rethink Home-Care after the Pandemic?" *Toronto Star*, contributor opinion, April 13. https://www.thestar.com/opinion/contributors/2020/04/13 /do-we-need-to-rethink-home-care-after-the-pandemic.html.

Lui, Lake. 2016. "Gender, Rural-Urban Inequality, and Intermarriage in China." *Social Forces* 95 (2): 639–662.

Lundberg, Shelly, and Robert A. Pollak. 2013. "Cohabitation and the Uneven Retreat from Marriage in the US, 1950–2010." National Bureau of Economic Research. https://doi.org /10.3386/w19413.

Lupica, Carina. 2016. "Paternity and Parental Leave in Latin America and the Caribbean. Essential Tools to Promote Greater Participation of Fathers in the Care of Children." *Masculinities and Social Change* 5 (3): 295–320.

Lustig, Nora, Valentina Martinez-Pabon, Federico Sanz, and Stephen Younger. 2020. *The Impact of COVID-19 Lockdowns and Expanded Social Assistance on Inequality, Poverty and Mobility in Argentina, Brazil, Colombia and Mexico.* Washington, DC: Center for Global Development. https://www.cgdev.org/publication/impact-covid-19-lockdowns-and-expanded-social -assistance-inequality-poverty-and-mobility.

Lutz, Helma. 2018. "Care Migration: The Connectivity between Care Chains, Care Circulation and Transnational Social Inequality." *Current Sociology* 66 (4): 577–589.

Lyttelton, Thomas, Emma Zang, and Kelly Musick. 2021. "Telecommuting and Gender Inequalities in Parents' Paid and Unpaid Work before and during the COVID-19 Pandemic." *Journal of Marriage and Family* 84 (1): 230–249.

MacDonald, Alistair. 2020. "Pandemic Hits Forgotten Profession: Special-Needs Careworkers." *Wall Street Journal*, June 11. https://www.wsj.com/articles/coronavirus-pandemic-pressures -special-needs-caregivers-11591867800.

MacLean, Nancy. 2017. *Democracy in Chains: The Deep History of the Radical Right's Stealth Plan for America.* New York: Viking.

Madgavkar, Anu, Olivia White, Mekala Krishnan, Deepa Mahajan, and Azcue Xavier. 2020. *COVID-19 and Gender Equality: Countering the Regressive Effects.* New York: McKinsey & Company.

Magongo, Bongani, Joshua Lam, Ignacio del Busto, Chris Chibwana, Lerato Remetse, Sindy Li, and Emily Coppel. 2020. "South Africa's Social Development Sector Response to COVID-19". National Development Agency Policy Brief. https://www.researchgate.net/publication /340647086_South_Africa_social_sector_responses_to_COVID-19_Policy_Brief.

Mahase, Elisabeth. 2020. "Covid-19: UK Government's Defense of Senior Aide Has Damaged Public and NHS Confidence, Say Experts." *BMJ-British Medical Journal* 369: m2109.

Malik, Rasheed. 2021. "Saving Child Care Means Preserving Jobs and Supporting Working Families and Small Businesses." Center for American Progress, January 13. https://www .americanprogress.org/article/saving-child-care-means-preserving-jobs-supporting -working-families-small-businesses/.

Maman, Daniel, and Zeev Rosenhek. 2007. "The Politics of Institutional Reform: The 'Declaration of Independence'of the Israeli Central Bank." *Review of International Political Economy* 14 (2): 251–275.

———. 2011. *The Israeli Central Bank: Political Economy, Global Logics and Local Actors*. New York: Routledge.

Manley, Melissa H., and Abbie E. Goldberg. 2021. "Consensually Nonmonogamous Parent Relationships during COVID-19." *Sexualities*, May 15. https://doi.org/10.1177/13634607211019356.

Marais, Hein. 2005. *Buckling: The Impact of AIDS in South Africa*. Pretoria: University of Pretoria Press.

Marchetti, Sabrina. 2016. "Citizenship and Maternalism in Migrant Domestic Work: Filipina Workers and Their Employers in Amsterdam and Rome." In *Paid Domestic Labour in Changing Europe: Questions of Gender Equality and Gendered Citizenship*, edited by B. Gullikstad, G. Kristensen, and P. Ringrose, 147–168. London: Palgrave Macmillan.

Marchetti, Sabrina, and Eileen Boris. 2020. "Migrant Domestic and Care Workers: High Risk but Low Protection." OpenDemocracy. https://www.opendemocracy.net/en/pandemic -border/migrant-domestic-and-care-workers-high-risk-low-protection/.

Marchetti, Sabrina, and Sara R. Farris. 2017. "From the Commodification to the Corporatization of Care: European Perspectives and Debates." *Social Politics* 24 (2–1): 109–131.

Marchetti-Mercer, Maria. 2012. "Those Easily Forgotten: The Impact of Emigration on Those Left Behind." *Family Process* 51 (3): 376–390.

Marchington, Mick. 2015. "Analysing the Forces Shaping Employee Involvement and Participation (EIP) at Organisation Level in Liberal Market Economies (LMEs)." *Human Resource Management Journal* 25 (1): 1–18. https://doi.org/10.1111/1748-8583.12065.

Marianno, Bradley D., Annie A. Hemphill, Ana Paula S. Loures-Elias, Libna Garcia, Deanna Cooper, and Emily Coombes. 2022. "Power in a Pandemic: Teachers' Unions and Their Responses to School Reopening." *AERA Open* 8 (1): 1–16.

Marr, Bernard. 2020. "Robots and Drones Are Now Used to Fight Covid-19." *Forbes*, March 18 https://www.forbes.com/sites/bernardmarr/2020/03/18/how-robots-and-drones-are -helping-to-fight-coronavirus/#35e6cca22a12.

Martínez Franzoni, Juliana. 2021a. "Los cuidados durante y después de pandemia en América Latina: ¿una emergencia con oportunidades?" In *Feminismo, políticas públicas e institucionalidad*, edited by Flavia Marco and Laura Pautassi, 123–154. Buenos Aires: Fundación Medife, Colección Cuidados.

Martínez Franzoni, Juliana. 2021b. "Understanding the State Regulation of Fatherhood in Latin America: Complementary versus Co-responsible." *Journal of Latin American Studies* 53 (3): 1–25.

Martínez Franzoni, Juliana, and Rosalía Camacho. 2007. "Equilibristas o malabaristas . . . , pero ¿con red? La actual infraestructura de cuidados en América Latina." In *Entre familia y trabajo: relaciones, conflictos y políticas de género en*, edited by María Antonieta Carbonero and Silvia Levín, 117–146. Barcelona: Ediciones Homo Sapiens.

Martin-Matthews, Anne, Joanie Sims-Gould, and John Naslund. 2010. "Ethno-cultural Diversity in Homecare Work in Canada: Issues Confronted, Strategies Employed." *International Journal of Ageing and Later Life* 5 (2): 77–101.

Massey, Douglas, Joaquín Arango, Graeme Hugo, Ali Kouaouci, Adela Pellegrino, and J. Edward Taylor. 1998. *Worlds in Motion: International Migration at the End of the Millennium*. Oxford: Oxford University Press.

Mauldin, Laura. 2021. "'If He Gets COVID, It's Over': I Talked to Spousal Caregivers during COVID, Here's What I've Learned." Caring Across Generations. https://caringacross.org /spousal-caregivers/.

———. 2022. "The Care Crisis Isn't What You Think—the American Prospect." The American Prospect, January 3. https://prospect.org/health/disability-care-crisis-isnt-what-you -think/.

Mauldin, Laura, and Robyn Lewis Brown. 2021. "Missing Pieces: Engaging Sociology of Disability in Medical Sociology." *Journal of Health and Social Behavior* 62 (4): 477–492. https:// doi.org/10.1177/00221465211019358.

Mauldin, Laura, Brian R. Grossman, Alice Wong, Sharon Barnartt, Jennifer Brooks, Angela Frederick, and Ashley Volion. 2020. "Disability as an Axis of Inequality: A Pandemic Illustration (Disability in Society)." *American Sociological Association* 48 (3): 15.

Mazzucato, Valentina. 2007. "Transnational Reciprocity: Ghanaian Migrants and the Care of Their Parents Back Home." In *Generations in Africa: Connections and Conflicts*, edited by Erdmute Alber, Sjaak van der Geest, and Susan R. Whyte, 91–109. Münster, Germany: LIT Verlag.

Mbonu, Ngozi C., Bart van den Borne, and Nanne K. De Vries. 2009. "Stigma of People with HIV/AIDS in Sub-Saharan Africa: A Literature Review." *Journal of Tropical Medicine*, August 16. https://doi.org/10.1155/2009/145891.

McCarthy, Joan, and Rick Deady. 2008. "Moral Distress Reconsidered." *Nursing Ethics* 15 (2): 254–262.

McCarthy, Niall. 2020. "U.S. Billionaire Wealth Surged since the Start of the Pandemic." *Forbes*, June 22. https://www.forbes.com/sites/niallmccarthy/2020/06/22/us-billionaire-wealth -surged-since-the-start-of-the-pandemic-infographic/?sh=6957461c3f8b.

McCully, Kirsty, and Katherine Ravenswood. 2020. "Unite against Covid-19: Kindness for Community Support Workers?" *Critical Solidarity* 19 (1): 4–6.

McDermott, Janie, and Annelies Goger. 2020. "The Heath Care Workforce Needs Higher Wages and Better Opportunities." Brookings Institution, *The Avenue* (blog), December 12. https:// www.brookings.edu/blog/the-avenue/2020/12/02/the-heath-care-workforce-needs -higher-wages-and-better-opportunities/.

McGarry, Brian E., Lori Porter, and David C. Grabowski. 2020. "Opinion | Nursing Home Workers Now Have the Most Dangerous Jobs in America: They Deserve Better." *Washington Post*, July 28. https://www.washingtonpost.com/opinions/2020/07/28/nursing-home -workers-now-have-most-dangerous-jobs-america-they-deserve-better/.

McGilton, Katherine S., Astrid Escrig-Pinol, Adam Gordon, Charlene H. Chu, Franziska Zúñiga, Montserrat Gea Sanchez, Veronique Boscart, Julienne Meyer, Kirsten N. Corazzini, Alessandro Ferrari Jacinto, Karen Spilsbury, Annica Backman, Kezia Scales, Anette Fagertun, Bei Wu, David Edvardsson, Michael J. Lepore, Angela Y. M. Leung, Elena O. Siegel, Maiko Noguchi-Watanabe, Jing Wang, and Barbara Bowers. 2020. "Uncovering the Devaluation of Nursing Home Staff during Covid-19: Are We Fueling the Next Health Care Crisis?" *Journal of the American Medical Directors Association* 21 (7): 962–965.

McIntosh, Kriston, Emily Moss, Ryan Nunn, and Jay Shambaugh. 2020. "Examining the Black–White Wealth Gap." Brookings, February 27. https://memphis.uli.org/wp-content/uploads /sites/49/2020/07/Examining-the-Black-white-wealth-gap.pdf.

McMullen, Jane. 2021. "Covid-19: Five Days That Shaped the Outbreak." *BBC News*, January 26. https://www.bbc.com/news/world-55756452.

MECON. 2020. Los cuidados, un sector económico estratégico. Medición del aporte del Trabajo doméstico y de cuidados unremunerated al Producto Interno Bruto. Ministerio de Economía, Buenos Aires, Argentina.

Meghani, Salimah H. 2004. "A Concept Analysis of Palliative Care in the United States." *Journal of Advanced Nursing* 46 (2): 152–161.

Mercadante, Sebastiano. 2020. "The Clash between Palliative Care and Covid-19." *Supportive Care in Cancer* 28 (12): 5593–5595.

Merli, Giovanna, M., and Alberto Palloni. 2006. "The HIV/AIDS Epidemic, Kin Relations, Living Arrangements, and the African Elderly in South Africa." In *Aging in Sub-Saharan Africa: Recommendations for Furthering Research*, edited by B. Cohen and J. Menken, 117–165. Washington, DC: The National Academies Press.

Merritt, Keri Leigh. 2017. *Masterless Men: Poor Whites and Slavery in the Antebellum South.* New York: Cambridge University Press.

Mertehikian, Yasmin, and Pilar Gonalons-Pons. 2022. "Work and Family Disadvantage: Mechanisms of Gender Gaps in Paid Work during the COVID-19 Pandemic." Working Paper, University of Pennsylvania Population Center. https://repository.upenn.edu/psc_publications/86/.

Mialkowski, Conrad. 2020. "Op Laser-JTFC Observations in Long Term Care Facilities in Ontario." http://www.documentcloud.org/documents/6928480-OP-LASER-JTFC-Observations-in -LTCF-in-On.html?_ga=2.89889304.2016270763.1600696512-1537114224.1592743338.

Michel, Sonya. 1999. *Children's Interests/Mothers' Rights: The Shaping of America's Child Care Policy.* New Haven: Yale University Press.

Michel, Sonya, and Ito Peng. 2012. "All in the Family? Migrants, Nationhood, and Care Regimes in Asia and North America." *European Journal of Social Policy* 22 (4): 406–418.

———, eds. 2017. *Gender, Migration and the Work of Care: A Multi-Scalar Approach to the Pacific Rim.* New York: McMillan-Palgrave.

Migration Policy Institute (MPI). 2020. "Immigrant Health-Care Workers in the United States." May 14. https://www.migrationpolicy.org/article/immigrant-health-care-workers-united -states-2018.

Ministry of Health. 2017. Guaranteed Hours Funding Framework (Transitional Arrangements for the Period 1 April 2017 to 30 June 2018). Wellington, New Zealand: Ministry of Health.

———. 2020. *COVID-19 in Health Care and Support Workers in Aotearoa New Zealand.* Wellington, New Zealand: Ministry of Health.

Mishel, Lawrence, Josh Bivens, Elise Gould, and Heidi Shierholz. 2012. *The State of Working America.* 12th ed. Ithaca, NY: Cornell University Press.

Mitchell, David T., and Sharon L. Snyder. 2015. *The Biopolitics of Disability: Neoliberalism, Ablenationalism, and Peripheral Embodiment.* Ann Arbor: University of Michigan Press.

Mohanty, Chandra Talpade. 2013. "Transnational Feminist Crossings: On Neoliberalism and Radical Critique." *Signs* 38 (4): 967–991. https://doi.org/10.1086/669576.

Mojtehedzadeh, Sara. 2021. "Long-Term-Care Homes Needed Staff during COVID-19. So They Turned to Gig Workers: Inside the 'Uber-ization' of Health Care." *Toronto Star*, March 19. https://www.thestar.com/news/gta/2021/03/19/long-term-care-homes-needed-staff-during -covid-19-so-they-turned-to-gig-workers-inside-the-uber-ization-of-health-care.html.

Mokomane, Zitha. 2013. "Social Protection as a Mechanism for Family Protection in Sub-Saharan Africa." *International Journal of Social Welfare* 22 (3): 248–259.

Molina, Natalia. 2011. "Borders, Laborers, and Racialized Medicalization Mexican Immigration and US Public Health Practices in the 20th Century." *American Journal of Public Health* 101 (6): 1024–1031.

Molinier, Pascale. 2012. "Care as Work: Mutual Vulnerabilities and Discrete Knowledge." In *New Philosophies of Labour: Work and the Social Bond*, edited by N. H. Smith and J. Deranty, 251–271. Boston, MA: Brill.

Montenovo, Laura, Xuan Jiang, Felipe Lozano Rojas, Ian M Schmutte, Kosali I Simon, Bruce A Weinberg, and Coady Wing. 2020. "Determinants of Disparities in Covid-19 Job Losses."

National Bureau of Economic Research Working Paper (27132). https://www.nber.org /papers/w27132.

Moore, Lisa. 2018. "Transformative Organizing in Precarious Times." *Critical Sociology* 44 (7–8): 1225–1234.

Moore, Mignon R., and Michael Stambolis-Ruhstorfer. 2020. "LGBT Sexuality and Families at the Start of the Twenty-First Century." *Annual Review of Sociology* 39 (1): 491–507.

Morel, Nathalie. 2015. "Servants for the Knowledge-Based Economy? The Political Economy of Domestic Services in Europe." *Social Politics: International Studies in Gender, State & Society* 22 (2): 170–192.

Morgan, Ivy, and Ary Amerikaner. 2018. *Funding Gaps: An Analysis of School Funding Gaps across the U.S. and within Each State.* Washington, DC: The Education Trust. https://edtrust.org /wp-content/uploads/2014/09/Funding-Gaps-2018-Report-UPDATED.pdf.

Moscrop, David. 2020. "In Canada, an Inspiring Movement Emerges in Response to the Coronavirus." *Washington Post*, March 24. https://www.washingtonpost.com/opinions/2020/03 /24/canada-an-inspiring-movement-emerges-response-coronavirus/.

Moyser, Melissa. 2017. *Women in Canada: A Gender-Based Statistical Report: Women and Paid Work.* Statistics Canada. https://www150.statcan.gc.ca/n1/en/pub/89-503-x/2015001/article /14694-eng.pdf?st=FwZRNFvM.

Mutler, Alison. 2020. "Romanian Migrants Get COVID-19 as Pandemic Exposes Bad Conditions for East European Workers." Radio Free Europe/Radio Liberty, May 30. https://www.rferl .org/a/romanian-migrants-get-covid-19-as-pandemic-exposes-bad-conditions-for-east -european-workers/30643195.html#:~:text=Hundreds%20of%20Romanian%20workers%20staged,they%20were%20working%20went%20bankrupt.

Myers, Kyle R., Wei Yang Tham, Yian Yin, Nina Cohodes, Jerry G. Thursby, Marie C. Thursby, Peter Schiffer, Joseph T. Walsh, Karim R. Lakhani, and Dashun Wang. 2020. "Unequal Effects of the COVID-19 Pandemic on Scientists." *Nature Human Behavior* 4: 880–883.

Nadasen, Premilla, and Tiffany Williams. 2014. "Valuing Domestic Work." Barnard Center for Research on Women, October 20. http://bcrw.barnard.edu/wp-content/nfs/reports/NFS5 -Valuing-Domestic-Work.pdf.

Nagasawa, Mark, and Kate Tarrant. 2020a. *Forgotten Frontline Workers: A Snapshot of Family Child Care and COVID-19 in New York.* CUNY, New York Early Childhood Professional Development Institute. https://educate.bankstreet.edu/sc/3.

———. 2020b. *Who Will Care for the Early Care and Education Workforce? COVID-19 and the Need to Support Early Childhood Educators' Emotional Well-Being.* CUNY, New York Early Childhood Professional Development Institute. https://educate.bankstreet.edu/sc/1.

Naples, Nancy A., Laura Mauldin, and Heather Dillaway. 2019. "From the Guest Editors: Gender, Disability, and Intersectionality." *Gender & Society* 33 (1): 5–18. https://doi.org/10.1177 /0891243218813309.

National Health Council. 2019. *About Chronic Diseases.* Washington, DC: National Health Council.

National Hospice and Palliative Care Organization (NHPCO). 2020. "Hospice Facts and Figures." Alexandria, VA: National Hospice and Palliative Care Organization.

Nazareno, Jennifer, Cynthia J. Cranford, Lolita Lledo, Valerie Damasco, and Patricia Roach. 2022. "Between Women of Color: The New Social Organization of Reproductive Labor." *Gender & Society* 36 (3): 342–367.

Nedelcu, Mihaela. 2017. "Transnational Grandparenting in the Digital Age: Mediated Co-Presence and Childcare in the Case of Romanian Migrants in Switzerland and Canada." *European Journal of Aging* 14 (4): 375–383.

Ne'eman, Ari. 2020. "Opinion | 'I Will Not Apologize for My Needs.'" *New York Times*, March 23. https://www.nytimes.com/2020/03/23/opinion/coronavirus-ventilators-triage-disability .html.

Nelson Joyce. 1995. "Dr. Rockefeller Will See You Now: The Hidden Players Privatizing Canada's Health Care System." *Canadian Forum* (January–February): 7–11.

Newmarker, Chris. 2020. "Trump Invokes Defense Product Act against Coronavirus." Massdevice, March 18. https://www.massdevice.com/breaking-trump-invokes-defense-pro duction-act-against-coronavirus/.

New York Times. 2020. "Biden Announces $775 Billion Plan to Help Working Parents and Caregivers." July 21. https://www.nytimes.com/2020/07/21/us/politics/biden-workplace-child care.html.

New Zealand Government. 2020. "How Government Works." https://www.govt.nz/browse /engaging-with-government/government-in-new-zealand/.

Nguyen, Long H., David A. Drew, Mark S. Graham, Amit D. Joshi, Chuan-Guo Guo, Wenjie Ma, Raaj S. Mehta, Erica T. Warner, Daniel R. Sikavi, and Chun-Han Lo. 2020. "Risk of COVID-19 among Front-Line Health-Care Workers and the General Community: A Prospective Cohort Study." *The Lancet Public Health* 5 (9): e475–e483.

Nielsen, Kim E. 2013. *A Disability History of the United States*. Boston: Beacon Press.

Novta, Natalija, and Joyce Wong. 2017. *Women at Work in Latin America and the Caribbean*. Washington, DC: International Monetary Fund.

Oburu, Paul O., and Kerstin Palmerus. 2005. "Stress Related Factors among Primary and Part Time Caregiving Grandmothers of Kenyan Grandchildren." *International Journal of Aging and Human Development* 65 (4): 273–282.

Office for National Statistics. 2020a. "Coronavirus (COVID-19) Related Deaths by Occupation, England and Wales: Deaths Registered up to and Including 20 April 2020." Statistical Bulletin. https://www.ons.gov.uk/peoplepopulationandcommunity/healthandsocialcare /causesofdeath/bulletins/coronaviruscovid19relateddeathsbyoccupationenglandandwa les/deathsregisteredbetween9marchand25may2020/pdf.

———. 2020b. "Parenting in Lockdown: Coronavirus and the Effects on Work-Life Balance." https://www.ons.gov.uk/peoplepopulationandcommunity/healthandsocialcare /conditionsanddiseases/articles/parentinginlockdowncoronavirusandtheeffectsonwor klifebalance/2020-07-22.

Oliver, Michael. 1998. "Theories of Disability in Health Practice and Research." *BMJ : British Medical Journal* 317 (7170): 1446–1449.

Ontario Government. 2020. "Ontario Provides $461 Million to Temporarily Enhance Wages for Personal Support Workers." News release, October 1. https://news.ontario.ca/en/release /58627/ontario-provides-461-million-to-temporarily-enhance-wages-for-personal -support-workers#quickfacts.

———. 2022a. "Ontario Releases 2021–22 Third Quarter Finances." News release, February 14. https://news.ontario.ca/en/release/1001603/ontario-releases-2021-22-third-quarter -finances.

———. 2022b. "Personal Support Workers and Direct Support Workers Permanent Compensation Enhancement Program." https://www.ontario.ca/page/personal-support-workers-and -direct-support-workers-permanent-compensation-enhancement-program#section-3.

Ontario Health Coalition. 2020. "Briefing Note: COVID-19 in Long-Term Care Litigation and Legal Actions." Ontario Health Coalition. https://www.ontariohealthcoalition.ca/wp -content/uploads/Final-Litigation-Report.pdf.

Organisation for Economic Co-operation and Development (OECD). 2014. *Migration Policy Debate: Is Migration Good for the Economy?* https://www.oecd.org/els/mig/OECD%20 Migration%20Policy%20Debates%20Numero%202.pdf.

———. 2015. *International Migration Outlook 2015*. https://www.oecd-ilibrary.org/social-issues -migration-health/international-migration-outlook-2015_migr_outlook-2015-en.

———. 2018. Diálogo de políticas sobre empoderamiento económico de las mujeres: recono-cimiento, redistribución y reducción del trabajo de cuidado no remunerado. Paris: OECD.

———. 2020a. *Net-Childcare Costs*. Paris: OECD.

———. 2020b. *Who Cares? Attracting and Retaining Care Workers for the Elderly*. Paris: OECD.

———. 2021. *The State of Global Education: 18 Months into the Pandemic*. Paris: OECD.

Ormseth, Matthew. 2020. "Northern California Official Ousted after Saying Elderly, Ill, Home-less Should Be Left to Die in Pandemic." *Los Angeles Times*, May 1. https://www.latimes .com/california/story/2020-05-01/northern-california-city-official-after-saying.

Ortiz, Isabel. 2020. "Neglected, Sacrificed: Older Persons during the Covid-19 Pandemic." Social Europe. https://www.socialeurope.eu/neglected-sacrificed-older-persons-during-the -covid-19-pandemic.

Ortiz, Isabel, and Matthew Cummins. 2013. "Austerity Measures in Developing Countries: Pub-lic Expenditure Trends and the Risks to Children and Women." *Feminist Economics* 19 (3): 55–81. https://doi.org/10.1080/13545701.2013.791027.

Ortiz, Isabel, and Matthew Cummings. 2022. *End Austerity: A Global Report on Budget Cuts and Harmful Social Reforms in 2022–25*. Eurodad, September 28. https://www.eurodad.org/end _austerity_a_global_report.

Ortiz, Isabel, and Thomas Stubbs. 2020. "Fighting Coronavirus: It's Time to Invest in Univer-sal Public Health." Opinion, Inter Press Service, March. https://www.ipsnews.net/2020 /03/fighting-coronavirus-time-invest-universal-public-health/.

Osborne, David, and Ted Gaebler. 1992. *Reinventing Government*. Boston: Addison-Wesley.

Our World in Data. n.d. "Coronavirus Pandemic Data Explorer." https://ourworldindata.org /coronavirus-data-explorer.

Oved, Marco Chown, Brenden Kennedy, Kenyon Wallace, Ed Tubb, and Andrew Bailey. 2020. "For-Profit Nursing Homes Have Four Times as Many Covid-19 Deaths as City-Run Homes, Star Analysis Finds." *Toronto Star*, May 8. https://www.thestar.com/business/2020/05/08 /for-profit-nursing-homes-have-four-times-as-many-covid-19-deaths-as-city-run-homes -star-analysis-finds.html.

Oxfam. 2020. *Care in the Time of Coronavirus: Why Care Work Needs to Be at the Centre of a Post-COVID-19 Feminist Future*. Oxford: Oxfam GB. https://oxfamilibrary.openrepository.com /bitstream/handle/10546/621009/bp-care-crisis-time-for-global-reevaluation-care -250620-en.pdf.

Oxfam, Promundo-US, and MenCare. 2020. *Caring under COVID-19: How the Pandemic Is—and Is Not—Changing Unpaid Care and Domestic Work Responsibilities in the United States*. Bos-ton: Oxfam.

Page, Joshua, Victoria Piehowski, and Joe Soss. 2019. "A Debt of Care: Commercial Bail and the Gendered Logic of Criminal Justice Predation." *RSF: The Russell Sage Foundation Jour-nal of the Social Sciences* 5 (1): 150–172.

Paikin, Steve. 2020. "To Win the COVID-19 War, We Need More Home-Care for Seniors." TVO, April 11. https://www.tvo.org/article/to-win-the-covid-19-war-we-need-more-home-care -for-seniors.

Palesy, Debra. 2018. "Developing Manual Handling Skills in Relative Social Isolation: A Case Study of Australian Home Care Workers." *Journal of Adult and Continuing Education* 24 (1): 37–57. https://doi.org/10.1177/1477971417707220.

Palesy, Debra, and Stephen Billett. 2017. "Learning Manual Handling without Direct Supervi-sion or Support: A Case Study of Home Care Workers." *Social Work Education* 36 (3): 273–288. https://doi.org/10.1080/02615479.2016.1218457.

Palmer, Elyane, and Joan Eveline. 2012. "Sustaining Low Pay in Aged Care Work." *Gender, Work & Organization* 19 (3): 254–275. https://doi.org/10.1111/j.1468-0432.2010.00512.x.

Pan American Health Organization (PAHO). 2020. *Epidemiological Update: COVID-19 among Healthcare Workers*. Relief Web, August 31. https://reliefweb.int/report/argentina/epide miological-update-covid-19-among-healthcare-workers-31-august-2020.

Pappa, Sofia, Vasiliki Ntella, Timoleon Giannakas, Vassilis G. Giannakoulis, Eleni Papoutsi, and Paraskevi Katsaounou. 2020. "Prevalence of Depression, Anxiety, and Insomnia among Healthcare Workers during the COVID-19 Pandemic: A Systematic Review and Meta-analysis." *Brain, Behavior, and Immunity* 88 (August): 901–907.

Pardee, Jessica, Jennifer Schneider, and Cindy Lam. 2021. "Childcare in COVID-19: Assessing Resilience of Service Critical Infrastructures." Paper presented at the 2021 IEEE International Symposium on Technologies for Homeland Security (HST), Boston, November 2021. https://doi.org/10.1109/HST53381.2021.9619835.

Parisotto, Aurelio, and Adam Elsheikhi. 2020. "COVID-19, Jobs and the Future of Work in the LDCs: A (Disheartening) Preliminary Account." ILO Working Paper 20. Geneva: ILO.

Parks, Jennifer, A. 2003. *No Place Like Home? Feminist Ethics and Home Health Care*. Bloomington: Indiana University Press.

Parreñas, Rhacel S. 2001. *Servants of Globalization: Migration and Domestic Work*. Stanford: Stanford University Press.

———. 2005. *Children of Global Migraion: Transnational Families and Gendered Woes*. Stanford: Stanford University Press.

———. 2012. "The Reproductive Labor of Migrant Workers." *Global Networks* 12 (2): 269–275.

———. 2015. *Servants of Globalization: Women, Migration, and Domestic Work*. 2nd ed. Stanford: Stanford University Press.

Pattison, Natalie. 2020. "End-of-Life Decisions and Care in the Midst of a Global Coronavirus (Covid-19) Pandemic." *Intensive & Critical Care Nursing* 58:102862-62. https://doi.org /10.1016/j.iccn.2020.102862.

Paul, Anju Mary. 2017. *Multinational Maids: Stepwise Migration in a Global Labor Market*. Cambridge, UK: Cambridge University Press.

Pautassi, Laura. 2007. "El cuidado como cuestión social desde un enfoque de derechos." *Serie Mujer y Desarrollo* N 87. Comisión Económica para América Latina y el Caribe, Santiago, Chile, October 2007.

Payne, Elizabeth. 2020. "Family Caregivers Will No Longer Be Locked Out of Long-Term Care during COVID Outbreaks." Ottawa Citizen. https://ottawacitizen.com/news/local-news /family-caregivers-will-no-longer-be-locked-out-of-long-term-care-during-covid-out breaks.

———. 2021. "'We Need Help': Home Care in Ontario—the Lynchpin of the Health Care System— Faces a Staffing Crisis." Ottawa Citizen, September 29. https://ottawacitizen.com/news /local-news/we-need-help-home-care-in-ontario-the-lynchpin-of-the-health-system -faces-a-staffing-crisis.

Pearson, Charlotte, and Julie Ridley. 2017. "Is Personalization the Right Plan at the Wrong Time? Re-Thinking Cash-for-Care in an Age of Austerity." *Social Policy & Administration* 51 (7): 1042–1059.

Peck, Emily. 2020. "The Economic Devastation of COVID-19 Is Hitting Women Particularly Hard." HuffPost. https://www.huffpost.com/entry/women-coronavirus-lost-jobs_n_5e90 a363c5b685fbc7d4a557?fbclid=IwARoFzINrPwcv1XfA_I7sdWmWLBIWu8AOrUHtxmoE4 LJ2DxJic9JP3cb-vwY&guccounter=1.

Pelizza, Annalisa, Stefania Milan, and Yoren Lausberg. 2021. "The Dilemma of Undocumented Migrants Invisible to Covid-19 Counting." In *COVID-19 from the Margins: Pandemic Invisibilities, Policies and Resistance in the Datafied Society*, edited by S. Milan, E. Treré, and

S. Masiero, 70–78. Amsterdam: Institute of Network Cultures. https://networkcultures
.org/wp-content/uploads/2021/02/Covid19FromTheMargins.pdf.

Pellandini-Simányi, Léna, Ferenc Hammer, and Zsuzsanna Vargha. 2015. "The Financializa-
tion of Everyday Life or the Domestication of Finance?" *Cultural Studies* 29 (5/6): 733–759.
https://doi.org/10.1080/09502386.2015.1017142.

Peng, Ito. 2017a. "Elderly Care Work and Migration: East and Southeast Asian Contexts."
Report to the UN Expert Group Meeting on Care and Older Persons: Links to Decent
Work, Migration and Gender, UN DESA, United Nations Headquarters, New York, December 5–7. https://www.un.org/development/desa/ageing/wp-content/uploads/sites/24
/2017/11/Peng-UN-Expert-Group-Meeting_Dec-5-7-final-Paper_4Dec.pdf.

———. 2017b. "Explaining Exceptionality: Care and Migration Policies in Japan and South
Korea." In *Gender, Migration, and the Work of Care: A Multi-Scalar Approach to the Pacific
Rim*, edited by S. Michel and I. Peng, 191–214. London: Palgrave Macmillan.

———. 2017c. *Transnational Migration of Domestic and Care Workers in Asia Pacific*. ILO. https://
www.ilo.org/global/topics/labour-migration/publications/WCMS_547228/lang—en
/index.htm.

———. 2021. "Systemic Resilience and Carework: An Asia-Pacific Perspective." MigResHub
Think Piece no. 7, Migration Policy Centre, RSCAS, European University Institute. https://
migrationpolicycentre.eu/docs/migreshub/MigResHub-think-piece-No7.pdf.

Peng, Ito, and Jiweon Jun. 2022. "Impacts of COVID-19 on Parents with Small Children in South
Korea: Survey Findings and Policy Implications." *International Journal of Care and Caring*
6 (1–2): 13–32. https://doi.org/10.1332/239788221X16330161584820.

Peng, Yinni, and Odalia M. H. Wang. 2013. "Diversified Transnational Mothering via Telecom-
munication: Intensive, Collaborative, and Passive." *Gender and Society* 27 (4): 491–513.

Penton, Mario. 2020. "Health Assistants in Miami without Coronavirus Protection." *Miami
Herald*, April 23. https://www.miamiherald.com/news/health-care/article242230736.html.

Petts, Richard J., Daniel L. Carlson, and Joanna R. Pepin. 2021. "A Gendered Pandemic: Childcare, Homeschooling, and Parents' Employment during COVID-19." *Gender, Work & Organization* 28 (S2): 515–534.

Pfau-Effinger, Birgit. 2005a. "Culture and Welfare State Policies: Reflections on a Complex
Interrelation." *Journal of Social Policy* 34 (1): 3–20. https://doi.org/10.1017/S004727940
4008232.

———. 2005b. "Welfare State Policies and Development of Care Arrangements." *European Societies* 7 (3): 321–347.

———. 2012. "Women's Employment in Institutional and Cultural Context." *International Journal of Sociology and Social Policy* 32 (9): 530–543.

———. 2014. "Explaining Differences in Women's Employment and Childcare across Six European Gender Arrangements." In *The Transformation of Care in European Societies*, edited
by M. León, 83–104. Basingstoke: Palgrave Macmillan.

Pfau-Effinger, Birgit, and Thorsten Euler. 2014. "Wandel der Einstellungen zu Kinderbetreuung
und Elternschaft in Europa—Persistenz kultureller Differenzen." *Soziale Welt* 20 (1):
175–193.

PHI International. 2020. "Direct Care Workers in the United States: Key Facts." https://www
.phinational.org/resource/direct-care-workers-in-the-united-states-key-facts/.

Picard, Andre. 2020. "Why Have We Neglected Home-Care?" *Globe and Mail*, opinion,
June 16, A1.

Pichler, Stefan, Katherine Wen, and Nicolas R. Ziebarth. 2020. "COVID-19 Emergency Sick Leave
Has Helped Flatten the Curve in the United States." *Health Affairs* 39 (12): 2197–2204.

Piepzna-Samarasinha, Leah Lakshmi. 2018. *Care Work: Dreaming Disability Justice*. Vancouver,
BC: Arsenal Pulp Press.

Pistor, Katharina. 2019. *The Code of Capital: How the Law Creates Wealth and Inequality.* Princeton, NJ: Princeton University Press.

Polanyi, Karl. (1944) 2001. *The Great Transformation.* Boston: Beacon Press.

Pollard, Martin. 2020. "Robot Designed in China Could Help Save Lives on Medical Frontline." *Reuters,* March 23. https://www.reuters.com/article/us-health-coronavirus-china-robot/robot-designed-in-china-could-help-save-lives-on-medical-frontline-idUSKBN21A0FY.

Poo, Ai-jen, and Palak Shah. 2020. "Health Care Workers Are the Future: Protect Their Rights." *New York Times,* June 24. https://www.nytimes.com/2020/06/24/opinion/sunday/corona virus-health-workers-nurses.html.

Posel, Dorrit, James A. Fairburn, and Frances Lund. 2004. "Labour Migration and Households: A Reconsideration of the Effects of the Social Pension on Labour Supply in South Africa." http://www.tips.org.za/files/Labour_Migration_and_Householdsposel_fairburn_lund.pdf.

Powell, Victoria D., and Maria J. Silveira. 2020. "What Should Palliative Care's Response Be to the Covid-19 Pandemic?" *Journal of Pain and Symptom Management* 60 (1): e1–e3.

Prasad, Vijay. 2019. "2.21 Aiming for the Hard Targets and Harm from Screening and Overdiagnosis with Dr. H. Gilbert Welch." *Plenary Session Podcast,* November 8. https://www.plenarysessionpodcast.com/.

Preiss, Joshua. 2021. *Just Work for All: The American Dream in the 21st Century.* New York: Routledge.

Price-Glynn, Kim, and Carter Rakovski. 2015. "The Best of Both Worlds? How Direct Care Workers Perceive Home Health Agencies and Long-Term Care Institutions." In *Caring on the Clock: The Complexities and Contradictions of Paid Care Work,* edited by Mignon Duffy, Amy Armenia, and Clare L. Stacey, 31–41. New Brunswick, NJ: Rutgers University Press.

Radbruch, Lukas, Felicia Marie Knaul, Liliana de Lima, Cornelis de Joncheere, and Afsan Bhadelia. 2020. "The Key Role of Palliative Care in Response to the Covid-19 Tsunami of Suffering." *The Lancet* 395 (10235): 1467–1469.

Ranney, Megan L., Valerie Griffeth, and Ashish K. Jha. 2020. "Critical Supply Shortages—the Need for Ventilators and Personal Protective Equipment during the Covid-19 Pandemic." *New England Journal of Medicine* 382 (18): e41.

Ravenswood, Katherine. 2020. "Low Staff Levels Must Be Part of Any Reviews into the Coronavirus Outbreaks in NZ Rest Homes." The Conversation. http://theconversation.com/low-staff-levels-must-be-part-of-any-reviews-into-the-coronavirus-outbreaks-in-nz-rest-homes-137764.

Ravenswood, Katherine, Julie Douglas, and Tanya Ewertowska. 2021. *The New Zealand Care Workforce Survey 2019.* Auckland, New Zealand: The New Zealand Work Research Institute.

Ravenswood, Katherine, and Candice Harris. 2016. "Doing Gender, Paying Low: Gender, Class and Work–Life Balance in Aged Care." *Gender, Work & Organization* 23 (6): 614–628. https://doi.org/10.1111/gwao.12149.

Ravenswood, Katherine, and Sarah Kaine. 2015. "The Role of Government in Influencing Labour Conditions through the Procurement of Services: Some Political Challenges." *Journal of Industrial Relations* 57 (4): 544–562. https://doi.org/10.1177/0022185615582238.

Ravenswood, Katherine, and Raymond Markey. 2018. "Gender and Voice in Aged Care: Embeddedness and Institutional Forces." *International Journal of Human Resource Management* 29 (5): 725–745. https://doi.org/10.1080/09585192.2016.1277367.

Rayner, Julie, and Daniel E. Espinoza. 2016. "Emotional Labour under Public Management Reform: An Exploratory Study of School Teachers in England." *International Journal of Human Resource Management* 27 (19): 2254–2274. https://doi.org/10.1080/09585192.2015.1093014.

Razavi, Shahra. 2007. "The Political and Social Economy of Care in Developing Countries: Conceptual Issues, Research Questions and Policy Options." Gender and Development Programme Paper, vol. 3. Geneva: UNRISD.

———. 2020. *Progress of the World's Women 2019–2020: Families in a Changing World.* New York: UNWomen.

Razavi, Shahra, and Silke Staab, eds. 2012. *Global Variations in the Political and Social Economy of Care: Worlds Apart.* New York: Routledge.

Reskin, Barbara E. 1988. "Bringing the Men Back In: Sex Differentiation and the Devaluation of Women's Work." *Gender & Society* 2 (1): 58–81.

———. 2012. "The Race Discrimination System." *Annual Review of Sociology* 38:17.

Reverby, Susan M. 1987. *Ordered to Care: The Dilemma of American Nursing, 1850–1945.* Cambridge: Cambridge University Press.

Rho, Hye Jin, Hayley Brown, and Shawn Fremstad. 2020. "A Basic Demographic Profile of Workers in Frontline Industries." Center for Economic and Policy Research. https://cepr.net/a-basic-demographic-profile-of-workers-in-frontline-industries/.

Richards, Neil, and William Smart. 2016. "How Should the Law Think about Robots?" In *Robot Law*, edited by R. Calo, A. M. Froomkin, and I. Kerr, 3–22. London: Edward Elgar.

Rico, María Nieves. 2014. El desafío de cuidar y ser cuidado en igualdad. Hacia el surgimiento de sistemas nacionales de cuidado. In *Pactos sociales para una protección social más inclusiva. Experiencias, obstáculos y posibilidades en América Latina y Europa*, edited by M. Hopenhayn, C. M. Valera, R. Martínez, M. N. Rico, and A. Sojo, 40–45. Serie Seminarios y Conferencias, No76 (LC/L.3820). Santiago, Chile: CEPAL.

Rico, María Nieves, and Flavia Marco Navarro. 2020. "La agenda pública de los cuidados en América Latina. Recorrido e interrogantes para una nueva estrategia." In *Crisis de cuidados, envejecimiento y políticas de bienestar en Cuba*, edited by E. Acosta, 35–68. Bogotá, Colombia: Universidad Sergio Arboleda.

Rico, María Nieves, and Claudia Robles. 2016. *Políticas de cuidado en América Latina: forjando la igualdad.* Serie Asuntos de Género, Santiago de Chile: CEPAL.

Rico, María Nieves, and Olga Segovia. 2017. *¿Quién cuida en la ciudad? Aportes para políticas urbanas de igualdad.* Libros de la Comisión Económica para América Latina y el Caribe N 150. Santiago, Chile.

Rivas, Lynn 2007. *Built to Last: Preventing Coalition Breakdowns.* PhD diss., University of California Berkeley.

Roberts, Dorothy E. 1997. "Spiritual and Menial Housework." *Yale Journal of Law and Feminism* 9 (51): 51–80.

Robinson, Fiona. 2011. *The Ethics of Care: A Feminist Approach to Human Security.* Philadelphia: Temple University Press, 2011.

Rogalewski, Adam, and Karol Florek. 2020. *The Future of Live-In Care Work in Europe: Report on the EESC Country Visits to the United Kingdom, Germany, Italy and Poland Following up on the EESC Opinion on "The Rights of Live-in Care Workers."* Brussels: European Economic and Social Committee. https://www.eesc.europa.eu/sites/default/files/files/report_on_the_eesc_country_visits_to_uk_germany_italy_poland_0.pdf.

Romero, Mary, and Nancy Pérez. 2016. "Conceptualizing the Foundation of Inequalities in Care Work." *American Behavioral Scientist* 60 (2): 172–188.

Rostgaard, Tine, and Anders Ejrnæs. 2020. "Denmark Country Note." In *International Review of Leave Policies and Research 2020*, edited by A. Koslowski, S. Blum, I. Dobrotić, G. Kaufman, and P. Moss, 221–234. http://www.leavenetwork.org/lp_and_r_reports/.

Ruggles, Steven, Sarah Flood, Ronald Goeken, Megan Schouweiler, and Matthew Sobek. 2022. IPUMS USA: Version 12.0 (dataset). Minneapolis, MN: IPUMS. https://doi.org/10.18128/D010.V12.0.

Ruiz, Neil G., Julian Menasce Horowitz, and Christine Tamir. 2020. *Americans Say They Have Experienced Discrimination Amid the COVID-19 Outbreak.* Washington, DC: Pew Research Center. https://www.pewsocialtrends.org/2020/07/01/many-black-and-asian-americans-say-they-have-experienced-discrimination-amid-the-covid-19-outbreak/.

Ruxandra, Paul. 2020. "Europe's Essential Workers: Migration and Pandemic Politics in Central and Eastern Europe during COVID-19." *European Policy Analysis* 6 (2): 238–263.

Sasser Modestino, Alicia. 2020. "Coronavirus Child-Care Crisis Will Set Women Back a Generation." *Washington Post*, July 29. https://www.washingtonpost.com/us-policy/2020/07/29/childcare-remote-learning-women-employment/.

Schmidt, Harald. 2020. "The Way We Ration Ventilators Is Biased—Not Every Patient Has a Fair Chance." *New York Times*, April 15. https://www.nytimes.com/2020/04/15/opinion/covid-ventilator-rationing-blacks.html.

Schober, Pia, Sonja Blum, Daniel Erler, and Thordis Reimer. 2020. "Germany Country Note." In *International Review of Leave Policies and Research 2020,* edited by A. Koslowski, S. Blum, I. Dobrotić, G. Kaufman, and P. Moss, 274–288. http://www.leavenetwork.org/lp_and_r_reports/.

Schulson, Michael. 2020. "It's Time to Rethink the Institutional Model for Elder Care: Is That Possible?" *Mother Jones*, June. https://www.motherjones.com/environment/2020/06/its-time-to-rethink-the-institutional-model-for-elder-care-is-that-possible/.

Schultz, Kai, and Suhasini Raj. 2020. "For Indian Women, the Coronavirus Economy Is a Devastating Setback." *New York Times*, June 9, A10.

Schwiter, Karin, Kendra Strauss, and Kim England. 2018. "At Home with the Boss: Migrant Live-in Caregivers, Social Reproduction and Constrained Agency in the UK, Canada, Austria and Switzerland." *Transactions of the Institute of British Geographers* 43 (3): 462–476.

Sedlak, Michael, and Steven Schlossman. 1987. "Who Will Teach? Historical Perspectives on the Changing Appeal of Teaching as a Profession." *Review of Research in Education* 14 (1): 93–131.

Seguino, Stephanie. 2020. "Engendering Macroeconomic Theory and Policy." *Feminist Economics* 26 (2): 27–61.

Sevenhuijsen, Selma. 2003. "The Place of Care: The Relevance of the Feminist Ethic of Care for Social Policy." *Feminist Theory* 4 (2): 179–197.

Sevilla, Almundena, and Sarah Smith. 2020. "Baby Steps: The Gender Division of Childcare during the COVID-19 Pandemic." *Oxford Review of Economic Policy* 36 (S1): S169–S186. https://doi.org/10.1093/oxrep/graa027.

Sevilla-Sanz, Almundena, Jose I. Gimenez-Nadal, and Cristina Fernandez. 2010. "Gender Roles and the Division of Unpaid Work in Spanish Households." *Feminist Economics* 16 (4): 137–184.

Shakespeare, Tom. 2013. "The Social Model of Disability." In *The Disability Studies Reader*, edited by L. J. Davis, 214–221. New York: Routledge.

Shapiro, Joseph P. 1994. *No Pity: People with Disabilities Forging a New Civil Rights Movement.* New York: Broadway Books.

Sharkey, Amanda, and Noel Sharkey. 2012. "Granny and the Robots: Ethical Issues in Robot Care for the Eldery." *Ethics and Information Technology* 14 (1): 27–40.

Sharpe, Marty. 2020. "Coronavirus Tracked: NZ's Latest Covid-19 Numbers." Stuff. https://www.stuff.co.nz/national/health/120667883/what-on-earth-is-going-on-with-ppe-gear-for-home-care-workers.

Shatzer, Jacob. 2013. "A Posthuman Liturgy? Virtual Worlds, Robotics, and Human Flourishing." *New Bioethics* 19 (1): 46–53.

Shi, Qiujie, Danny Dorling, Guangzhong Cao, and Tao Liu. 2020. "Changes in Population Movement Make COVID-19 Spread Differently from SARS." *Social Science & Medicine* 255:113036. https://doi.org/10.1016/j.socscimed.2020.113036.

Sibai, Abla M., Aline Semaan, Aline Tabbara, and Anthony Rizk. 2017. "Ageing and Health in the Arab Region: Challenges, Opportunities and the Way Forward." *Population Horizons* 14 (2): 73–84.

Siegler, Eugenia L., Sonam D. Lama, Michael G. Knight, Evelyn Laureano, and M. Carrington Reid. 2015. "Community-Based Supports and Services for Older Adults: A Primer for Clinicians." *Journal of Geriatrics* 2105: 678625. https://doi.org/10.1155/2015/678625.

Singer, Merrill. 2009. *Introduction to Syndemic: A Critical Systems Approach to Public and Community Health.* San Francisco: Jossey-Bass.

Sins Invalid. 2019. *Skin Tooth and Bone: The Basis of Movement Is Our People.* 2nd ed. Berkeley, CA: Sins Invalid.

Sinsky, Christine A., Roger L. Brown, Martin J. Stillman, and Mark Linzer. 2021. "COVID-Related Stress and Work Intentions in a Sample of US Health Care Workers." *Mayo Clinic Proceedings: Innovations, Quality & Outcomes* 5 (6): 1165–1173.

Slack, Donovan, and Dinah Voyles Pulver. 2020. "US Never Spent Enough on Emergency Stockpile, Former Managers Say." *USA Today,* March 27. https://www.usatoday.com/story/news/investigations/2020/03/27/u-s-never-spent-enough-emergency-stockpile-former-managers-say/2915567001/.

Smit, Ria. 2001. "The Impact of Labor Migration on African Families in South Africa: Yesterday and Today". *Journal of Comparative Family Studies* 32 (4): 533–548.

Smith, Anja, Rose T. Peter, Shivani Ranchhod, Dave Strugnell, and Jodi Wishnia. 2020. "The Economy-Linked Impact of COVID-19 on Mortality and Health: Early Learnings For South Africa's Coronavirus-Linked Recession." Technical Report, July. https://doi.org/10.13140/RG.2.2.20284.67205.

Smith, Catherine, H. Dickinson, Nicole Carey, and Gemma Carey. 2020. "The Challenges and Benefits of Stewarding Disruptive Technology." In *The Palgrave Handbook of the Public Servant,* edited by H. Sullivan, H. Dickinson, and H. Henderson, 1–17. Basingstoke: Palgrave MacMillan.

Smith, Sheila, and Maribel Granja. 2021. Early Childhood Education throughout the COVID-19 Pandemic: The Experiences of Arkansas Educators. New York: National Center for Children in Poverty.

Smith, Yves. 2019, "Why Hospitals Never Have Enough Nurses: The Explanatory Power of 'Prasad's Law' of Wealth Concentration." naked capitalism, December. https://www.nakedcapitalism.com/2019/12/why-hospitals-never-have-enough-nurses-the-explanatory-power-of-prasads-law-of-wealth-concentration.html?emci=645dcb4d-a41a-ea11-828b-2818784d6d68&emdi=9ad0501f-b61a-ea11-828b-2818784d6d68&ceid=3918525.

Sparrow, Robert, and Mark Howard. 2017. "When Human Beings Are Like Drunk Robots: Driverless Vehicles, Ethics, and the Future of Transport." *Transportation Research Part C: Emerging Technologies* 80 (July): 206–215.

Spaull, Nic, and Servaas Van der Berg. 2020. "Counting the Cost: COVID-19 School Closures in South Africa and Its Impact on Children." *South African Journal of Childhood Education* 10 (1): a924. https://doi.org/10.4102/ sajce.v10i1.924.

Ssengonzi, R. 2009. "The Impact of HIV and AIDS on the Living Arrangements and Well-Being of Elderly Caregivers in Rural Uganda." *AIDS Care* 21 (3): 309–314.

Staab, Silke. 2012. "Maternalism, Male-Breadwinner Bias, and Market Reform." *Social Politics* 19 (3): 299–332.

———. 2020. "Covid-19 Sends the Care Economy Deeper into the Crisis Mode." UN Women, April 22. https://data.unwomen.org/features/covid-19-sends-care-economy-deeper-crisis-mode.

Stacey, Clare. 2011. *The Caring Self: The Work Experiences of Home-Care Aides.* Ithaca: Cornell University Press.

Stack, Megan K. 2020. "A Sudden Coronavirus Surge Brought Out Singapore's Dark Side." *New York Times*, May 20. https://www.nytimes.com/2020/05/20/magazine/singapore-corona virus.html.

Stage, Helena B., Joseph Shingleton, Sanmitra Ghosh, Francesca Scarabel, Lorenzo Pellis, and Thomas Finnie. 2020. "Shut and Re-open: The Role of Schools in the Spread of COVID-19 in Europe." medRxiv, June 24. https://www.medrxiv.org/content/10.1101/2020.06.24 .20139634v1.

Stankiewicz, Kevin. 2020. ".Boston Dynamics' Dog-Like Tobot Spot Is Being Used on Corona-virus Social Distancing Patrol." CNBC, May 15. https://www.cnbc.com/2020/05/15/boston -dynamics-dog-like-robot-spot-used-on-social-distancing-patrol.html.

Star Staff. 2020. "Today's Coronavirus News." *Toronto Star*, October 1. https://www.thestar.com /news/canada/2020/10/01/coronavirus-updates-covid-19-canada-ontario-toronto-gta -oct-1-2020.html.

Statistics Canada, n.d. *Census Profile, 2016 Census*. https://www12.statcan.gc.ca/census-recense ment/2016/dp-pd/prof/details/page.cfm?Lang=E&Geo1=PR&Code1=01&Geo2=PR&Code2 =01&SearchText=Canada&SearchType=Begins&SearchPR=01&B1=Immigration%20and%20 citizenship&TABID=1&type=0.

Statistics New Zealand. n.d. "Population." https://www.stats.govt.nz/topics/population.

Stiglitz, Joseph. 2009. "The Global Crisis, Social Protection and Jobs." *International Labor Review* 148:1–13.

Stokes, Jeffrey E., and Sarah E. Patterson. 2020. "Intergenerational Relationships, Family Care-giving Policy, and COVID-19 in the United States." *Journal of Aging and Social Policy* 32 (4): 416–424.

Stolberg, Sheryl Gay. 2020. "Trump Allies Got Medicine Unavailable to Others." *New York Times*, December 23. https://www.nytimes.com/2020/12/09/us/politics/trump-corona virus-treatments.html.

Stoyles, Megan. 2017. "Micare Launches Aged Care Robot to Benefit Workers." Australian Age-ing Agenda, November 22. https://www.australianageingagenda.com.au/2017/11/22/micare -launches-aged-care-robot-benefit-workers/.

Stramondo, Joseph. 2020. "COVID-19 Triage and Disability: What NOT to Do." Bioethics.Net, March. http://www.bioethics.net/2020/03/covid-19-triage-and-disability-what-not-to-do /?fbclid=IwAR1h8RcueMcdn6spIPnhjVXz0Sno8-ir2LfUwCB5aeSobzdEK9XNbpLU8yM.

Struthers, James. 2017. "Home, Hotel, Hospital, Hospice. Conflicting Images of Long-Term Res-idential Care in Ontario, Canada." In *Care Home Stories. Aging, Disability, and Long-Term Residential Care Aging Studies*, edited by S Chivers and U. Kriebernegg, 283–301. Bielefeld, Germany: Transcript Verlag.

Sun, Ken Chih-Yan. 2012. "Fashioning Reciprocal Norms of Elder Care: A Case of Immigrants in the U.S. and Their Parents in Taiwan." *Journal of Family Issues* 33 (9): 1240–1271.

———. 2014. "Transnational Healthcare Seeking: How Aging Taiwanese Return Migrants Think About Homeland Public Benefits." *Global Networks* 14 (4): 533–550.

———. 2020. "Constructing Networks of Elder Care across Borders: The Experiences of Taiwan-ese Immigrants in the US and Their Parents in the Homeland." In *Aging and Elder Care in East Asia: Beyond Filial Piety*, edited by Jeanne L. Shea and Hong Zhang, 166–190. New York: Berghahn.

———. 2021. *Time and Migration: How Long-Term Taiwanese Migrants Negotiate Later-Life*. Ithaca, NY: Cornell University Press.

Suskind. Dana. 2020. "Universal Child Care Was Provided during World War II. We Need It Again during This Pandemic—and Beyond." *Chicago Tribune*, May 5, updated November 19. https://napavalleyregister.com/opinion/columnists/universal-child-care-was-provided

-during-world-war-ii-we-need-it-again-during-this/article_a82e311a–42c2-5fc4-80fa
-cddf87e9fef4.html.

Swinth, Kirsten. 2018. *Feminism's Forgotten Fight: The Unfinished Struggle for Work and Family*. Harvard, MA: Harvard University Press.

Tarrant, Kate, and Mark Nagasawa. 2020. *New York Early Care and Education Survey: Understanding the Impact of COVID-19 on New York Early Childhood System*. New York: New York Early Childhood Professional Development Institute.

Thai, Hung Cam. 2014. *Insufficient Funds: The Culture of Money in Low-Wage Transnational Families*. Stanford: Stanford University Press.

Therborn, Goran. 2004. *Between Sex and Power: Family in the World, 1900–2000*. London: Routledge.

Thomas, Carol. 2007. *Sociologies of Disability and Illness: Contested Ideas in Disability Studies and Medical Sociology*. New York: Palgrave.

Thompson, Nicole. 2022. "Staffing Shortages Hitting Beleaguered Ontario Home-Care Sector." *Toronto Star*, January 24. https://www.thestar.com/news/canada/2022/01/24/staffing-shortages-hitting-beleaguered-home-care-sector-organization-says.html.

Thomson, Rosemarie Garland. 1997. *Extraordinary Bodies: Figuring Physical Disability in American Culture and Literature*. New York: Columbia University Press.

Tippet, Krista, 2020 "This Is Our (Caring) Revolution." On Being (transcript), April 2. https://onbeing.org/programs/ai-jen-poo-this-is-our-caring-revolution/.

Trappenburg, Margo, and Gercoline Van Beek. 2019. "'My Profession Is Gone': How Social Workers Experience De-professionalization in the Netherlands." *European Journal of Social Work* 22 (4): 676–689.

Travers, Jasmine L., Anne M. Teitelman, Kevin A. Jenkins, and Nicholas G. Castle. 2020. "Exploring Social-Based Discrimination among Nursing Home Certified Nursing Assistants." *Nursing Inquiry* 27 (1): e12315.

The Treasury. 2020. *Half Year Ecomomic and Fiscal Update 2020*. Wellington, New Zealand: The New Zealand Treasury, December 16. https://treasury.govt.nz/publications/efu/pre-election-economic-and-fiscal-update-2020.

Trevedei, Anjani. 2020. "The Robots-Are-Taking-Our-Jobs Threat Gets Real." *Financial Review*, May 21. https://www.afr.com/technology/the-robots-are-taking-our-jobs-threat-gets-real-20200521-p54v7x.

Triandafyllidou, Anna and Sabrina Marchetti. 2014. "Europe 2020: Addressing Low Skill Labour Migration at Times of Fragile Recovery." Robert Schuman Centre for Advanced Studies Research Paper No. RSCAS. https://cadmus.eui.eu/bitstream/handle/1814/31222/RSCAS_PP_2014_05.pdf?sequence=1.

———. 2017. *Employers, Agencies and Immigration: Paying for Care*. New York: Routledge.

Tronto, Joan C. 2013. *Caring Democracy: Markets, Equality and Justice*. New York: NYU Press.

———. 2015. "Democratic Caring and Global Care Responsibilities." In *Ethics of Care: Critical Advances in International Perspective*, edited by T. Brannelly, L. Ward, and N. Ward, 21–30. Bristol: Policy Press.

———. 2017. "There Is an Alternative: Homines Curans and the Limits of Neoliberalism." *International Journal of Care and Caring* 1 (1): 27–43. https://doi.org/10.1332/239788217x14866281687583.

———. 2020. *¿Riesgo o cuidado?* Ciudad Autónoma de Buenos Aires: Fundación Medifé Edita.

True, Sarah, Juliette Cubanski, Rachel Garfield, Matthew Rae, Gary Claxton, Priya Chidambaram, and Kendal Orgera. 2020. "COVID-19 and Workers at Risk: Examining the Long-Term Care Workforce." KFF. https://www.kff.org/coronavirus-covid-19/issue-brief/covid-19-and-workers-at-risk-examining-the-long-term-care-workforce/.

Tsaplina, Marina, and Joseph A. Stramondo. 2020. "#WeAreEssential: Why Disabled People Should Be Appointed to Hospital Triage Committees." The Hastings Center. https://www .thehastingscenter.org/weareessential-why-disabled-people-should-be-appointed-to -hospital-triage-committees/.

Tungohan, Ethel. 2020. "Filipino Healthcare Workers during COVID-19 and the Importance of Race-Based Analysis." Broadbent Institute. https://www.broadbentinstitute.ca/filipino _healthcare_workers_during_covid19_and_the_importance_of_race_based_analysis.

Turcotte, Martin, and Katherine Savage. 2020. "The Contribution of Immigrants and Population Groups Designated as Visible Minorities to Nurse Aide, Orderly and Patient Service Associate Occupations." Statistics Canada, June. https://www150.statcan.gc.ca/n1/pub/45 -28-0001/2020001/article/00036-eng.htm.

Turkle, Sherry. 2017. *Alone Together: Why We Expect More from Technology and Less from Each Other.* New York: Basic Books.

Twigg, Julia. 2000. *Bathing: The Body and Community Care.* London: Routledge.

UK Women's Budget Group. 2020. *Creating a Caring Economy: A Call to Action.* https://wbg.org .uk/analysis/creating-a-caring-economy-a-call-to-action-2/.

United Nations (UN). 2019a. *Living Arrangements of Older Persons around the World.* New York: United Nations.

———. 2019b. *World Population Ageing 2019: Highlights.* New York: United Nations.

———. 2020. *Policy Brief: Education during COVID-19 and Beyond.* New York: United Nations.

United Nations Development Programme and United Nations Women (UNDP, UN Women). 2020. *COVID-19 Global Gender Response Tracker.* https://data.undp.org/gendertracker/.

United Nations Educational, Scientific and Cultural Organization (UNESCO). 2020a. *From COVID-19 Learning Disruption to Recovery: A Snapshot of UNESCO's Work in Education in 2020.* Paris: UNESCO.

———. 2020b. *Responding to COVID-19: Education in Latin America and the Caribbean.* Santiago, Chile: UNESCO.

United Nations Educational, Scientific and Cultural Organization and International Labour Organization (UNESCO and ILO). 2020. *Supporting Teachers in Back-to-School Efforts: Guidance for Policy-Makers.* Geneva: UNESCO and ILO.

United Nations Entity for Gender Equality and the Empowerment of Women (UN Women). 2015. *Progress of the World's Women 2015–2016: Transforming Economies, Realizing Rights.* New York: UN Women.

———. 2017. *Progress of Women in Latin America and the Caribbean: Transforming Economies, Realizing Rights. Companion Report to the Progress of the World's Women 2015–2016.* New York: UN Women.

———. 2020a. *Covid-19 and Its Economic Toll on Women: The Story Behind the Numbers.* New York: UN Women.

———. 2020b. *COVID-19 and the Care Economy: Immediate Action and Structural Transformation for a Gender-Responsive Recovery.* New York: UN Women.

———. 2020c. *Whose Time to Care? Unpaid Care and Domestic Work during COVID-19.* New York: UN Women.

———. 2020d. *Women as Drivers of Economic Recovery and Resilience during COVID-19 and Beyond.* New York: UN Women.

———. n.d. *Policy Brief no. 2: Women Migrant Workers' Contributions to Development.* New York: UN Women.

United Nations High Commissioner for Refugees and International Organisation for Migration (UNHCR & IOM). 2020. "COVID-19 and Mixed Population Movements: Emerging Dynamics, Risks and Opportunities: A UNHCR/IOM Discussion Paper." https://data2 .unhcr.org/en/documents/details/76474.

Valli, Linda, and Daria Buese. 2007. "The Changing Roles of Teachers in an Era of High-Stakes Accountability." *American Educational Research Journal* 44 (3): 519–558.

Vandemeulebroucke, Tijs, Bernadette Dierckx de Casterlé, and Chris Gastmans. 2018. " How Do Older Adults Experience and Perceive Socially Assistive Robots in Aged Care: A Systematic Review of Qualitative Evidence." *Aging and Metal Health* 22 (2): 149–167.

Van Houtven, Courtney Harold, Nicole DePasquale, and Norma B. Coe. 2020. "Essential Long-term Care Workers Commonly Hold Second Jobs and Double-or Triple-Duty Caregiving Roles." *Journal of the American Geriatrics Society* 68 (8): 1657–1660.

van Wynsberghe, Aimee. 2015. *Healthcare Robots: Ethics, Design and Implementation*. Abingdon: Ashgate Publishing.

———. 2016. "Service Robots, Care Ethics, and Design." *Ethics Information Technology* 18:311–321.

Verbeek, Hilde, Debby L. Gerritsen, Ramona Backhaus, Bram S. de Boer, Raymond T. C. M. Koopmans, and Jan P. H. Hamers. 2020. "Allowing Visitors Back in the Nursing Home during the Covid-19 Crisis: A Dutch National Study into First Experiences and Impact on Well-Being." *Journal of the American Medical Directors Association* 21 (7): 900–904.

Verick, Sher. 2014. "Female Labor Force Participation in Developing Countries." *IZA World of Labor* 2014: 87. https://doi.org/10.15185/izawol.87.

Vermund, Sten H., Emily K. Sheldon, and Mohsin Sidat. 2015. "Southern Africa: The Highest Priority Region for HIV Prevention and Care Interventions." *Current HIV/AIDS Reports* 12 (2): 191–195.

Visagie, Justin, and Ivan Turok. 2021. "Rural–Urban Inequalities Amplified by COVID-19: Evidence from South Africa." *Area Development and Policy* 6 (1): 1–13. https://doi.org/10.1080/23792949.2020.1851143.

Vogtman, Julie. 2017. *Undervalued: A Brief History of Women's Care Work and Child Care Policy in the United States*. Washington, DC: National Women's Law Center.

Wallace, Cara L., Stephanie P. Wladkowski, Allison Gibson, and Patrick White. 2020. "Grief during the Covid-19 Pandemic: Considerations for Palliative Care Providers." *Journal of Pain and Symptom Management* 60 (1): e70–e76.

Walsh, Katie, and Lena Näre, eds. 2016. *Transnational Migration and Home in Older Age*. New York: Routledge.

Ward, Lizzie, Mo Ray, and Denise Tanner. 2020. "Understanding the Social Care Crisis in England through Older People's Lived Experiences." In *Care Ethics, Democratic Citizenship and the State*, edited by P. Urban and L. Ward, 219–239. Basingstoke: Palgrave Macmillan.

White, Alan. 2016. *Shadow State: Inside the Secret Companies That Run Britain*. London: Oneworld.

White House. 2021. Executive Order: A Proclamation on the Suspension of Entry as Immigrants and Non-Immigrants of Certain Additional Persons Who Pose a Risk of Transmitting Coronavirus Disease. January 25, 2021. https://www.whitehouse.gov/briefing-room/presidential-actions/2021/01/25/proclamation-on-the-suspension-of-entry-as-immigrants-and-non-immigrants-of-certain-additional-persons-who-pose-a-risk-of-transmitting-coronavirus-disease/.

Whiteside, Heather. 2016. "Neoliberalism as Austerity: The Theory, Practices and Purpose of Fiscal Restraint since the 1970s." In *Handbook of Neoliberalism*, edited by S. Springer, K. Birch, and J. MacLeavy, 361–369. New York: Routledge.

Whittington, Charlie, Katalina Hadfield, and Carina Calderón, C. 2020. *The Lives and Livelihoods of Many in the LGBTQ Community Are at Risk amidst COVID-19 Crisis*. Washington, DC: Human Rights Campaign Foundation. https://www.hrc.org/resources/the-lives-and-livelihoods-of-many-in-the-lgbtq-community-are-at-risk-amidst.

Wieler, Lothar, Ute Rexroth, and René Gottschalk. 2020. "Emerging COVID-19 Success Story: Germany's Strong Enabling Environment." Our World in Data. https://ourworldindata.org/covid-exemplar-germany.

Wilkinson, Adrian, Tony Dundon, Jimmy Donaghey, and Richard B. Freeman. 2014. "Employee Voice: Bridging New Terrains and Disciplinary Boundaries." In *Handbook of Research on Employee Voice*, edited by A. Wilkinson, J. Donaghey, T. Dundon, and R. B. Freeman, 2–18. Cheltenham, UK: Edward Elgar Publishing.

Williams, Fiona. 2018. "Care: Intersections of Scales, Inequalities and Crises." *Current Sociology* 66 (4): 547–561.

Williams, Fiona, and Deborah Brennan. 2012. "Care, Markets and Migration in a Globalising World: Introduction to the Special Issue." *Journal of European Social Policy* 22 (4): 355–362.

Williams Fiona, and Anna Gavanas. 2008. "The Intersection of Childcare Regimes and Migration Regimes: A Three-Country Study." In *Migration and Domestic Work: A European Perspective on a Global Theme*, edited by L. Helma, 13–28. Surrey: Ashgate.

Williamson, John, and Myhill Marion 2008. "Under 'Constant Bombardment': Work Intensification and the Teachers' Role." In *Teaching: Professionalization, Development and Leadership*, edited by D. Johnson and R. Maclean, 25–43. New York: Springer Dordrecht.

Wilson, Jim. 2020. "Trudeau Pushes for 10 Days' Paid Sick Leave for All Workers." HRReporter, May 26. https://www.hrreporter.com/focus-areas/compensation-and-benefits/trudeau -pushes-for-10-days-paid-sick-leave-for-all-workers/329931.

Winters, Jeffrey A. 2010. *Oligarchy*. New York: Cambridge University Press.

Wired.com. 2020 "The Covid-19 Pandemic Is a Crisis That Robots Were Built For." Wired.com, March 3. https://www.wired.com/story/covid-19-pandemic-robots/.

Wolbring, Gregor. 2008. "The Politics of Ableism." *Development* 51 (2): 252–258. https://doi.org /10.1057/dev.2008.17.

———. 2020. "COVID-19, Its Aftermath and Disabled People: What Is the Connection to Ethics?" *International Journal of Disability, Community & Rehabilitation* 18 (1). http://www.ijdcr .ca/VOL18_01/articles/wolbring.shtml.

Wolfe, Julia, Jori Kandra, Lora Engdahl, and Heidi Shierholz. 2020. *Domestic Workers Chartbook*. Washington, DC: Economic Policy Institute. https://www.epi.org/publication /domestic-workers-chartbook-a-comprehensive-look-at-the-demographics-wages -benefits-and-poverty-rates-of-the-professionals-who-care-for-our-family-members-and -clean-our-homes/.

Wolin, Sheldon S. 2008. *Democracy Incorporated: Managed Democracy and the Specter of Inverted Totalitarianism*. Princeton, NJ: Princeton University Press.

Wong, Alice. 2020. "Freedom for Some Is Not Freedom for All." Disability Visibility Project, June 7. https://disabilityvisibilityproject.com/2020/06/07/freedom-for-some-is-not-free dom-for-all/.

Wong, Kimberly. 2020. *The Improved Labour Market Performance of New Immigrants to Canada, 2006–2019*. Research Report 2020–03. Ottawa: Centre for the Study of Living Standards. http://www.csls.ca/reports/csls2020–03.pdf.

Wooten, Melissa E., and Enobong H. Branch. 2012. "Defining Appropriate Labor: Race, Gender, and Idealization of Black Women in Domestic Service." *Race, Gender & Class* 19 (3): 292–308.

World Bank. 2012. *Latin America and the Caribbean Poverty and Labor Brief, August 2012: The Effect of Women's Economic Power in Latin America and the Caribbean*. Washington, DC: World Bank.

———. 2018. *Moving for Prosperity: Global Migration and Labor Markets*. Washington, DC: World Bank. https://www.worldbank.org/en/research/publication/moving-for-prosperity.

———. 2020. "World Bank Predicts Sharpest Decline of Remittances in Recent History." April 22. https://www.worldbank.org/en/news/press-release/2020/04/22/world-bank -predicts-sharpest-decline-of-remittances-in-recent-history.

World Health Organization (WHO). 2000. *Community Home Based Care: Family Caregiving. Caring for Family Members with HIV/AIDS and Other Chronic Illnesses: The Impact on Older Women and Girls.* A Botswana Case Study. Geneva: WHO.

———. 2017. *Women on the Move: Migration, Care and Health.* Geneva: WHO.

———. 2020a. "Archived: WHO Timeline—COVID-19." June 27. https://www.who.int/news/item/27-04-2020-who-timeline—covid-19.

———. 2020b. "#China Has Reported to WHO a Cluster of #pneumonia Cases—with No Deaths—in Wuhan, Hubei Province: Investigations Are Underway to Identify the Cause of This Illness." @WHO. https://twitter.com/WHO/status/1213523866703814656.

———. 2020c. "Keep Health Workers Safe to Keep Patients Safe: WHO." News item. https://www.who.int/news/item/17-09-2020-keep-health-workers-safe-to-keep-patients-safe-who.

———. 2020d. *State of the World's Nursing 2020.* Geneva: WHO.

———. 2021a. *The Impact of COVID-19 on Health and Care Workers: A Closer Look at Deaths.* Geneva: WHO.

———. 2021b. "World Health Statistics 2021: A Visual Summary." https://www.who.int/data/stories/world-health-statistics-2021-a-visual-summary.

———. 2022. WHO Coronavirus (COVID-19) Dashboard. https://covid19.who.int.

Wusu, Onipede, and Uche C. Isiugo-Abanihe. 2006. "Interconnection among Changing Family Structure, Childbearing, and Fertility Behavior among the Ogo, Southern Western Nigeria: A Qualitative Study." *Demographic Research* 14 (8): 139–156.

Yarris, Kristine Elizabeth. 2017. *Care across Generations: Solidarity and Sacrifice in Transnational Families.* Stanford: Stanford University Press.

Yerkes, Mara A., Birgit Pfau-Effinger, and Wim van Lancker. 2022. "Trajectories of Modernization of Parenting Leave Policies within Continental Europe: Similarities and Unexpected Differences." In *Research Handbook on Leave Policy*, edited by I. Drobrotić, S. Blum, and A. Koslowski, 219–231. London: Edward Elgar.

Zalev, Marcia. 2020. "Home-Care Next on Ford's Privatization Hit List: Ontario Changed, and Ford Changed with It, Cohn." *Toronto Star*, June 20.

Zamarro, Gema, and María J. Prados. 2021. "Gender Differences in Couples' Division of Childcare, Work and Mental Health during COVID-19." *Review of Economics of the Household* 19 (1): 11–40.

Zechner, Minna. 2017. "Transnational Habitus at the Time of Retirement." *Identities* 24 (5): 573–589.

Zelnick, Jennifer. 2015. "Part of the Job? Workplace Violence and Social Services." In *Caring on the Clock: The Complexities and Contradictions of Paid Care Work*, edited by Mignon Duffy, Amy Armenia, and Clare L. Stacey, 104–116. New Brunswick, NJ: Rutgers University Press.

Zhou, Muzhi, Ekaterina Hertog, Kamila Kolpashnikova, and Man-Yee Kan. 2020. "Gender Inequalities: Changes in Income, Time Use and Well-Being Before and during the UK COVID-19 Lockdown." *SOCArxiv.* https://doi.org/10.31235/osf.io/u8ytc.

Zhou, Yanqiu Rachel. 2012. "Space, Time, and Self: Rethinking Aging in the Contexts of Immigration and Transnationalism." *Journal of Aging Issues* 26 (3): 232–242.

Zinchuk, Brian. 2020. "NDP Promises 700 Home-care Workers to Help out Seniors." *Toronto Star*, October 6. https://www.thestar.com/news/canada/2020/10/06/ndp-promises-700-home-care-workers-to-help-out-seniors.html.

NOTES ON
CONTRIBUTORS

ODICHINMA AKOSIONU is a PhD candidate in the health economics track of the Health Services Research, Policy and Administration Program at the University of Minnesota, School of Public Health (UMN-SPH). Her research area is in the economics of aging, investigating how structural racism and discrimination shape the experiences and health outcomes of older adults receiving long-term services and supports. Prior to the PhD program, she worked as a Human Services Program consultant with the Minnesota Department of Human Services. Odi holds a master's degree in public health from UMN-SPH and a bachelor's degree in human biology from the University of California, San Diego.

AMY ARMENIA is a professor of sociology at Rollins College. She has published research on childcare, care work, and family leave in *Work and Occupations*, the *Journal of Family Issues*, and *Social Science Research*. She was coeditor of *Caring on the Clock: The Complexities and Contradictions of Paid Care Work*. She recently has completed comparative research with Mignon Duffy on the paid care sector for UN Women. Dr. Armenia has been involved in the Carework Network since its inception, serving as a member of the steering committee for six years and chairing the organizing committee for two conferences.

PAT ARMSTRONG is a distinguished research professor in sociology at York University and fellow of the Royal Society of Canada. Focusing on the fields of social policy, of women, work, feminist theory, and the health and social services, she has published widely in academic and nonacademic venues. Framed by feminist political economy and focused on making change for social justice, her research has long been collaborative, in partnership with community and union groups. She was principal investigator of a ten-year Social Sciences and Humanities Research Council–funded project, Reimagining Long-Term Residential Care: An International Study of Promising Practices, and on two current SSHRC projects, Changing Places: Unpaid Work in Public Places and COVID and Families.

ORLY BENJAMIN, DPhil Oxford, is a professor at the sociology and anthropology department and at the Gender Studies program, Bar-Ilan University. Her articles appeared in the *Sociological Review*, *Sociological Perspectives*, and more. She chairs the European Sociological Association research network on gender relations in the

247

labor market and the welfare state. Her book *Feminism, Family and Identity in Israel: Women's Marital Names* (with Michal Rom) introduces her theory on couples' negotiation, and her book *Gendering Israel's Outsourcing: The Erasure of Employees' Caring Skills* introduces a feminist perspective on public procurement in welfare, education, and health care services.

CINDY L. CAIN is an assistant professor of sociology at the University of Alabama at Birmingham. Her research examines end-of-life care practices, care worker well-being, and changes to the institution of medicine. She is particularly interested in using sociological perspectives to understand the intended and unintended consequences of attempts to improve health care. Her research has been published in *Journal of Health and Social Behavior, Sociology of Health and Illness, Human Relations, JAMA Internal Medicine, Journal of Pain and Symptom Management*, and *Palliative Medicine*.

CYNTHIA J. CRANFORD is an associate professor of sociology at the University of Toronto. Dr. Cranford's recent research compares the social organization of in-home personal elder care and disability support. She is the author of *Home Care Fault Lines: Understanding Tensions and Creating Alliances*, and her work on care has also been published in *Critical Sociology, Labor Studies Journal, Sociological Theory, Work, Employment and Society*, and several edited volumes.

HELEN DICKINSON is professor of public service research and director of the Public Service Research Group at the School of Business, University of New South Wales, Canberra. Her expertise is in public services, particularly in relation to topics such as governance, policy implementation, and stewardship of Fourth Industrial Revolution technologies. Helen has published eighteen books and over seventy peer-reviewed journal articles on these topics and is also a frequent commentator within the mainstream media. She has worked with a range of different levels of government, community organizations, and private organizations in Australia, the UK, New Zealand, and Europe on research and consultancy programs.

JANETTE DILL is an associate professor in the School of Public Health at the University of Minnesota. Her research focuses on the organization of work, particularly in the health care sector, and the intersection of gender and carework. Her current research examines job quality in the health care sector for adults without a college degree and the challenges of reorganizing work in primary health care clinics. She has published in many public health and sociology journals, including *Gender & Society, Social Science and Medicine*, and *Work, Employment & Society*, and her research has been featured in the *New York Times, The Atlantic*, the *Harvard Business Review*, and other press outlets.

FRANZISKA DORN is a PhD candidate at the Department of Economics and a research assistant in statistics at the University of Goettingen, Germany. Her research focuses on time and income inequality, carework, and the interrelation between environmental degradation and inequality.

MIGNON DUFFY is an associate professor and chair of the sociology department at University of Massachusetts Lowell. Her scholarship is focused on the intersections of paid carework with gender, race, citizenship, and class inequalities. Her book, *Making Care Count: A Century of Gender, Race and Paid Care Work*, was published by Rutgers University Press in 2011. She also coedited a collection focused on paid care workers entitled *Caring on the Clock: The Complexities and Contradictions of Paid Care Work* (Rutgers, 2015). Her research has also appeared in journals such as *Gender & Society* and *Social Problems*, and she has played a leadership role in the international Carework Network.

THURID EGGERS is a doctoral research fellow at the University of Hamburg, Germany. Her research focuses on comparative welfare state analysis as well as on institutional and cultural explanations of change in European long-term care policies. Her most recent publication has appeared in *Ageing & Society* and *American Behavioral Scientist*.

VALERIA ESQUIVEL is an employment policies and gender specialist at the International Labour Office, based in Geneva. Her latest publications have focused primarily on care policies and care workers. She has coauthored the reports *Innovations in Care: New Concepts, New Actors, New Policies* and *Care Work and Care Cobs for the Future of Decent Work*. She has also coedited two *Gender & Development* issues, the first devoted to the Sustainable Development Goals and the other to Beijing +25. Her current work focuses on the intersections of gender, employment, and macroeconomics.

NANCY FOLBRE is professor emerita of economics and director of the Program on Gender and Care Work at the University of Massachusetts Amherst, with a longstanding interest in the economics of care.

LEILA GAUTHAM is a PhD candidate at the Department of Economics, University of Massachusetts Amherst. Her research focuses on the intersections of gender, care, and development.

PILAR GONALONS-PONS is an assistant professor in the Department of Sociology at the University of Pennsylvania. Her work focuses on the political economy of reproductive labor and economic inequality. She uses quantitative methods and cross-national comparative data to examine how work, families, and public policies structure economic inequalities, with a particular focus on the organization and gendering of reproductive labor, both paid and unpaid. Her work has appeared in the *American Sociological Review, Demography, Social Problems, Social Science Research*, and the *RSF: Russell Sage Foundation Journal of the Social Sciences*.

CHRISTOPHER GRAGES is a postdoctoral researcher at the University of Hamburg, Germany. He was a visiting scholar at UC Berkeley and at Aalborg University, Denmark, and earned his PhD at the University of Hamburg. He is currently working in the EU H2020-funded project EUROSHIP (Closing Gaps in European Social

Citizenship). His research revolves around comparative welfare state research and comparative political economy with a specific focus on institutional and cultural change in European social policies and the marketization of social services. His most recent publication has appeared in *Ageing & Society* and *American Behavioral Scientist*.

AMEETA JAGA is an associate professor of organizational psychology in the School of Management Studies at the University of Cape Town. In spring 2020, she was a Mandela Mellon Fellow at the Hutchins Centre for African and African American Research, Harvard University. Her research focuses on the work–family interface relating to culture, race, class, and gender, and more recently she is using Southern Theory to prioritize context in work–family research while underlining global inequalities in knowledge production. Her current research projects deal with understanding how gender equality (via breastfeeding at work) is understood in twenty-first-century South Africa.

J'MAG KARBEAH is a PhD candidate in the University of Minnesota School of Public Health's Division of Health Policy Management, studying health services research, policy, and administration. She is also a predoctoral trainee in the Minnesota Population Center's Population Health Sciences program. Her research analyzes the impact of structural racism on maternal and child health inequities. Her scholarship has done this by examining alternative perinatal care models to address inequities in access and quality that Black birthing people face, and acknowledging and challenging how anti-Black racism is perpetuated through public health and medical institutions.

JULIE KASHEN is a senior policy advisor at the National Domestic Workers Alliance (NDWA) and the director of Women's Economic Justice at The Century Foundation. With more than two decades forwarding work and care issues in federal and state government and through advocacy, Julie has contributed to three major pieces of national legislation. As labor policy adviser to the late senator Edward M. Kennedy (D-MA), she worked on the first national paid sick days bill. As policy director of the Make It Work campaign, she drafted a visionary child care proposal, the principles of which were incorporated into the Child Care for Working Families Act. As senior adviser to NDWA, she led work to introduce the national Domestic Workers Bill of Rights. As deputy director of policy for Senator Jon Corzine (D-NJ), she helped New Jersey become the second state to adopt paid family and medical leave. Julie holds a master's in public policy from Harvard University's Kennedy School of Government and a bachelor's from the University of Michigan.

JANNA KLOSTERMANN is a feminist sociologist and long-term care scholar exploring the politics of care through narrative, ethnographic and arts-based research. "What about the limits of care?" is a question central to her work. She is an assistant professor in the Department of Sociology at the University of Calgary, and a member of the Changing Places: Unpaid Work in Public Places research team.

MARTHA MACDONALD is a professor and past chair in the Department of Economics, Sobey School of Business, Saint Mary's University, Canada, where she teaches courses in labor economics, social policy, and women and the economy. Recent research has focused on long-term care, precarious work, and income security policy. She is a past president of the International Association for Feminist Economics.

SABRINA MARCHETTI is an associate professor in sociology at University Ca' Foscari in Venice. She is currently the principal investigator of the European Research Group Starting Grant project DomEQUAL: Paid Domestic work and Global Inequalities (2016–2021), which looks at India, the Philippines, Taiwan, Ecuador, Colombia, Brazil, Germany, Italy, and Spain (see www.domequal.eu). Her books are *Black Girls: Migrant Domestic Workers and Colonial Legacies* and *Employers, Agencies and Immigration: Paying for Care* (with Anna Triandafyllidou). Her most recent books are *Domestic Work and Migration* and *Global Domestic Workers: Intersectional Inequalities and Struggles for Rights*.

JULIANA MARTÍNEZ FRANZONI is a professor at the School of Political Science and a researcher at the Center for Research and Political Studies (El Centro de Investigación y Estudios Políticos) at the University of Costa Rica. She holds a PhD in sociology from the University of Pittsburgh. Her research has addressed welfare regimes, care policy, and social policy formation in Latin America. Her latest book is *The Quest for Universal Social Policy: Actors, Ideas and Architectures*, coauthored with Diego Sánchez-Ancochea. She is a coeditor of *Social Politics, International Studies in Gender, State and Society* and leads the Latin American network for the analysis of social policy (www.PolSoc.org).

LAURA MAULDIN is an associate professor of women's, gender, and sexuality studies and human development and family sciences at the University of Connecticut. A sociologist of health, illness, and disability, much of her work bridges disability studies and medical sociology. She is author of the book *Made to Hear: Cochlear Implants and Raising Deaf Children* and has published in such journals as *Social Science and Medicine, Science, Technology and Human Values, Sociology of Health and Illness*, and *Disability Studies Quarterly*.

MERITA MESIÄISLEHTO is a senior researcher at the Social Policy Unit of the Finnish Institute for Health and Welfare. Her research focuses on poverty and inequalities and welfare state outcomes on socially and economically disadvantaged groups. She has written several articles on the situation of domestic and care workers and the role of institutions in shaping their position in the labor markets. Her PhD thesis is titled "The layers of Inequality in Paid Domestic Labour: A Global Study on Domestic Workers and Precarious Work."

ZITHA MOKOMANE is an associate professor in the Department of Sociology at the University of Pretoria, South Africa. Professor Mokomane has extensive research, policy, and programmatic expertise in the fields of family studies, with specific interest in the work–family interface, childcare, and elder care. She has researched and published widely in these areas. Her current research projects deal with the development of informal and community-based care systems for older people in Africa.

LAURA C. PAUTASSI is a researcher for the Scientific and Technical Research Council (Consejo de Investigaciones Científicas y Técnicas), a tenured researcher at the Ambrosio Gioja Legal and Social Research Institute (Instituto de Investigaciones Jurídicas y Sociales A. Gioja), and a professor at the University of Buenos Aires/UBA Law School, Buenos Aires, Argentina. She is the director of the Social Rights and Public Policy Interdisciplinary Working Group (http://www.dspp.com.ar/).

ITO PENG is a Canada Research Chair in global social policy at the University of Toronto. She is a world authority on global social policy, specializing in gender, migration, and care policies. She has written extensively on social policies and political economy of care in East Asia. Her current research includes The Care Economy: Gender-Sensitive Macroeconomic Models for Policy Analysis and Care Economies in Context: Towards Sustainable Social and Economic Development (http://cgsp.ca/). Her recent book, coedited with Sonya Michel, is called *Gender, Migration and the Work of Care: A Multi-Scalar Approach to the Pacific Rim*.

BIRGIT PFAU-EFFINGER is a research professor for cultural and institutional change at the University of Hamburg, Germany. She was a professor at universities in Berlin, Jena, and Southern Denmark, a visiting professor at universities in Barcelona, Aalborg, and Tampere, and an honorary professor at the University of Southern Denmark. Her main fields of research include historical and cross-national comparative research about culture and welfare states, family policies, gender and the work–family relationship, and labor markets. She has published numerous articles in international scientific journals and published books with international publishers.

KIM PRICE-GLYNN is associate professor of sociology at the University of Connecticut. She is coeditor of the Carework in a Changing World series (Rutgers University Press) with Mignon Duffy and Amy Armenia. She has published work on gendered organizations and paid and unpaid care with New York University Press, *Gender & Society*, *Sociology of Health & Illness*, as well as other journals and the edited volume *Caring on the Clock*. Her current study (under contract with Rutgers University Press) explores the dimensions of parenting groups' carework that demonstrate both barriers and possible solutions to more equitable and transformative care practices. She is an active member and past cochair of the Carework Network.

JOHANNA S. QUINN is an assistant professor of sociology at Fordham University. Her work examines schools as workplaces and focuses on the organization of race, class, care, and gender in producing and ameliorating workplace and educational inequalities. Her research appears in *Gender, Work and Organizations*, *Research in Human Development*, *Applied Developmental Science*, and the *Journal of Early Adolescence*.

KATHERINE RAVENSWOOD is an associate professor of employment relations at Auckland University of Technology. She has held appointments with a number of academic and industry boards and organizations, such as the Caring Counts Coalition (New Zealand Human Rights Commission) and working parties on community support with the New Zealand Ministry of Health. Katherine focuses on high-quality research that has strong links with the community and industry. Her research focuses on the examination of power, gender, and diversity in the employment relationship, with a specific focus on carework regimes; gender and employee well-being; and inequality, power, and voice at work.

MARÍA NIEVES RICO is an Argentine social anthropologist at the Universidad de Rosario Nacional de Rosario, Argentina, with a master's degree in development sociology from Instituto de Sociologia del Area Iberica in Madrid, España, urban development from Instituto Nacional de Administración Local, Madrid, España, and international relations from Instituto Complutense de Estudios Internacionales, Madrid, España. She completed her doctoral studies in sociology at Universidad Complutense de Madrid, España. Rico worked as a United Nations official between 1992 and 2020. She is a former director of the Division for Gender Affairs and the Division for Social Development of the Economic Commission for Latin America and the Caribbean. A specialist in social policies with a gender and human rights perspective, she is the author of books and articles on family relationships, care, violence against women, urban development, and other topics. She has served as a guest professor at universities in Argentina, Chile, Ecuador, Spain, and Mexico and currently works as an independent consultant.

VEENA SIDDHARTH blends human rights perspectives with economic and policy analysis to forge unconventional alliances for social change. Organizations that she has worked for include the World Bank, Human Rights Watch, Oxfam International, Planned Parenthood, and United Nations Development Programme. She has an MSc in quantitative research methods and evaluation from University College London and a master's in public policy from Harvard University. She is currently a doctoral student at the University of Costa Rica researching care and attitudes toward working mothers in Central America. She started her career as a Peace Corps Volunteer working with women farmers in rural Nepal.

CATHERINE SMITH is a lecturer at the Melbourne Graduate School of Education at the University of Melbourne on the lands of the Wurundjeri peoples. Her research focuses on care ethics and social justice in the nexus of evidence-informed policy and practice and concentrates particularly on equity and well-being in the use of digital and robotic technologies. In her thirty years as an educator, Catherine has developed and delivered school and tertiary-level courses, as well as executive and professional education in policy reform in Canada, Guinea-Bissau, the UK, Australia, and Indonesia. She is committed to universal design, choice, and equitable access in education in physical and digital spaces.

KEN CHIH-YAN SUN is an assistant professor of sociology and criminology at Villanova University. His research interests include families, migration, life stage, inequalities, and globalization. He published his works in *Journal of Marriage and Family*, *Global Networks*, *Sociological Forum*, *Qualitative Sociology*, *Ethnic and Racial Studies*, *Journal of Ethnic and Migration Studies*, *Identities*, *Journal of Family Issues*, and *Current Sociology*. His book on how long-term migrants negotiate later life is titled *Time and Migration: How Long-Term Taiwanese Migrants Negotiate Later Life*.

JOAN C. TRONTO is professor emerita of political science at the City University of New York and the University of Minnesota. She is the author of many works on care ethics, including *Moral Boundaries: A Political Argument for an Ethics of Care* and *Caring Democracy: Markets, Equality and Justice*.

INDEX

Page numbers in italics refer to figures and tables.

ableism, 45–52; and health care system, 48–49
"ablenationalism," 49
Abramowitz, Sharon A., 98
Ackerly, Brooke, 12
activism, 50–51
Africa: demographic trends, 94–95; elder care in South Africa, 96–101; NEP+ (Ethiopia), 99
AIDS epidemic, 95, 98
Akosionu, Odichinma, 3, 8, 193
American Association of People with Disabilities, 51
Amnesty International, 76
anxiety among health care workers, 76, 97, 108
Aotearoa/New Zealand, 183–190
Arai, Hidenori, 177
Argentina: wages for health care workers, 77; women's unpaid work, 67
Armstrong, Pat, 3, 8–9, 101
artificial intelligence, 180–181. *See also* robot technology
Asian women: in domestic work, 86; in health care sector, 38; occupational distribution, 29; and unpaid childcare, 89–90
Australia: COVID case rates, 183; Human Rights Commission, 179; Royal Commissions on healthcare, 177–178

Balaz, Joyce, 161
Benjamin, Orly, 4, 112
Bennie, Garth, 186
Black women: in domestic work, 86, 193–194; in health care jobs, 36–44; and unpaid childcare, 89–90
Borenstein, Jason, 181
Brewster, Amanda L., 99
burnout among health care workers, 61, 76, 87, 89, 128

Cahn, Naomi, 14
Cain, Cindy L., 4, 159, 160
Canada: home care in Ontario, 161–167; schools, 77; supplemental pay policy, 117–127, 118–125; wages for carework, 33
Canada Health Act, 54
Canadian Armed Forces, 53
Canadian Charter of Rights and Freedoms, 59
capitalism, predatory, 13. *See also* wealth-care
Carbone, June, 14

care: definitions of, 182; as family responsibility, 14–15; individual contrasted with collective responsibility, 192–193; as "investment," 14; paid contrasted with unpaid, 53–60
Care and Support Workers Act (2017), 185
"care arrangement" approach, 92, 152–155
Care Can't Wait Coalition, 195
"care circulation," 102, 108
Care Collective, The, 12
care infrastructure, U.S., 191–198; benefits of quality system, 195–198
"caremongering," 176
care robots, 176–182
"carewashing," 12
carework: gender redistribution of unpaid carework, 32–33; labor market valuation of, 30–31; as private concern, 22; reorganization of, 24–25; "retraditionalization" of roles, 25; three Rs of unpaid carework, 31–32; undervaluation of, 19; wage adjustments, 33
care workers: compensation, 195–196; during economic recovery, 80–81; in education, 79; employee voice, 183–190, 189; gendered inequalities, 200; global connections, 187–188; home-based care and domestic workers, 78–79; institution-based contrasted with home-based, 77–78; invisibility of, 14, 20, 27, 62, 67, 184–185, 200; undervaluation of, 193–194
Caring for Those Who Care (UNI Global Union), 188
cash transfers, 23, 24, 25, 98, 140
Center for Public Representation, 49
Centers for Medicare & Medicaid Services (CMS), 169, 172
Central Bank of Israel, 146–148
Chami, Ralph, 34
childcare: familial contrasted with non-familial, 112; policies in Europe, 151–158, 153; professionalization of, 86; racialization of workforce, 83–84, 84; unpaid, 89–92, 91
childcare workers: challenges faced during pandemic, 85–87; contrasted with elementary teachers during pandemic, 82–93; family childcare, 85; racism and devaluation of work, 86
children and adolescents, welfare of, 73–74
Chile, 22, 68

Chinese immigrants in U.S., 105
Chu, Ruby, 106–107
citizenship, 135–136; and division of labor, 163; duties of, 15–16
Clair, Robin P., 145
collective bargaining. See unionization
collective contrasted with individual responsibility for care, 192–193
communication technology, 105–106, 116
Community Based Health Insurance, Ethiopia, 99
community-based support and services (CBSS) model, 98–101, 100
congregate care settings, 45, 47; contrasted with home care, 47, 48; group homes, 48. See also long-term care (LTC) settings; nursing homes
Costa Rica, 22, 69
COVID-19 pandemic: COVID-deniers, 16; responsibility and blame, 11; timeline, 1–2
Cranford, Cynthia J., 4, 47, 50, 159, 160
Creative Teamwork (Armstrong & Lowndes), 53
Crenshaw, Kimberlé, 42–43
Crip Fund, 51

death and dying. See end-of-life considerations
Deetz, Stanley A., 145
deinstitutionalization, 49
democracy, managed, 17
Democracy in Chains (MacLean), 15
"democratic caring," 162, 166
Denmark, childcare policy, 153, 155–156
depression among health care workers, 76, 170
Dickinson, Helen, 4, 159, 160
Dill, Janette, 3
disability, 45–52; disability activism, 50–51; disability analytics, 45–46; social model of, 46
Disability and the Politics of Care (Kelly), 50
Disability Justice Culture Club, 51
domestic abuse and violence, 66, 70, 147
domestic workers, 37, 78–79; in Europe, 135; in Latin America, 21
Dorn, Franziska, 4, 111
drones, 179. See also robot technology
Duffy, Mignon, 3

Ebola epidemic, 95, 98
Economic Commission for Latin America and the Caribbean, 67
economic remittances, 31, 34–35n5, 104, 105
education: care workers in, 79; of children during pandemic, 69; disinvestment in, 14; education levels and care workers, 21, 26n5, 41; Head Start and pre-Kindergarten, 83, 85, 86, 87, 90, 196; online classes, 69, 74, 79, 82, 87; primary school teachers, 87–89
Eggers, Thurid, 4, 25, 92, 112
Eisler, Riane, 67
elder care: in South Africa, 96–101; for transnational families, 103–104
Elson, Diane, 31–32
employee voice, 188–190, 189
employment recovery, 73

end-of-life considerations, 168–175; support for care workers, 171–174
England, childcare policies, 154–155, 157
equipment shortages, 15, 116, 172
Esquivel, Valeria, 3, 62, 63
essential workers, 59, 61, 68; definitions of "essential work," 115, 126; supplemental pay for, 111, 115–128; teachers as, 79
ethical concerns, 159, 173–175, 179, 182
Europe: childcare policies, 151–158, 153; migrant workforce, 134–141, 137, 138; shortage of care workers, 29
European Commission guidelines (March 2020), 136
European Economic and Social Committee, 135
European Labour Force Survey, 136
European Parliament, 135

facial coverings, 79, 169, 170, 172
family caregiving, 55–58; policies in Europe, 151–158, 153; transnational, 102–109
Federal Canada Health Act, 162–163
femininity index, 67, 72n3
financial crisis (2008) and care infrastructure, 80–81
Floyd, George, 36
Folbre, Nancy, 4
food security, 98, 99, 144
for-profit care contrasted with nonprofit, 173
fragmentation of care, 78, 192–193
France, 77, 139
Frankfurt, Harry, 12–13
frontline care workers, 27. See also essential workers
future planning: care infrastructure in U.S., 194–198; care robots, 181–182; for economic recovery, 196; importance of interconnected systems, 174–175; South Africa, 97–99

Gautham, Leila, 4
gender: gender-blind responses to COVID-19, 23–24; gender discrimination, challenges to, 183–190; gender inequities, 20, 30, 89–90, 151, 158, 200; gender inequities in Israel, 143–150; gender regimes, 188–189; and racial inequities in healthcare, 37–41, 38, 39, 40; and redistribution of unpaid carework, 32–33; and responses to COVID-19 pandemic, 23–24; UN Women's 2017 regional report on Latin America, 20–23
Gentilini, Ugo, 138–139
Germany: childcare policy, 154, 155, 156–157; supplemental pay policy, 117–127, 118–125
Glenn, Evelyn Nakano, 54
global interdependence, 27–29, 29; and migration, 30–31
Goldberg, Abbie E., 90
Gonalons-Pons, Pilar, 3, 62, 63
Grages, Christopher, 4, 25, 92, 112
grandchildren, elders' care for, 62–63. See also multigenerational households
group homes, 48. See also congregate care settings
Guaranteed Hours Funding Framework (2017), 185

Hanson Robotics, 180
Harding, Rosie, 182
Harrington, Brooke, 14
hazard pay, 4, 117, *118*, *119*, 126, 128. *See also* supplemental pay for essential workers
Head Start and pre-Kindergarten, 83, 85, 86, 87, 90, 196
health and safety guidelines for infection control, 43, 187, 190
health care: health care assistants and collective voice, 189–190; symbolic valuing of workers, 174; workers, 74–77, *75*; workers and COVID infection rates, 76; workers and moral stress, burnout and attrition, 128, 172–173; workers and personal risk, 171–172; workers blamed as vectors of disease, 41; workers in multiple settings, 126, 164–165; workforce in crisis, 177–178; working conditions, 43
high-risk categories, 45–46
Hispanic women: in domestic work, 86; in health care sector, 38; and unpaid childcare, 89–90
HIV infections, 95, 98
home and community-based services (HCSBs), 48, 49
Home and Community Support Settlement Act (2016), 185
home care: contrasted with congregate care settings, 47, 48; in Ontario, Canada, 161–167; vulnerability of, 68; workers, 50; workers as personal support workers, 161
home confinement, 66. *See also* lockdowns
home health aides, 47
hospice and palliative care, 168–173
Howard, Ayanna, 181
Human Rights Commission (Australia), 179

ILO (International Labour Organization). *See* International Labour Organization (ILO)
Income Defense Industry, 14
Indigenous and local knowledge, 98
individual responsibility for care, 192–193
infection control, 43, 187, 190
infection rates for health care workers, 27, 48, 56, 76–77
infrastructure: and ableism, 49, 52; care infrastructure in U.S., 191–198; and elder care, 97–98, 101; investment in, 32, 36, 43; social infrastructure, 19, 25, 32–34, 178
injustice: in distribution of care, 11–12; frameworks and patterns, 12; wealth-care as injustice, 13–14, 15–17
International Domestic Workers' Federation, 141
International Labour Organization (ILO), 28, 31, 76, 94, 140; Convention C-189 (2011), 33, 135; 2018 report, 1
intersectionality, 192; approach to Latin American situation, 66–67; COVID-19 as health crisis and economic crisis, 73–81; gender and race, 42–43
invisibility: of Black women workers, 37; of carework, 14, 20, 27, 62, 67, 184–185, 200; of housekeeping positions, 41; lack of data and statistics, 136

isolation, social, 62, 99, 180, 182
Israel and marginalized advocacy for care, 143–150; Central Bank of Israel, 146–148; Ministry of Finance, 148–150; Ministry of Welfare, 145–146
Italy, 76–77, 136, 137, 139, 140, 141

Jaga, Ameeta, 3, 62
Japan, 177
Jones, Janelle, 191
justice, crisis of, 11

Kaine, Sarah, 190
Karbeah, J'Mag, 3
Kashen, Julie, 4, 37, 159, 160
Kelly, Christine, 50
Klostermann, Janna, 3, 8–9, 101

labor organization. *See* unionization
labor policies, 112
Latin America: carework in the economy, 67; response to COVID-19, 19–25; and right to care, 65–72
Latina women. *See* Hispanic women
Lazar, M., 145
Leiblfinger, Michael, 140
Lemieux, Pierre, 15
Lewis, Talila, 46–47
LGBTQ parents, 90
Lin, Jacob, 107–108
local and Indigenous knowledge, 98
lockdowns, 62, 66; Aotearoa/New Zealand, 185–186; in Israel, 143–144; South Africa, 96
long-distance family dispersal. *See* transnational family caregiving
long-term care (LTC) settings, 27; care workers, 77–78; for-profit, 78; long-term residential care (LTRC), 162, 164; workers' wages, 41. *See also* congregate care settings; nursing homes
Lundberg, Shelly, 14

MacDonald, Martha, 4
MacLean, Nancy, 15
Maman, Daniel, 148
"managed democracy," 17
Manley, Melissa H., 90
Marchetti, Sabrina, 4, 111, 112
Marchington, Mick, 189
marketization. *See* privatization
Markey, Raymond, 188
Martínez Franzoni, Juliana, 3, 8
masks, 79, 169, 170, 172
Massey, Douglas, 109
maternalism, 22
maternity leave, 21
Mauldin, Laura, 3, 8, 184
means-testing for supplemental pay, 126
Medicaid, 43, 48, 169, 193; and congregate care residents, 49
medical ethics, 173–175. *See also* ethical concerns
Medicare, 169
Mesiäislehto, Merita, 4, 111, 112

migrant workers: in Canada, 165; care workers and domestic workers, Europe, 134–141, *137*, *138*; employment standards, 33–34; and transnational caregiving, 102–109
migration, 27–34; immigrants in U.S., 28; migration policies, 112, 141
military contractors, 13
military support for long-term care, 58
Mill, John Stuart, 12
minimum wage, 43
Ministry of Finance, Israel, 148–150
Ministry of Welfare, Israel, 145–146
Mitchell, David T., 48
Mokomane, Zitha, 3, 62
Money Follows the Person, 49
multigenerational households, 62–63, 94–95, 96

National Council of Independent Living, 51
National Domestic Workers Alliance, 191, 192
neoliberalism, 30, 31, 46, 66–67, 143, 178; and privatization of care, 54–56, 58, 59–60
NEP+ (Ethiopia), 99
New Deal and racism, 47, 52n2, 194
New Zealand (Aotearoa), 183–190
#NoBodyIsDisposable, 51
nurses: gender and racial biases, 23, *40*, 68, 75; global shortage of, 128; and supplemental pay policies, *124*, *125*; vulnerability during pandemic, 172; workplace stress, 42, 128
nursing homes: deaths in Ontario, Canada, 53; for-profit, 55–56, 59; need for structural change, 58–59; required reporting on COVID cases, 172; unpaid family care of residents, 56–58. *See also* congregate care settings; long-term care (LTC) settings

Oligarchy (Winters), 14
Oliver, Michael, 46
online teaching, 69, 74, 79, 82, 87–88, 93n1
Ontario, Canada, and long term care, 53–60
Organization for Economic Cooperation and Development, 79

palliative care and hospice, 168–173
parental leave, 22, 32, 155–158
paternity leave, 22, 32
Pautassi, Laura C., 3, 12, 24, 61, 62, 63, 134, 187
Peck, Emily, 150
Peng, Ito, 3, 8, 184, 187, 200
Pfau-Effinger, Birgit, 4, 25, 92, 112, 152
planning. *See* future planning
Polanyi, Karl, 15–16
Pollack, Dr. Marjorie, 1–2
Pollak, Robert A., 14
Poo, Ai-jen, 192
Portugal, *137*, 139
poverty, 41–42, 65, 66–67
PPE (personal protective equipment), shortages of, 15, 43, 144, 165, 169–170, 172, 186, 187
"predatory capitalism," 13
Preiss, Joshua, 13
privatization, 30; of care, 53–56, 58; of care in Aotearoa/New Zealand, 184; of early years childcare, 86–87, 92; of government

functions, 13; of home care in Canada, 163; of medical service in Italy, 76–77
ProMed (medical surveillance system), 1

quality of life, 48, 168, 170, 171
queer families, 90
Quinn, Johanna S., 3, 62, 63

racial inequities, 88; in COVID rates, 116–117; disparities in infection and mortality, 36; in employment, 161, 162–165; in healthcare, 37–41, *38*, *39*, *40*; racialized economic inequality, 90
racism: in Roosevelt's New Deal, 47–48, 52n2; structural, 36. *See also* slavery, legacy of
rationed care and "triage plans," 48, 51
rationing of resources, 172–173. *See also* PPE (personal protective equipment), shortages of
Ravenswood, Katherine, 4, 159, 160, 188, 190
remittances, 31, 34–35n5, 104, 105
remote learning, 69, 74, 79, 82, 87–88, 93n1
residence permits, 135, 136, 139, 141
Richards, Neil, 178
Rico, María Nieves, 3, 12, 24, 61, 62, 63, 134, 187
"right to care," 53–54, 56, 60, 65–72; regression in, 69–70
robot technology, 176–182
Romania, 106, 134–135, *137*, 141
Roosevelt, Eleanor, 197
Rosenhek, Zeev, 148

scarcity myth, 192–193
school closures, 73–74, 79, 82; primary schools, 87–89; South Africa, 97. *See also* online teaching
separation of families. *See* transnational family caregiving
"shadow state," 13
sick leave, 43–44, 197
Siddharth, Veena, 3, 8
single parents, 86, 90
Sins Invalid, 51
Skin, Tooth, and Bone (Sins Invalid), 51
slavery, legacy of, 13, 37, 86, 193. *See also* racial inequities; racism
Smart, William, 178
Smith, Catherine, 4, 159, 160
Snyder, Sharon L., 48
social care (support for daily activities), 56, 59, 99, 162–163
social distancing, 61, 96–97, 116, 156
social infrastructure, 19, 25, 32–34, 178
social isolation, 62, 99, 180, 182
socially assistive robots (SARs), 178–179
social protection programs, 22, 24–25, 71, 78, 94, 98, 138–139
social workers, 76; in Israel, 143, 145–146
South Africa, elder care, 96–101
Spain, 29, 135, *137*, 139, 140, 141
stimulus packages, 81
structural racism, 36–44
Sun, Ken Chih-Yan, 3, 62

supplemental pay for essential workers, 111, 115–128, *118–125*; means-testing for, 126
syndemic, COVID-19 as, 12, 61–62, 64, 65–72; postsyndemic scenarios, 70–72

Taylor, Breonna, 36
teachers: primary school, 87–89; teacher morale, 88–89; unionization, 88–89
telework, 68–69, 79
Temporary Wage Enhancement (Ontario, Canada), 164
three Rs of unpaid carework, 31–32
transnational family caregiving, 62, 102–109
travel bans, 62, 97
"triage plans" and rationed care, 48, 51
Tronto, Joan C., 2–3, 7, 66, 112, 134, 159–160, 162, 166, 190
Tudo, Flavius, 106
Turkle, Sherry, 182

undocumented workers, 135–136, 139
UNI Global Union campaign, 188
unionization: community-level unionism for home care workers, 165–167; of nursing homes, and COVID mortality rates, 173; unions as collective voice, 188; and worker bargaining power, 116
universalizing approach to disability analytics, 46

UN Women's 2017 regional report on Latin America, 20–23
Uruguay, 22
U.S. Heroes Act, 117
utilitarianism, 173

vaccines: vaccination rates, 71; vaccine development, 70; vaccine distribution, 199
van Wynsberghe, Aimee, 178
ventilators, shortages of, 15, 173
visitation, limits placed on, 170–171

wealth-care, 11–17, 112, 190; alternatives to, 16–17
wealth managers, 14, 17n3
welfare states and childcare policy in Europe, 151–158, *153*
White, Alan, 13
WHO (World Health Organization) and COVID-19 timeline, 1–2
Winters, Jeffrey, 14
Wolin, Sheldon, 16–17
women: gender distribution in health care workforce, 75; gender distribution in home-based care, 78–79; and labor market uncertainty, 68; participation in labor market, 19, 20; and poverty in Latin America, 67–68; and role in family-based care, 55–58; and traditional sexual division of labor, 66
work-family conflicts, 62, 88–90, 92, 151